Endoscopic Diagnosis of Esophageal Carcinoma for ESD

Tsuneo Oyama
Editor

Endoscopic Diagnosis of Esophageal Carcinoma for ESD

Springer

Editor
Tsuneo Oyama
Director of Endoscopy
Saku Central Hospital Advanced Care Center
Saku
Nagano
Japan

Based on a translation from the Japanese language edition: ESD no tameno shokudo-gan jutuzen shindan by Prof. Tsuneo Oyama Copyright © Nankodo co., ltd., 2017 All Rights Reserved.
ISBN 978-981-32-9029-7 ISBN 978-981-32-9030-3 (eBook)
https://doi.org/10.1007/978-981-32-9030-3

This Springer imprint is published by the registered company Springer Nature Singapore Pte Ltd.
The registered company address is: 152 Beach Road, #21-01/04 Gateway East, Singapore 189721, Singapore

Preface

We, at Saku Central Hospital Division of Endoscopy, use magnifying endoscopy for all of our endoscopic evaluations. It is our routine practice to perform white light imaging, followed by NBI observation, and finally with magnifying NBI to consider histological structures. Our diagnoses are based on endoscopic findings, confirmed by biopsies. And our endoscopists themselves review all the biopsy microslides, and all of the histological findings are compared with the endoscopic images.

Markings for ESD are routinely performed with magnifying endoscopes. And, immediately following each ESD, the resected specimen is spread, pinned, and examined under the stereotypic microscope for image documentations. Furthermore, the resected specimen is observed with magnifying NBI to determine how to slice the specimen for histological evaluation. After formalin fixation of the specimen, each endoscopist who has performed ESD must slice the fixed specimen for microslides, make histological diagnosis of the prepared microslides, and prepare histological mapping of the fixed specimen. At our ESD conferences, preoperative diagnoses are evaluated with utmost scrutiny for accuracy, based on comparative evaluations of pre-ESD endoscopic images, post-ESD stereotypic microscope images, and histological images of the resected lesion.

Based on our prior experiences, we published in 2010 the Japanese edition of *Endoscopic Diagnosis of Superficial Gastric Cancer for ESD*, which to date has undergone fourth printing, and was translated and published in Chinese and English editions as well. English publications (related to GI endoscopy) are many but often coming short in endoscopic image quality, likely due to the fact that endoscopes are generally considered as tools for obtaining biopsies, not as tools for making diagnoses in many countries. We are indeed pleased that our English edition of *Endoscopic Diagnosis of Superficial Gastric Cancer for ESD*, utilizing high-quality endoscopic images and explaining relationships between the magnified endoscopic images and the histological images, is well accepted internationally. Early diagnosis of esophageal cancer is difficult, representing one of the more difficult cancers to treat. But superficial esophageal cancer cases are increasingly diagnosed in recent years. The classification of esophageal cancer introduced in 2014 and published in 2017 by the Japan Esophageal Society had significantly improved magnified endoscopic diagnoses of esophageal squamous cell cancer cases. And yet, it remains difficult to perform accurate endoscopic diagnoses of invasion depths of esophageal cancers.

We have come to publish this time *Endoscopic Diagnosis of Esophageal Cancer for ESD*. The contributing authors are all former trainees of the Department of Gastroenterology of Saku Central Hospital and the newly formed Division of Endoscopy at Saku Medical Center, who all have come to study together in the Oyama school and graduated. This textbook shows the results of their continuing efforts in practicing what they have learned in the Oyama school, studying each precious cases.

Saku Central Hospital was divided and relocated, creating the new Division of Endoscopy at Saku Central Hospital Advanced Care Center consisting of Drs. Akiko Takahashi, Nobukazu Yorimitsu, and myself. With only three of us, we are now performing over 300 ESD and LECS cases yearly, as well as histological preparations, diagnosis, and mapping. Our skills have inevitably been sharpened and improved. In closing this preface, I thank my two colleagues for their efforts in preparation of this publication while maintaining the rigorous daily clinical duties.

May 20, 2017, prior to the 71st Japan Esophageal Society annual meeting in Saku.

Saku, Nagano, Japan Tsuneo Oyama

The original version of this book was revised: Copyright comment has been updated. The correction to this book can be found at https://doi.org/10.1007/978-981-32-9030-3_30

Contents

Part I Basic Knowledge of Diagnostic Endoscopy of ESD for Esophagus Cancer

1 **Basic Structure of Esophageal Cancers** 3
Tsuneo Oyama

2 **Indications for Endoscopic Resections** 7
Nobukazu Yorimitsu and Tsuneo Oyama

3 **Diagnosis of Lateral Margins** 13
Akiko Takahashi and Tsuneo Oyama

4 **Diagnosis of Invasion Depths** 21
Tsuneo Oyama and Shigetaka Yoshinaga

Part II Diagnosis and Treatment of Each Carcinoma Type

5 **Type 0-Is Esophageal Cancer** 43
Manabu Takeuchi

6 **Type 0-Ip Esophageal Cancer** 47
Manabu Takeuchi

7 **Type 0-Isp Esophageal Cancer** 51
Manabu Takeuchi

8 **Type 0-IIa Esophageal Cancer: First Case** 55
Dai Hirasawa

9 **Type 0-IIa Esophageal Cancer: Second Case** 59
Dai Hirasawa

10 **Type 0-IIb Esophageal Cancer: First Case** 63
Nobukazu Yorimitsu

11 **Type 0-IIb Esophageal Carcinoma: Second Case** 69
Nobukazu Yorimitsu

12 **Type 0-IIc Esophageal Carcinoma: First Case** 75
Dai Hirasawa

13 **Type 0-IIc Esophageal Carcinoma: Second Case** 79
Dai Hirasawa

14 **Type 0-III Esophageal Carcinoma** 85
Shinichi Furutachi

15 **Large Superficially Spreading Esophageal Carcinoma** 91
Manabu Takeuchi

Part III Practices

16 Question 1: What Is the Invasion Depth? 101
Kotaro Shibagaki

17 Question 2: What Is the Invasion Depth? 109
Tokuma Tanuma

18 Question 3: What Is the Invasion Depth? 117
Shinichi Furutachi

19 Question 4: What Is the Invasion Depth? 125
Keita Funakawa

20 Question 5: What Is the Invasion Depth? 133
Keita Funakawa

21 Question 6: What Is the Histological Type? 141
Tadashi Miike

22 Question 7: What Is the Histological Type? 151
Toshiyuki Kubo

23 Question 8: What Is the Histological Type? 159
Takaaki Kishino

24 Question 9: What Is the Histological Type? 169
Kotaro Shibagaki

25 Question 10: What Is the Diagnosis? 179
Ryutaro Furukawa

26 Question 11: What Is the Diagnosis? 187
Shinichiro Takeda

27 Question 12: What Is the Diagnosis? 195
Nobukazu Yorimitsu

28 Question 13: What Is the Diagnosis? 203
Yoko Kitamura

29 Question 14: What Is the Diagnosis? 211
Shinichi Furutachi

Correction to: Endoscopic Diagnosis of Esophageal Carcinoma for ESD C1

Editor and Contributors

Editor

Tsuneo Oyama, M.D., Ph.D. Department of Endoscopy, Saku Central Hospital Advanced Care Center, Saku, Japan

Translator

Toyomi Fukushima, M.D., M.P.H., F.A.C.P. Division of Digestive Diseases and Clinical Nutrition, Kobe Adventist Hospital, Hyogo, Japan

Contributors

Keita Funakawa, M.D. Department of Gastroenterology, Kagoshima City Hospital, Kagoshima, Japan

Ryutaro Furukawa, M.D. Department of Endoscopic Medicine, Saku Central Hospital Advanced Care Center, Saku, Japan

Shinichi Furutachi, M.D. Department of Gastroenterology, Okayama Medical Center, National Hospital Organization, Okayama, Japan

Dai Hirasawa, M.D. Department of Gastroenterology, Sendai Kosei Hospital, Sendai, Miyagi, Japan

Takaaki Kishino, M.D. Department of Gastroenterology, Nara City Hospital Center for Digestive Diseases, Nara, Japan

Yoko Kitamura, M.D. Department of Gastroenterology, Nara City Hospital Center for Digestive Diseases, Nara, Japan

Toshiyuki Kubo, M.D. Department of Gastroenterology and Hepatology, Sapporo Medical University School of Medicine, Sapporo, Hokkaido, Japan

Tadashi Miike, M.D. Department of Gastroenterology, Miyazaki University School of Medicine, Miyazaki, Japan

Tsuneo Oyama, M.D., Ph.D. Department of Endoscopy, Saku Central Hospital Advanced Care Center, Nagano, Japan

Kotaro Shibagaki, M.D. Department of Endoscopic Diagnosis and Therapeutics, Shimane University School of Medicine Hospital, Matsue, Shimane, Japan

Akiko Takahashi, M.D. Department of Endoscopy, Saku Central Hospital Advanced Care Center, Nagano, Japan

Shinichiro Takeda, M.D. Department of Gastroenterology, Matsudo City Hospital, Matsudo, Japan

Manabu Takeuchi, M.D., Ph.D. Department of Gastroenterology, Nagaoka Red Cross Hospital, Niigata, Japan

Tokuma Tanuma, M.D. Center for Digestive Diseases, Teine Keijinkai Hospital, Sapporo, Hokkaido, Japan

Nobukazu Yorimitsu, M.D. Department of Endoscopy, Saku Central Hospital Advanced Care Center, Nagano, Japan

Shigetaka Yoshinaga, M.D. Division of Endoscopy, National Cancer Research Center Central Hospital, Tokyo, Japan

Part I

Basic Knowledge of Diagnostic Endoscopy of ESD for Esophagus Cancer

1 Basic Structure of Esophageal Cancers

Tsuneo Oyama

1.1 Basic Structure of Esophageal Mucosa

The basic structures of esophageal squamous cell epithelia and gastric or intestinal epithelia vary greatly. The stomachs and intestines consist of glandular epithelia, with cells aligned in one row forming papillary and tubular structures (Fig. 1.1). Blood vessels run in the interstitial spaces.

On the other hand, the squamous epithelia show overwrapping squamous cells above the basement membrane and the lamina propria between the basement membrane and the muscularis mucosa (Fig. 1.2). Parts of the basement mem-

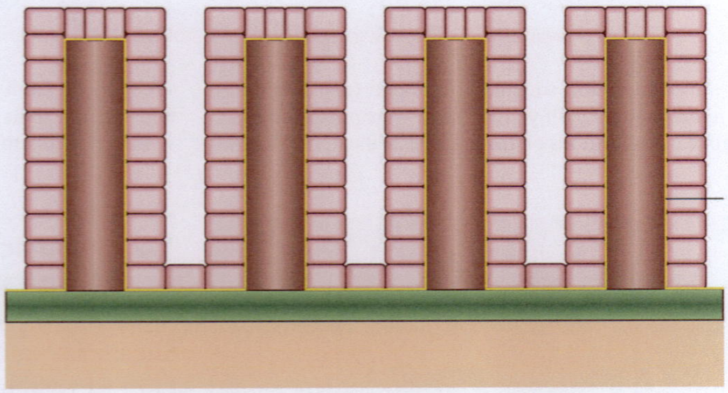

Fig. 1.1 Structure of glandular epithelia (explanations on the right side of the figure), mucosal epithelium, lamina propria, muscularis mucosa, submucosa

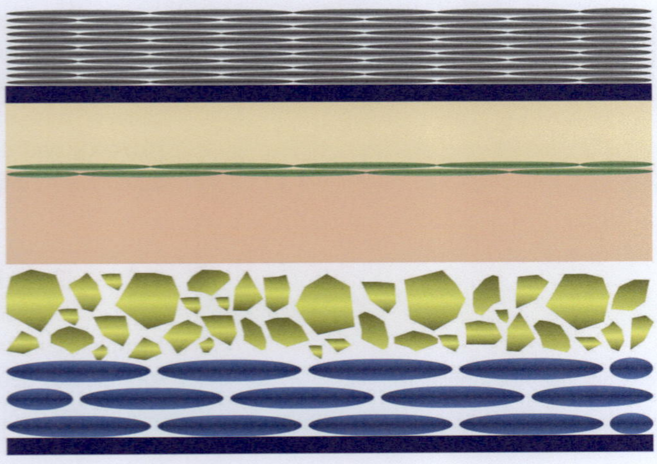

Fig. 1.2 Structure of squamous epithelia (explanations on the right side of the figure), mucosal epithelium, basement membrane, lamina propria, muscularis mucosa, submucosa, muscularis propria, serosa

T. Oyama (✉)
Department of Endoscopy, Saku Central Hospital Advanced Care Center, Nagano, Japan
e-mail: oyama@coral.ocn.ne.jp

T. Oyama (ed.), *Endoscopic Diagnosis of Esophageal Carcinoma for ESD*, https://doi.org/10.1007/978-981-32-9030-3_1

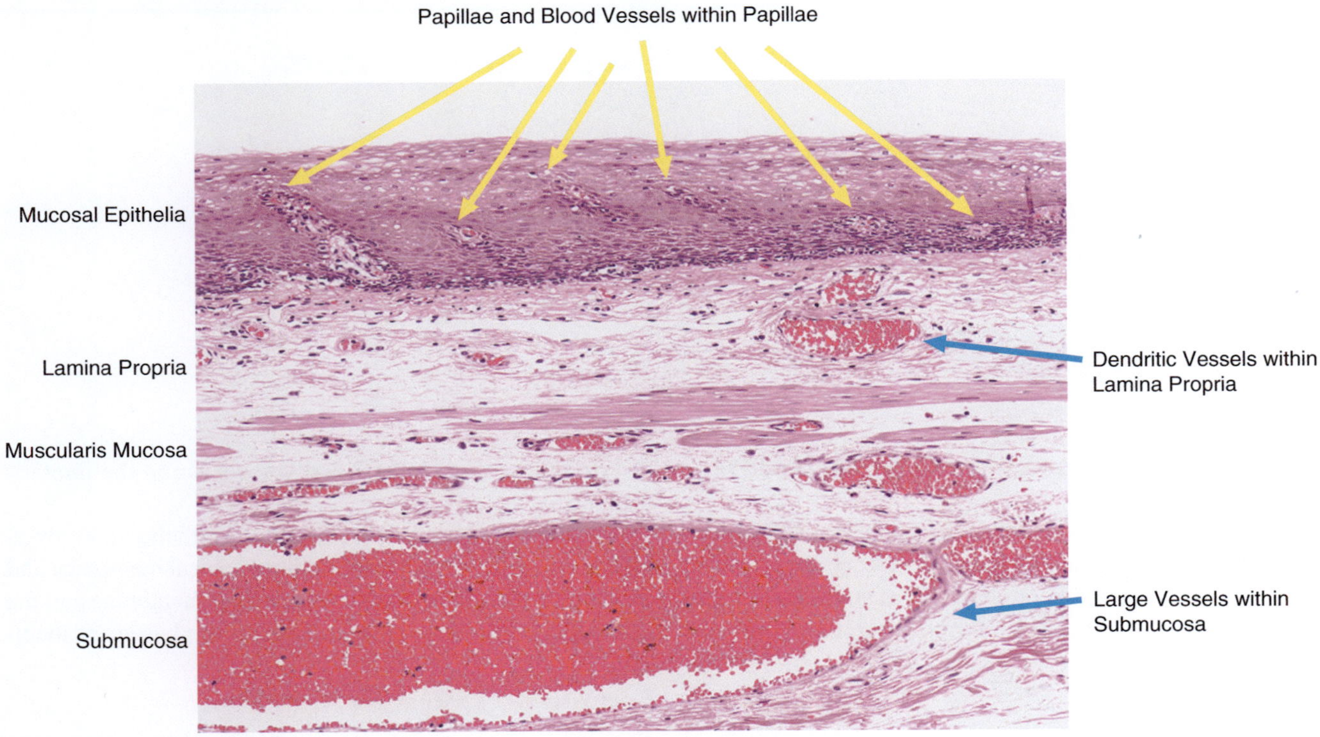

Fig. 1.3 Vascular structure within squamous epithelia (explanation on the top side of the figure marked with yellow lines) → papillae and blood vessels within papillae, (explanations on the left side of the figure), mucosal epithelia, lamina propria, muscularis mucosa, submucosa, (explanations on the right side of the figure marked with blue lines), dendritic vessels within lamina propria, large vessels within the submucosa

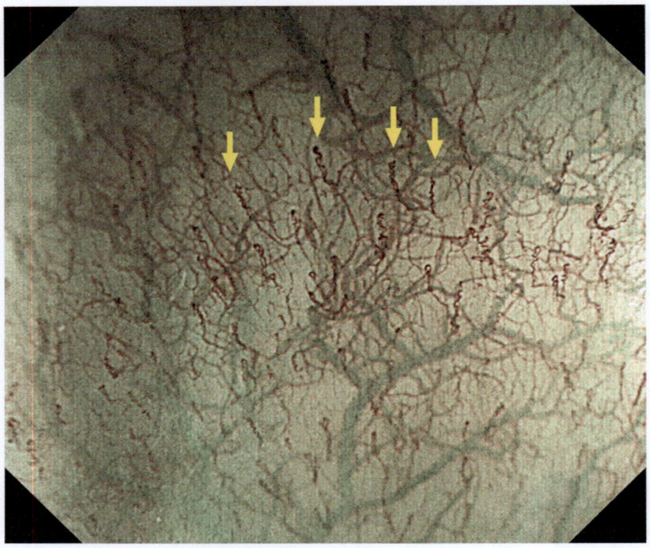

Fig. 1.4 Microvessels with loop-like formations

brane form papilla by extending upward (Fig. 1.3). Inside these papilla are seen loop forming blood vessels called intrapapillary capillary loop (IPCL) [1]. IPCL can be observed by NBI magnification imaging as loop forming microvessels branching from the dendritic vessels within the lamina propria (Fig. 1.4).

1.2 Basic Structure of Esophageal Squamous Cancer

Squamous cell carcinomas arise in mucosal epithelia (T1a-EP) and invade into the lamina propria (T1a-LPM) and the submucosa (T1b-SM) (Fig. 1.5). With T1a-EP~LPM, the lymph node metastases are 0% but with T1a-MM and deeper show lymph node invasions. The author with 22 collaborating facilities enlisted 664 cases of T1a-MM and T1b-SM1 cancers and showed lymph node involvement in 9.3% (41/440) and 19.6% (44/224) [2]. Therefore, preoperative diagnosis of depth of invasion is important.

1.3 Subclassifications of T1b-SM [3]

Lymphatic metastases occur with increased frequencies with submucosal depth of invasion. The submucosal layer can be subdivided by three and classified into SM1, 2, 3 in surgically resected specimens. However, this classification cannot be used with endoscopically resected specimens as the lesions are resected mid-level of the submucosa. Therefore, for endoscopically resected specimens, invasion depths are measured as distance from the muscularis mucosa and notified as T1b-SM1 for lesions with invasion depths of 200 μm or less and T1b-SM2 for those 201 μm and above, without T1b-SM3 (Fig. 1.5).

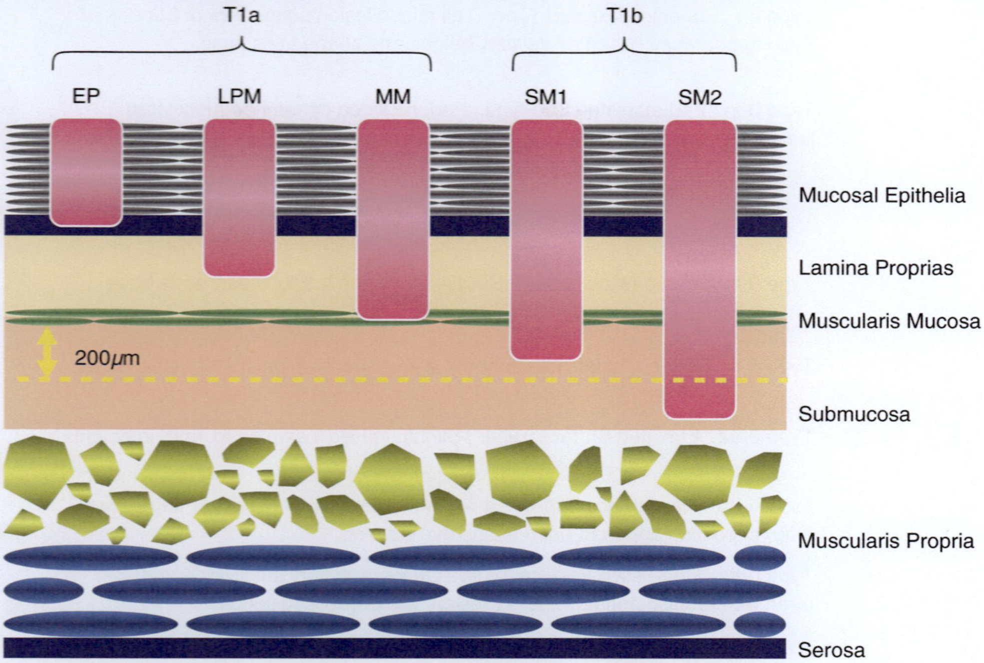

Fig. 1.5 Esophageal squamous cell carcinoma with different depths of invasion (explanation of the right side of the figure), mucosal epithelia, lamina propria, muscularis mucosa, submucosa, muscularis propria, serosa

Table 1.1 Description rule for esophageal squamous cell cancers

T1a	EP (epithelial), LPM (lamina propria), MM (muscularis mucosa)
T1b	SM (submucosa)
Superficial cancers	T1a + T1b
Early cancers	T1a

For both superficial and early cancers, lymph node metastasis is not required for inclusion or exclusion

Table 1.2 Morphological classification (superficial type and advanced types)

Type 0	Superficial type
Type I	Raised type
Type 2	Limited ulceration type
Type 3	Infiltrated ulceration type
Type 4	Diffuse infiltration type
Type 5	Unclassifiable type

1.4 Superficial Caners and Early Cancers [3]

Esophageal cancers with depths of invasion within the mucosal layers are defined as early esophageal cancer regardless of the status of lymphatic metastases. And those with the depths of invasion down to the submucosal layers are defined as superficial esophageal cancer regardless of the status of lymphatic metastases (Table 1.1).

1.5 Morphological Type Classifications [3]

The "Japanese Classification of Esophageal Cancer" classifies morphological types to Type 0 to 5. Lesions with visually estimated depths of invasion down to the submucosal layer are considered as "superficial types," and those with visually estimated depths of invasion beyond the muscularis propria are considered as "advanced types."

"Superficial types" are noted as Type 0 and subclassified into Type 0-I, 0-II, and 0-III. "Advanced types" are subclassified as four basic types (Type 1, 2, 3, and 4). Those which cannot be expressed in either of the four basic types or their combinations are classified as Type 5 (Table 1.2, Fig. 1.6).

0-I and 0-IIa are both elevated-type lesions, but cancers with lesion height up to 1 mm are classified as 0-IIa and those above 1 mm in height as 0-I. But to accurately diagnose the 1 mm lesion height with endoscopy is difficult, and lesion height varies easily with degrees of air insufflation. Lesions should be observed with sufficient air insufflation to achieve more objective height assessment and accurate morphological type classification.

Type 0-I Superficial Raised Type: Tall raised lesion suggestive of Superficial Type appearance based on its size, height, and shape at its base.

Type 0-Ip Pedunculated Sub-type: Pedunculated or semi-pedunculated lesion narrowest at its base.

Type 0-Is Sessile (wide-based): Sessile tall raised lesion widest at its base.

Type 0-II Surface Type: Lesion without prominent elevations or depressions.

Type 0-IIa Elevated Surface Type: Slightly raised lesion up to 1mm in height.

Type 0-IIb Flat Surface Type: Lesion without visible elevation or depression, often becoming apparent upon Iodine dye staining.

Type 0-IIc Depressed Surface Type: Lesion with very shallow depression, often with reddish appearance. “Erosion” like depressed lesion.

Type 0-III Superficial Depressed Type: More depressed than 0-IIc forming ulceration deeper than the level of muscularis mucosa.

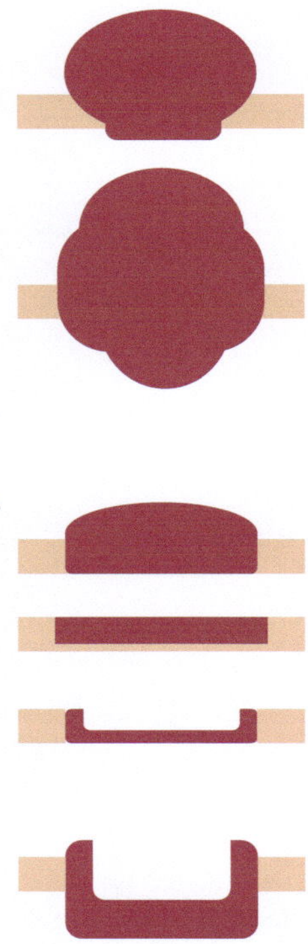

Fig. 1.6 Subclassification for superficial type (Type 0)

References

1. Inoue H, et al. Ultra-high magnification endoscopic observation of carcinoma in situ of the esophagus. Dig Endosc. 1997;9:16–8.
2. Oyama T, et al. The 46th esophageal dye study group questionnaire report—characteristics of m3-sm1 esophageal cancers with metastasis. Stomach Intestines. 2002;37:71–4.
3. Japan Esophageal Society. Japanese classification of esophageal cancer 11th edition Part I, II and III. Esophagus. 2017;14(1):1–65.

2 Indications for Endoscopic Resections

Nobukazu Yorimitsu and Tsuneo Oyama

Endoscopic therapies for early esophageal cancers include endoscopic submucosal resection (EMR), EMR-tube method [1], two-channel method [2], and EMR-C method [3], all developed during the 1990s. But, for larger lesions, these resulted in multiple-piece resections with increased risks of local recurrences, making it more difficult to accurately evaluate resected specimens.

In 2000, endoscopic submucosal dissection (ESD) for early esophageal cancer was reported [4], making it possible to resect larger lesions of any size and shape as one piece. Esophageal ESD resulted in greater single-piece resection rates than EMR, with equal rates of complications and long-term prognoses [5], becoming approved as a new procedure reimbursed by the Japanese national health plan.

According to the Guidelines for Diagnosis and Treatments of Carcinoma of the Esophagus (third edition) [6] published in April of 2012 by the Japan Esophageal Society, the following algorithm of esophageal cancer treatments (Fig. 2.1) is described, recom-

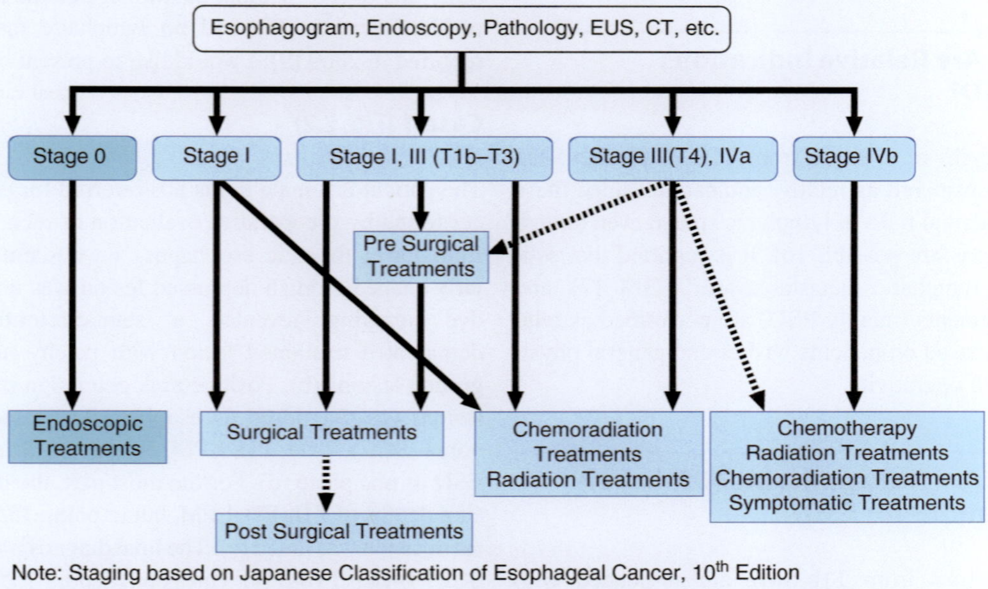

Fig. 2.1 Algorithm for esophageal cancer treatments

N. Yorimitsu · T. Oyama (✉)
Department of Endoscopy, Saku Central Hospital Advanced Care Center, Nagano, Japan
e-mail: oyama@coral.ocn.ne.jp

T. Oyama (ed.), *Endoscopic Diagnosis of Esophageal Carcinoma for ESD*, https://doi.org/10.1007/978-981-32-9030-3_2

mending endoscopic therapies only for Stage 0, which is T1a lesions with cN0.

2.1 What Are Appropriate Indications for ESD?

Lesions with depths of invasion of EP or LPM, with very rare lymph node metastases and acceptable cure rates [6], are considered appropriate indications for endoscopic treatments. Although for superficially spreading cancer with diameter greater than 5 cm, depth of invasion may reach deeper levels at multiple locations, very careful assessments of invasion depths are required. For lesions resulting in greater than two-thirds the circumferential resection, there are increased risks of stricture formations post-mucosal resections, and adequate preoperative explanations of risks and stricture prevention measures are recommended [6]. For lesions resulting in greater than two-thirds the circumferential resection, endoscopic treatments are not included in absolute indication but as relative indications according to the second edition of the guidelines because of significant risks of post-resection stricture formations, but such restrictions are removed in the third edition of the guidelines.

2.2 What Are Relative Indications for ESD?

Lesions with depths of invasion from T1a-MM~sT1b-SM1 with cN0 are considered as relative indications since these lesions carry potential risks of lymphatic spread even though mucosal resections are possible [6]. It is reported that estimated rates of lymphatic metastases are 7–20% [7], and endoscopic treatments (mainly ESD) are performed as relative indications based on patients wishes and general physical conditions for operativity.

2.3 What Are Nonapplicable (Off-Label) Indications for ESD?

Depths of invasions from T1b-SM2 are associated with approximately 50% rates of metastases. Therefore, even superficial cancers with these criteria should be treated as advanced cancers (invading deeper than muscularis mucosa) [6] and would be nonapplicable (off-label) indications for endoscopic resection.

2.4 What Are the Issues Regarding Lesions with Relative Indications?

Lesions diagnosed as T1a-MM or T1b-SM1, without lymph node metastasis considered as relative indications for endoscopic resections. However, if the final diagnosis of invasion depths post-endoscopic resections is T1b-SM1, additional treatments such as surgical resection and chemoradiation need to be considered [6]. Therefore, preoperative diagnoses of lesions with T1a-MM and T1b-SM1 are both considered as relative indications for endoscopic resections, but postoperative diagnoses of invasion depths of T1a-MM and T1b-SM1 differ in requirements for additional treatments.

Since T1b-SM1 is reported to have lymph node metastases of 15–20% [7, 8], carrying out surgical treatments for all cases would result in possible 80% over surgery.

On the other hand, risk factors for lymphatic metastases for lesions T1a-MM and T1b-SM1 are Type 0-I, Type 0-III, and diameters greater than 50 mm, by visual assessment, and lymphatic vessel invasions, poorly differentiated histology, and INF-b, c by histological assessments. Those lesions without these factors are reported to have lymphatic metastases rates of only 4.2% [7]. The author and colleagues have followed patients with T1b-SM1 lesions with negative margins, negative lymphatic involvements, and invasion pattern other than INF-c without additional treatments according to patients' wishes. We had no lymphatic metastases when reported in 2009 [9]. I would like to present one such case.

Case 1 (Fig. 2.2)

The patient is a male in his 80s referred for esophageal cancer found by preoperative evaluation of rectal cancer. In the right lower thoracic esophagus, a well-demarcated irregularly shaped reddish depressed lesion was noted (a). Iodine dye spraying revealed a semi-circumferential well-demarcated unstained lesion with patchy unstained background lesions (b). Positive pink color sign is noted (c). The lesion was diagnosed as esophageal squamous cell carcinoma (SCC), 0-IIc, T1a-LPM, 50 mm, Lt, Rt and resected by ESD as one piece (d). For the most part, the lesion had invasion depths of T1b-EP~LPM, but in point, 155 μm submucosal invasion was noted (e). The final diagnosis was esophageal SCC, 0-IIc, T1b-SM1 (invasion depth: 155 μm, invasion width: 190 μm, INFa), ly(−),v(−), HM0, LM0, 56 × 39 mm in 60 × 53 mm, Lt, Rt (f). The patient was explained of the result and did not wish additional treatments, and was followed with periodic observation only. No recurrence was noted until his death from lung cancer 8 years from the ESD.

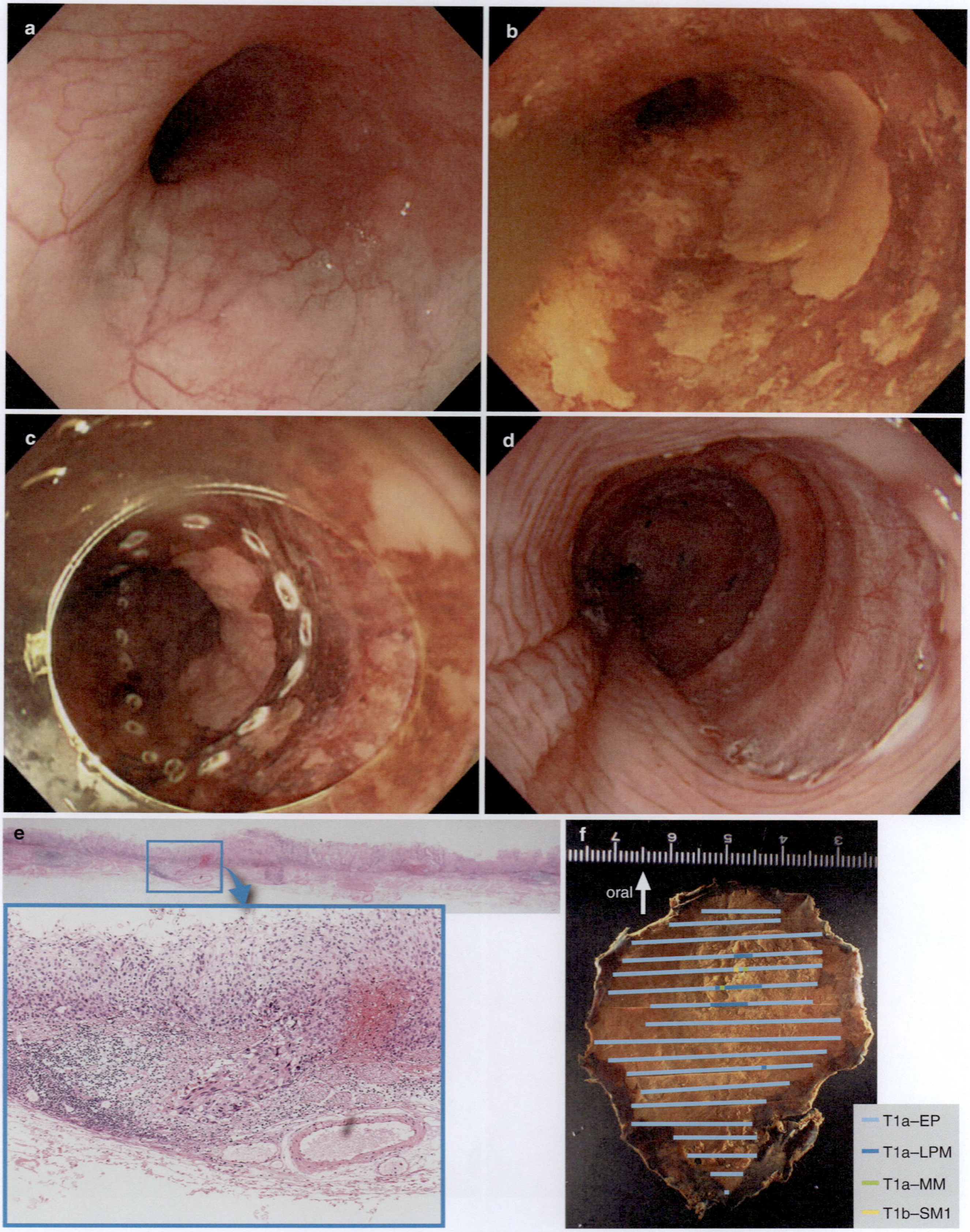

Fig. 2.2 Case 1

Among lesions with T1a-MM and T1b-SM1, if it becomes possible to accurately select the high-risk group for lymphatic metastases, it would help selecting cases for additional treatments. This presents further studies. Even those without high risks of recurrences, it is important to screen every half year with esophagogastroduodenoscopy (EGD), endoscopic ultrasound (EUS), and CT.

2.5 Problems Relating to Post-ESD Esophageal Stenosis

Although greater than three-fourths the circumferential resection is listed as a risk factor for esophageal strictures, it became known in recent years that steroid injection or oral administration can prevent esophageal strictures.

As to steroid injections, Hashimoto and colleagues have reported the effectiveness of steroid injections for semi-circumferential ESD greater than three-fourths the circumference, providing triamcinolone injections on the 3rd, the 7th, and the 10th day post-ESD, reducing stricture formation rates from 75% to 19%, without adverse events [10]. Hanaoka and colleagues also reported single-dose injection of triamcinolone post-ESD greater than three-fourths the circumference, reducing stricture formation rates from 66% to 10%, with post-procedure complication rate of 7% including one case of bleeding and one case of submucosal injury [11].

As to oral steroid administration, Yamaguchi and colleagues reported the use of oral prednisolone administration for after ESD of greater than three-fourths the circumference, reducing stricture formation rates from 31.8% to 5.3% 3 months post-ESD without adverse events [12].

However, it is known that delayed perforation post-steroid injection, severe infections, psychosis, or diabetes with oral steroid administrations can occur. The author and colleagues have used triamcinolone injections for stricture prophylaxis because of concerns for systemic side effects of oral steroid administrations.

Case 2 (Fig. 2.3)

The patient is a male in his 60s without chief complaints, found to have an esophageal cancer by screening endoscopy and referred for treatment. In the anterior mid thoracic esophagus, a clearly demarcated reddish shallowly depressed lesion extending to both right and left lateral walls was noted. The depressed area was flat without irregular elevations or depressions showing reasonable extension with air inflation (a). NBI observation revealed a brownish area (BA) with clear demarcation (b). NBI magnification observation revealed dilated, tortuous, looping vessels with irregular calibers and shapes, considered as Type B1 blood vessels. Iodine dye spray revealed a clearly demarcated unstained semi-circumferential lesion (c). The lesion was diagnosed as esophageal SCC, T1a-LPM, 0-IIc, 60 mm, M5, 11/12th circumference. Full circumferential ESD was performed (d). Immediately following ESD, triamcinolone injections totaling 50 mg were injected into 25 places (e). The lesion was removed in tubular form in one piece (f). The final diagnosis was esophageal SCC, 0-IIc, T1a-EP, ly(−), v(−), HM0, LM0, 67 × 57 mm in 70 × 62 mm, Mt., circ (g). On the 7th day, the 11th day, the 16th day, the 21th day, and the 28th day

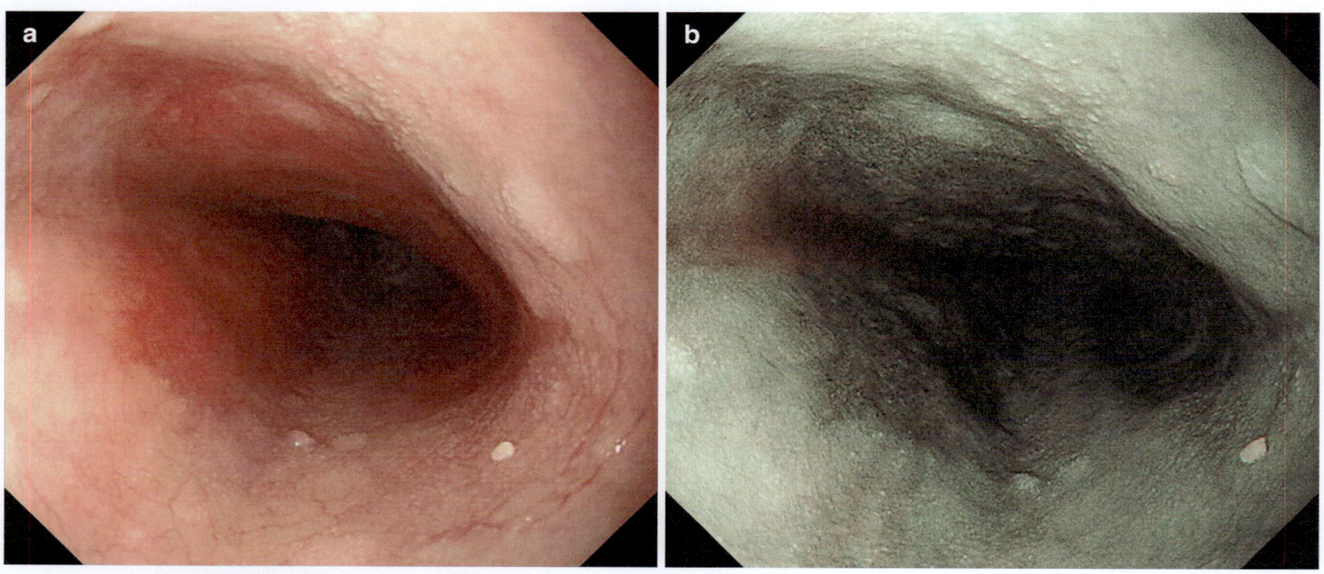

Fig. 2.3 Case 2

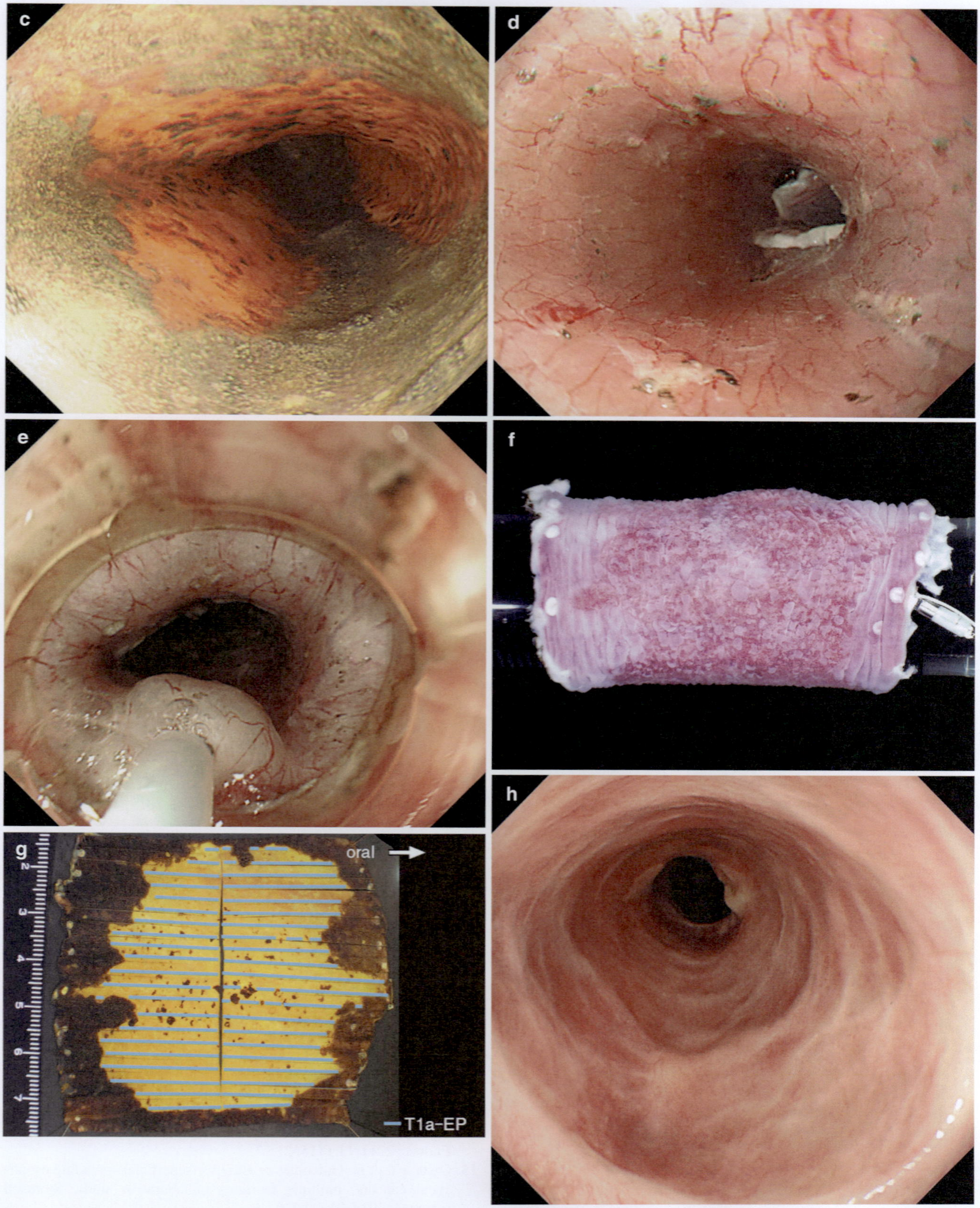

Fig. 2.3 (continued)

post-ESD, additional injections of triamcinolone 50 mg were provided. No stricture needing balloon dilation was formed. ESD ulceration was fully healed with complete epithelialization post-135th day (h).

But for superficially spreading cancers, 41% of the final diagnosis for ESD performed esophageal cancers are T1a-MM~T1b-SM2 [13], with high possibilities for requiring additional treatments. But chemoradiation treatment cannot be started until ESD ulceration completely is scarred and may cause delay in treatment up to 3 months. And chemoradiation carries a risk of stenosis. Therefore, it is important to inform the patients ahead of time of possibilities of recommending surgical resections if final diagnoses require additional treatments.

2.6 Summary

With improving endoscopic imaging qualities and better diagnostic technologies, more esophageal cancers are found at earlier stages and treated endoscopically for cure. On the other hand, there remain issues to be solved regarding additional treatments for lesions with T1a-MM to T1b-SM1. Detailed endoscopic observations, accurate endoscopic diagnoses, and histological diagnoses need to be accumulated to clarify histological and endoscopic features of lesions requiring additional treatments.

Column: Prophylaxis of ESD-Related Stenosis

Common prophylactic methods for stenosis post fully circumferential esophageal ESD are oral steroid use or topical steroid injections. However, oral steroid use may result in worsening of diabetes, psychological conditions, or infections, and the author and my colleagues use steroid injections.

We use triamcinolone 50 mg/5 mL solution and inject 2 mg at a time to total of 25 places. It is important to inject into the submucosa as injections into the muscularis mucosa may result in delayed perforations. To ensure safety of injections, it is important to dissect not to expose the muscularis mucosa maintaining the level of dissection at about one-third into the submucosal layer. It is also important to use 1.8 mm long needle rather than 4 mm long needle. In the case of fully circumferential resections of more than 5 cm in length, we perform injections of 100 mg (2 mg × 50places) for the initial session.

For semi-circumferential resections, stenosis can be prevented in most cases with injections immediately following ESD. However, for fully circumferential resections, endoscopic evaluations are required in 2 weeks following ESD.

If no stenosis is noted, additional 50 mg of triamcinolone is injected using 4 mm long injection needle, with shallow injections into the ulcer base directing needles in parallel fashion to the muscle layer, as intramuscular injections may result in delayed perforations.

If stenosis is noted, a 12–15 mm dilation balloon is used to dilate with very diligent care slowly inflating at 2 atm/min rate to 8 atm over 4 min. After the balloon is removed post-dilation, 50 mg of triamcinolone is injected in the submucosa. Too shallow an injection may leak out, while too deep an injection may puncture the muscle layer. Success of stenosis prevention depends on the technique of sure injections into the submucosa.

References

1. Makuuchi H, et al. Practical descriptions of endoscopic mucosal resection for early esophageal cancers, EEMR-tube method. Stomach Intestine. 1993;28:153–9.
2. Monma K, et al. Practical descriptions of endoscopic mucosal resection for early esophageal cancers, two channel method. Stomach Intestine. 1993;28:141–51.
3. Inoue H, et al. Practical descriptions of endoscopic mucosal resection for early esophageal cancers, two channel method. Stomach Intestine. 1993;28:153–9.
4. Oyama T, et al. Endoscopic submucosal dissection of early esophageal cancer. Clin Gastroenterol Hepatol. 2005;3(7 Suppl 1):S67–70.
5. Kitamura Y, et al. Outcomes of m1 and m2 esophageal cancers post ESD. Stomach Intestine. 2007;42:1323–9.
6. Japan Esophageal Society, editor. Guidelines for diagnosis and treatments of carcinoma of the esophagus 2012. Tokyo: Kanehara Publishing; 2012.
7. Oyama T, et al. The 46th Esophageal Dye Study Group questionaire report—characteristics of m3-sm1 esophageal cancers with metastasis. Stomach Intestine. 2002;37:71–4.
8. Yoshida S. Endoscopic treatment in junction with consideration for surgical resection -esophageal cancers. Dig Endosc. 1997;9:380–5.
9. Oyama T, et al. Outcomes of ESD for esophageal SCC, focusing on T1a-MM and SM1. Stomach Intestine. 2009;44:405–16.
10. Hashimoto S, et al. The efficacy of endoscopic triamcinolone injection for the prevention of esophageal stricture after endoscopic submucosal dissection. Gastrointest Endosc. 2011;74:1389–93.
11. Hanaoka N, et al. Intralesional steroid injection to prevent stricture after endoscopic submucosal dissection for esophageal cancer; a controlled prospective study. Endoscopy. 2005;37:1111–5.
12. Yamaguchi N, et al. Usefulness of oral prednisolone in the treatment of esophageal stricture after endoscopic submucosal dissection for superficial esophageal squamous cell carcinoma. Gastrointest Endosc. 2011;73:1115–21.
13. Oyama T, et al. Outcomes of ESD for superficial spreading esophageal cancers, multiple facilities collaborative study. Stomach Intestine. 2014;49:1182–9.

3 Diagnosis of Lateral Margins

Akiko Takahashi and Tsuneo Oyama

Diagnosis of lateral margins for esophageal squamous cell cancers (SCC) is based on white light imaging (WLI), narrowband imaging (NBI), and iodine dye spraying, especially important in determining resection margins. It is easy when the three modalities of white light imaging, narrowband imaging, and iodine dye spraying have a matching diagnosis, but the three modalities do not necessarily match always. This chapter explains how to make a generalized diagnosis based on features of each modality.

3.1 White Light Imaging (WLI)

For diagnosis of lateral margins with white light imaging, differences in height, color tone, and vascular visibility should be noted.

Depression

For SCC, depressed lesions are more frequently noted, and difference in levels must be observed. Observation with full inflation of air makes the difference in levels less noticeable (Fig. 3.1a), and observation with underinflation of air is necessary (Fig. 3.1b).

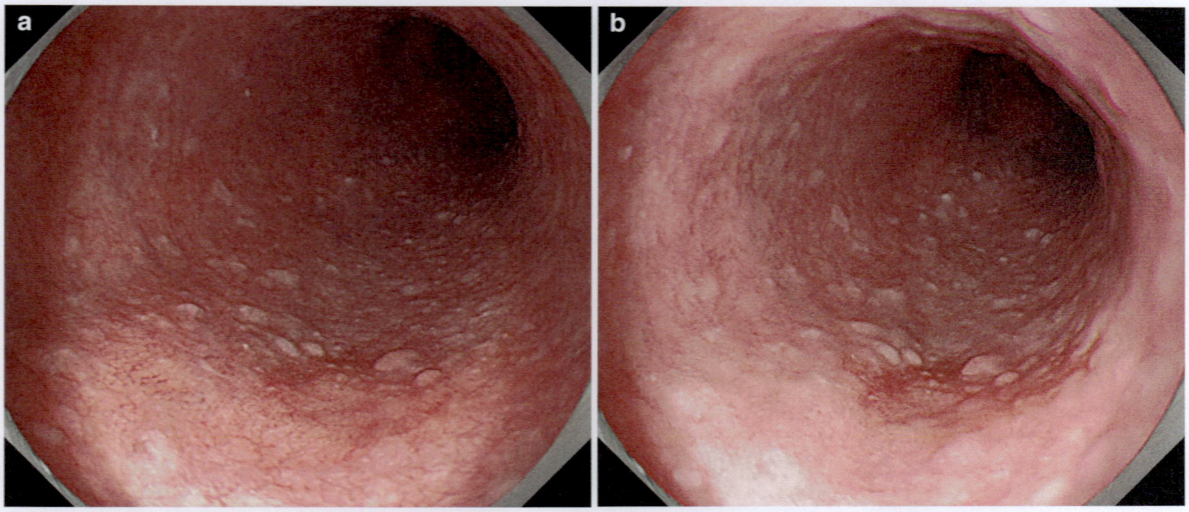

Fig. 3.1 Difference in levels with white light observation

A. Takahashi · T. Oyama (✉)
Department of Endoscopy, Saku Central Hospital Advanced Care Center, Nagano, Japan
e-mail: oyama@coral.ocn.ne.jp

T. Oyama (ed.), *Endoscopic Diagnosis of Esophageal Carcinoma for ESD*, https://doi.org/10.1007/978-981-32-9030-3_3

Color Tone

Adhesion of necrotic materials may appear as a discolored raised lesion (Fig. 3.2a). This can be easily washed off, and it is important to observe after sufficient washing (Fig. 3.2b). It is more common to observe redness with SCC, but inflammation may also appear reddish. For such cases, it is helpful to note evenness of reddish coloration and demarcations. Reddish color noted with cancer appears even with clear demarcations (Fig. 3.3), while inflammation appears with varied degrees of redness with unclear demarcations (Fig. 3.4a). This inflammatory change disappeared with the use of PPI (proton pump inhibitor). It is also helpful to use magnified imaging discussed later (Chap. 4) in differentiating cancer from inflammation.

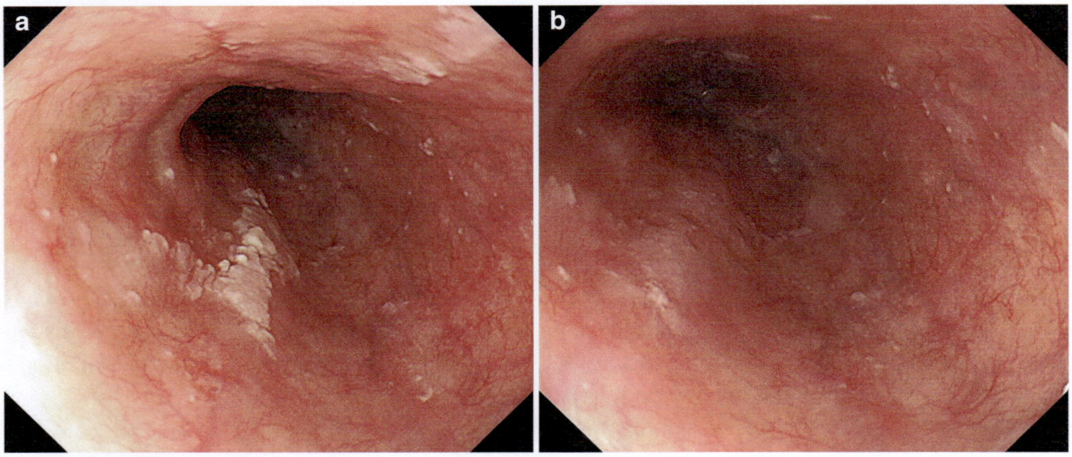

Fig. 3.2 Color tone (discoloration) under white light imaging

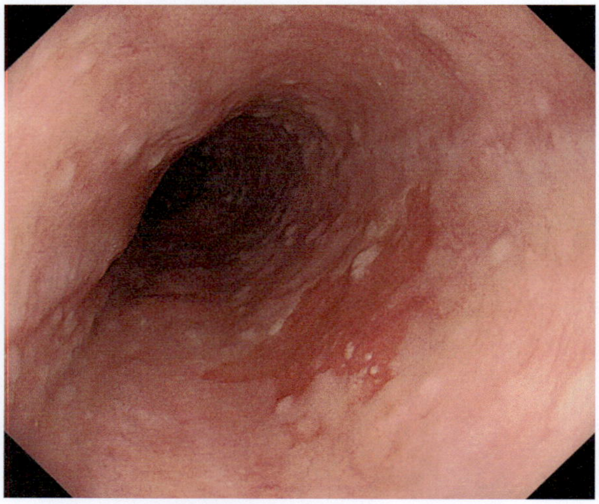

Fig. 3.3 Color tone (even redness) under white light imaging

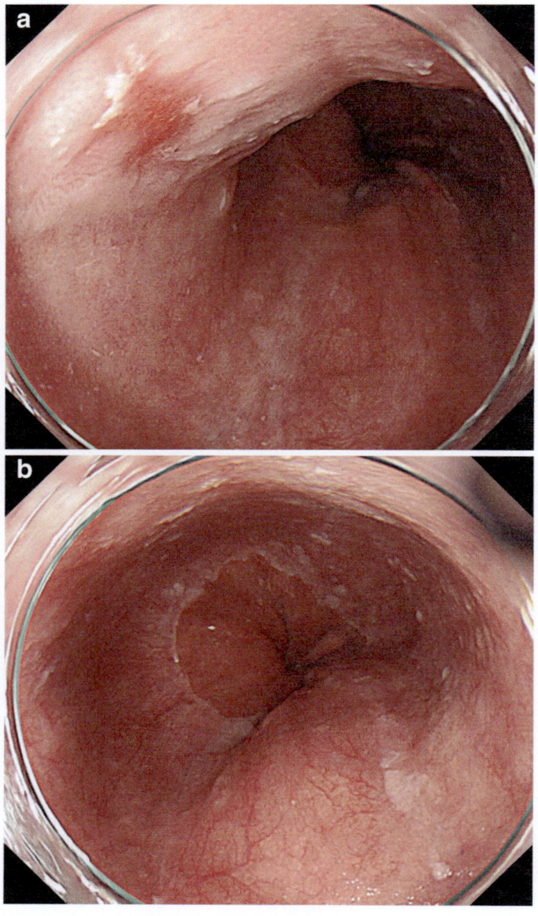

Fig. 3.4 Color tone (varied degrees of redness with unclear demarcations) under white light imaging

Vascular Visibilities

Submucosal blood vessels are observed beneath the normal mucosa, but vascular visibilities disappear in the cancerous mucosa (Fig. 3.5a, b). But this finding is only seen with inflation of full air and less distinct with reduced air inflation (Fig. 3.5c). It is thus important to adjust air inflation for careful evaluation.

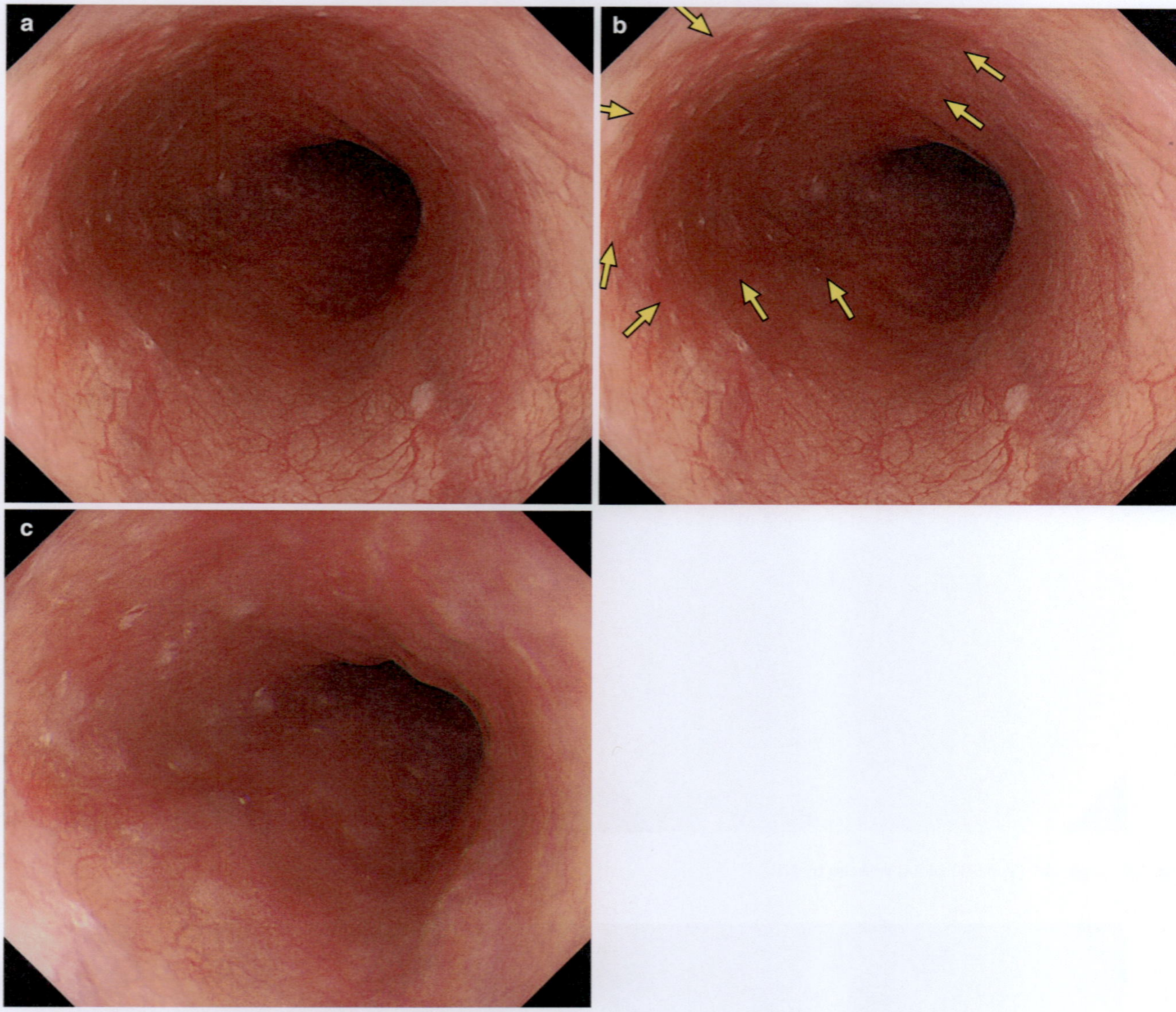

Fig. 3.5 Vascular visibilities under white light observation

3.2 NBI Observation

There are two types of brownish areas (BA), dark BAs and light BAs. Dark BA lesions are easier to diagnose as SCC (Fig. 3.6), while it is harder to diagnose light BA lesions as neoplastic or not. Magnification imaging is useful for evaluating light BA lesions. If noted with Type B1 blood vessels (Fig. 3.7a), the lesion can be diagnosed SCC (Fig. 3.7b). On the other hand, if a light BA lesion (Fig. 3.8a) is noted with subepithelial capillary network (SECN) (Fig. 3.8b), it can be diagnosed as simple epithelial atrophy.

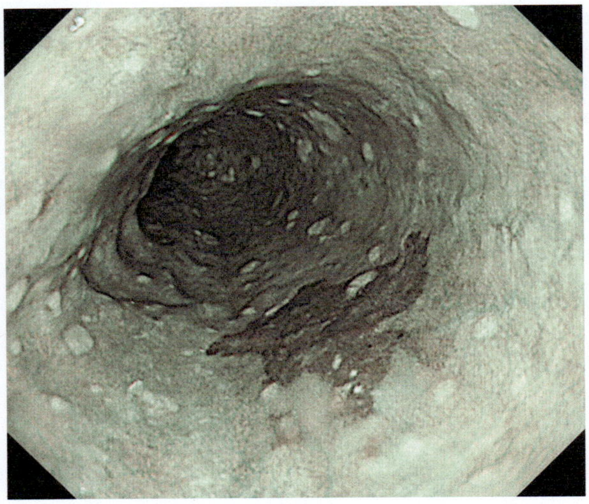

Fig. 3.6 Dark BA noted by NBI

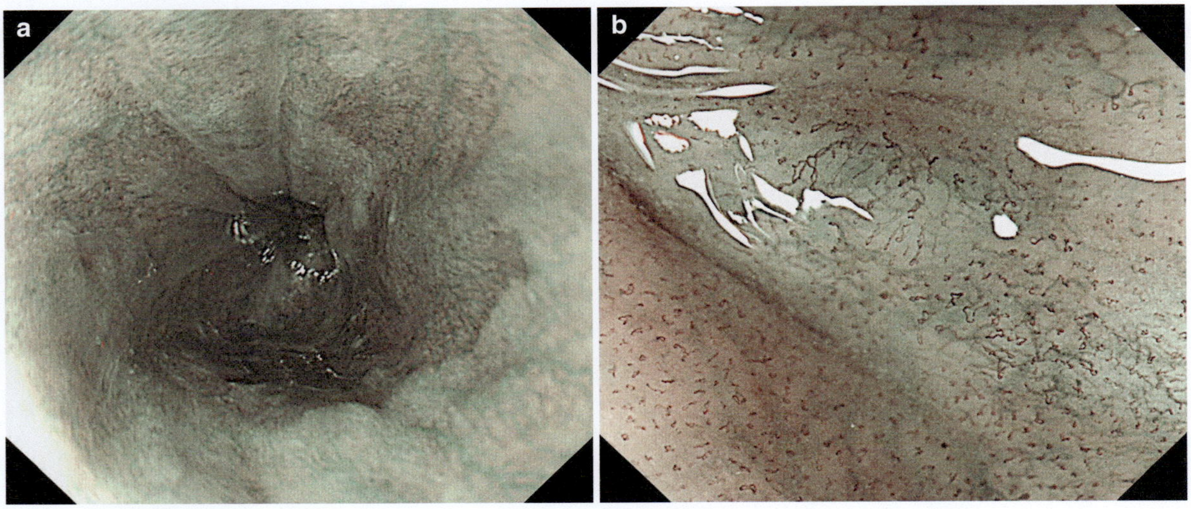

Fig. 3.7 Light BA (Type B1 blood vessels) by NBI

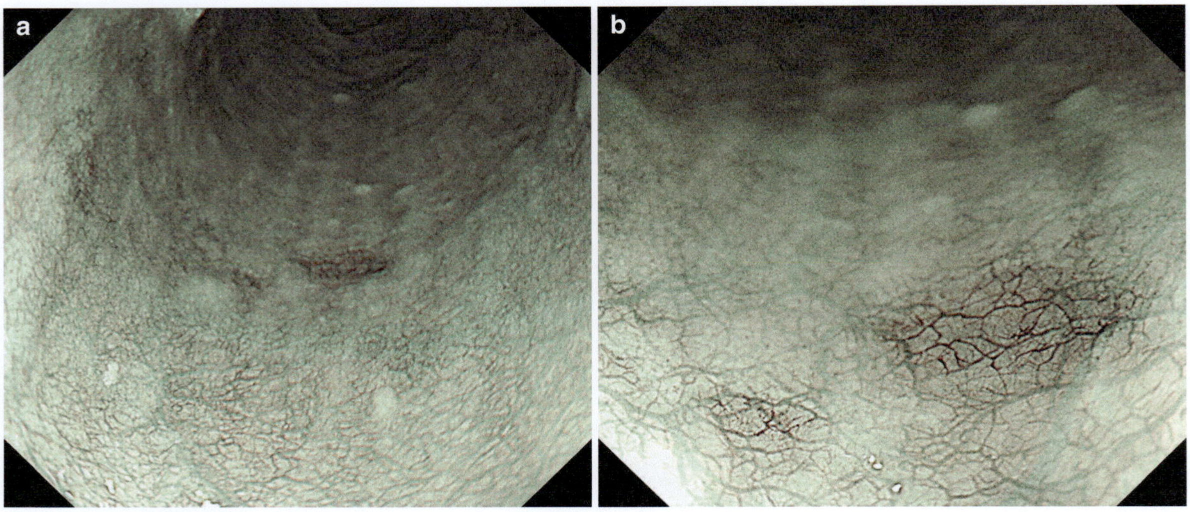

Fig. 3.8 Light BA (SECN) by NBI

3.3 Iodine Dye Staining

Iodine dye is caustic and with higher concentration can result in surface layer sloughing. Therefore, use of 1.5–3% iodine solution should be avoided. The author and colleagues use 0.75% iodine solution. If iodine dye staining is not sufficient, it can be stained the second time (Fig. 3.9 (a) iodine dye staining the first time, (b) iodine dye staining the second time).

Shortly after iodine dye staining, the unstained area turns pink in color, which is described as "pink color sign" [1]. With NBI, the change is described as "metallic color sign" [2] useful in distinguishing SCC from nonneoplastic lesions. When lightly stained with iodine, it is often difficult to distinguish neoplastic from nonneoplastic lesions. But "pink color sign" and "metallic silver sign," when positive, indicate a diagnosis of tumor and, when negative, a diagnosis of nontumor.

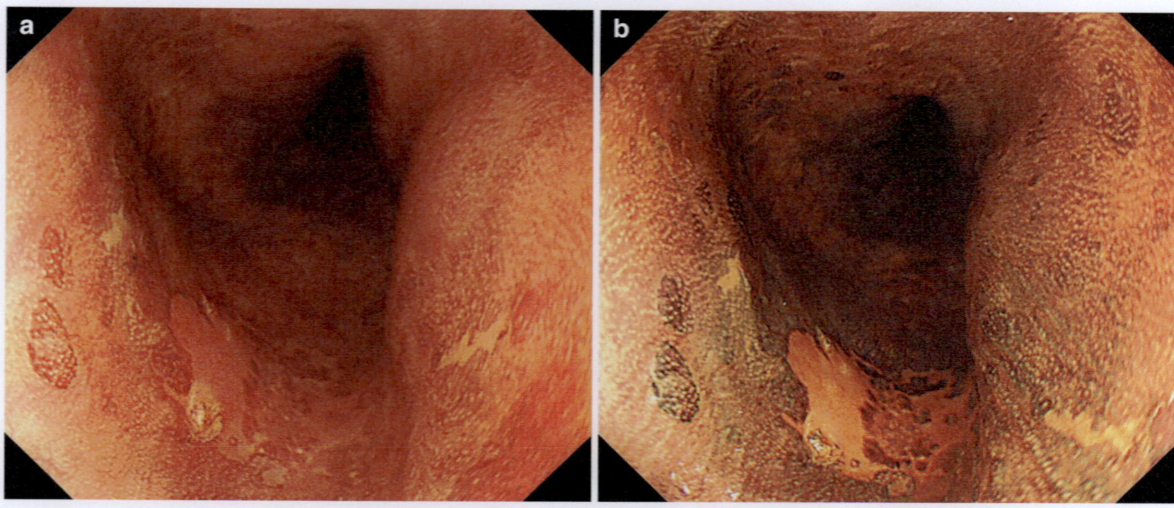

Fig. 3.9 Iodine dye staining (first and second time)

Case 1: A Case of Useful Pink Color Sign and Metallic Silver Sign

Lightly staining area with iodine dye (Fig. 3.10a, b): The area marked with a yellow arrow shows positive pink color and metallic silver signs indicating diagnosis of SCC. The area marked with a green arrow shows negative pink color and metallic silver signs indicating nontumor.

As mentioned above, iodine dye is highly caustic; iodine dye staining to T1a-EP~LPM SCC lesions may result in surface sloughing and epithelialization of the tumor with nontumor squamous cells. This leads to temporary shrinkage of the unstained area, necessitating scheduling of ESD to be 1 month or more from the date of the last iodine staining [3].

Column: Merits and Demerits of Iodine Dye Staining

Iodine dye staining is the most sensitive method for determining lateral margins of SCC.

However, its highly caustic nature may cause sloughing of the mucosal layer. This may lead to the replacement of the superficial cancer with nontumor squamous cell epithelium turning superficial cancer to basal layer-type cancer. Iodine dye staining should be limited to minimum as second iodine dye staining will reduce unstained areas.

It is possible to confirm diagnosis of SCC with NBI showing BA and NBI magnification showing Type B1 blood vessels. Ideally, preoperative diagnosis can be performed with WLI, NBI + NBI magnification alone, and the initial iodine dye staining should be reserved for the day of ESD.

When T1b is suspected, it is necessary to immediately perform ESD. But if T1a-EP~LPM is suspected, the disease will not advance in 2–3 months. Therefore, for cases referred after iodine staining, if the depth of invasion is T1a-EP~LPM, it is safer to perform ESD after about 3 months of waiting.

(Tsuneo Oyama)

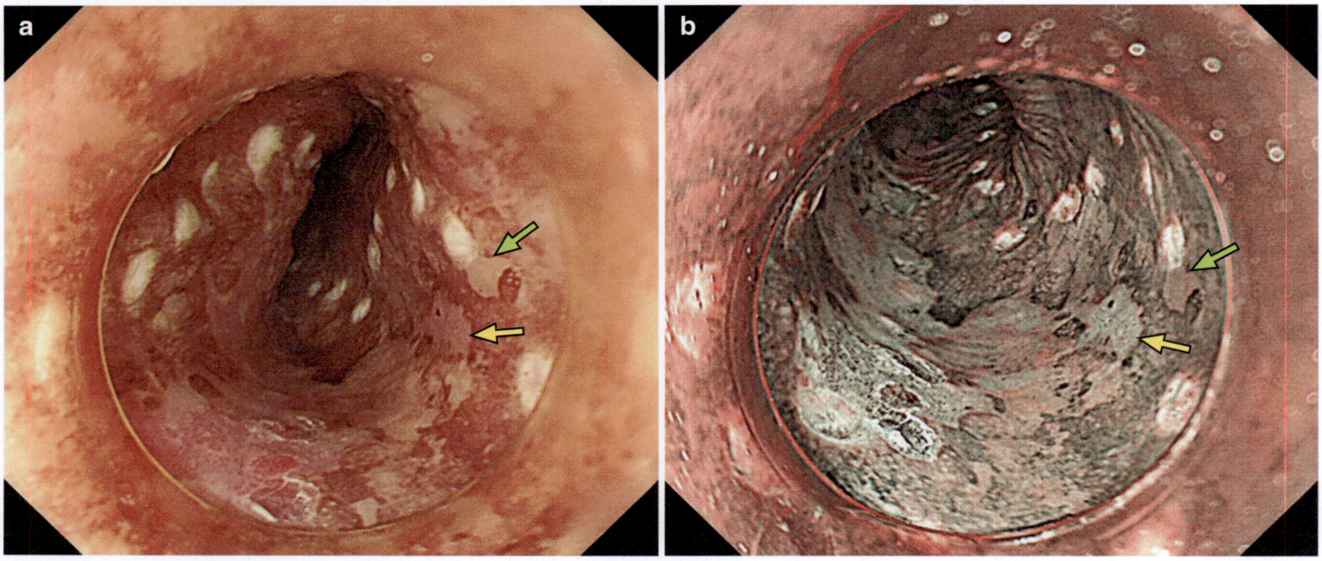

Fig. 3.10 Case 1

Case 2: A Case of Reduced Lesion Size After Iodine Staining

The first iodine staining revealed a clearly demarcated unstained area (Fig. 3.11a). ESD was scheduled 1 month later revealing a different unstained lesion pattern (Fig. 3.11b). Even the use of 0.75% iodine dye requires caution.

In this case, markings were placed carefully comparing the pre-ESD images with the initial iodine dye spray images of the lesion with surrounding darkly staining glycogenic acanthosis as reference points to completely remove the initially unstained target lesion. (Fig. 3.11c, at the time of markings; Fig. 3.11d, after markings; (e) resected specimen. Five arrows of varied colors are matched with corresponding reference points.)

Histopathologically, carcinoma was noted in the basal squamous cell layer of the stained area also (Fig. 3.11f). Mapping of the lesion on the resected specimen revealed widely formed basal layer-type cancer, extending the unstained area (g: light blue lines show T1a-LPM, dotted lines show basal layer type cancer, red line shows the section f).

As basal layer-type cancers formed by preoperative iodine dye staining are iodine dye stainable, these lesions may not to be diagnosable at the time of ESD. Decision to even cancel ESD is important if iodine staining imaging on the day of ESD differs greatly from the preoperatively obtained images.

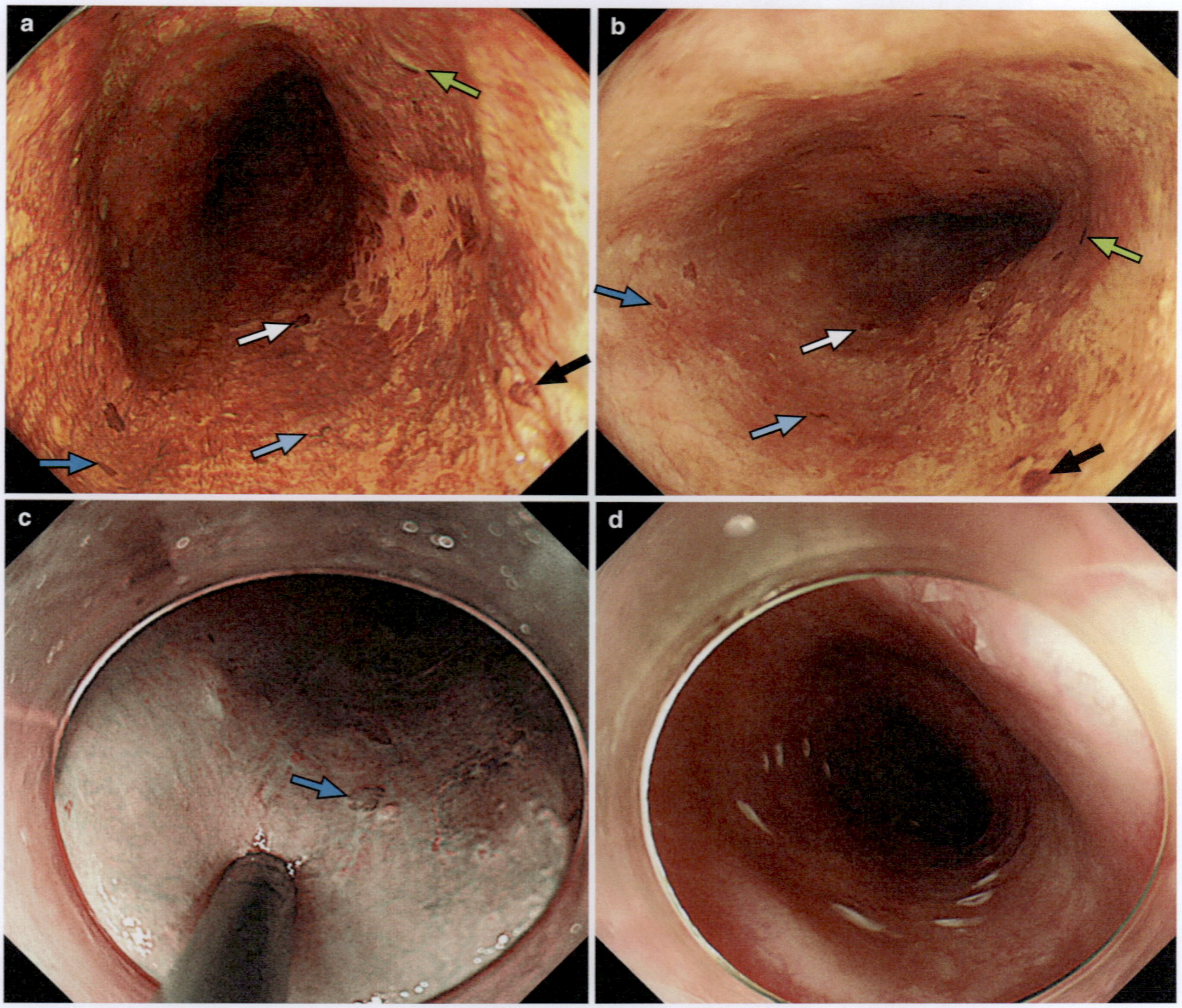

Fig. 3.11 Case 2. A case of reduced lesion size after iodine staining. (**a**) The initial iodine staining. (**b**) The second iodine staining (1 month later). (**c**) At the time of marking. (**d**) After marking. (**e**) Resected specimen. (**f**) Histopathological image (section f). (**g**) Lesion mapping (red line shows section f)

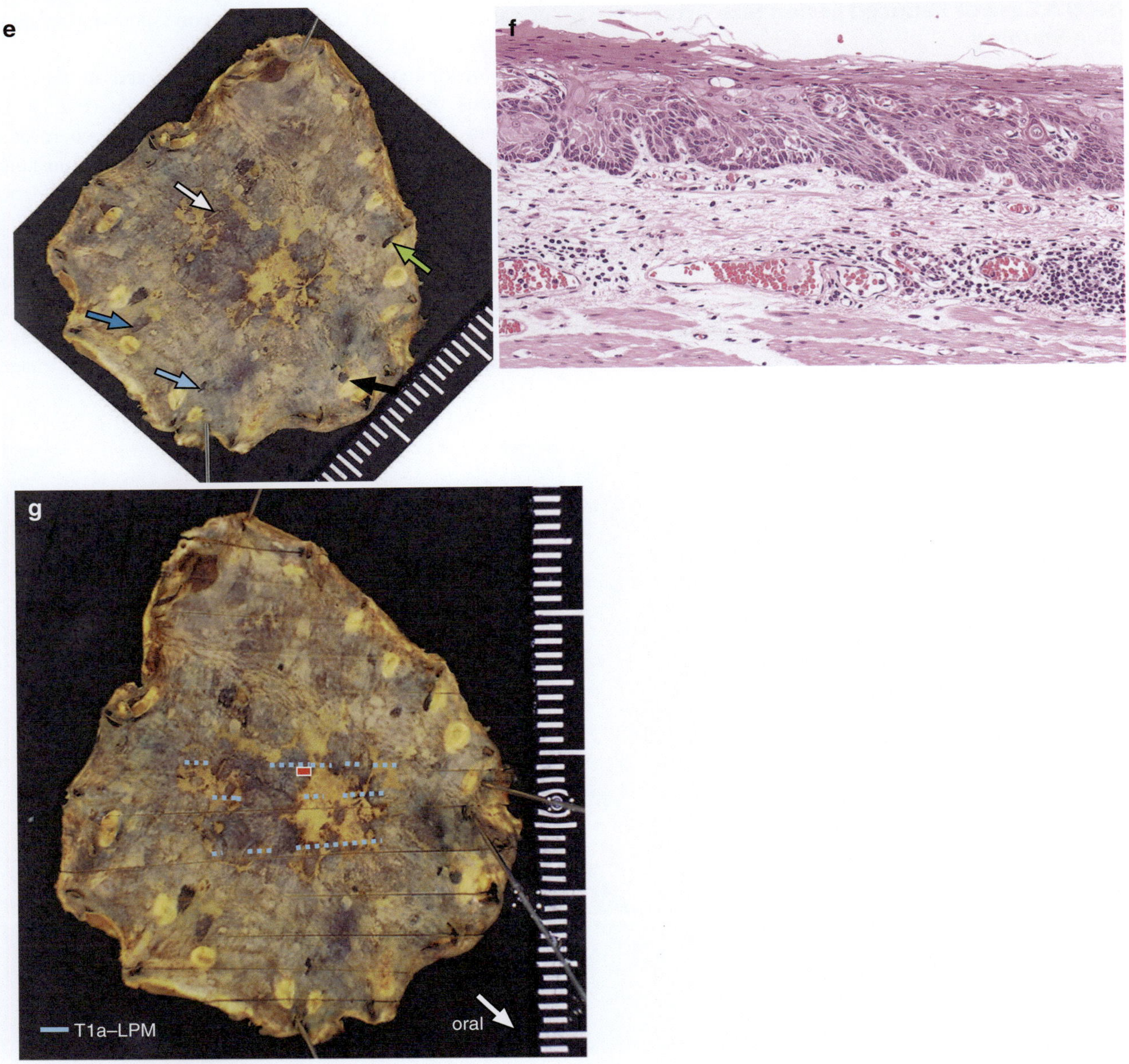

Fig. 3.11 (continued)

3.4 Summary

Features of white light imaging, NBI magnification imaging, and iodine dye staining method in diagnosis of lateral margins are summarized. The basis of determination of lateral margins is iodine dye staining method, and it is desirable to perform the first iodine dye staining on the day of ESD, as surface mucosal sloughing of the lesion may be induced by iodine dye staining. And in the case of unclear lateral margins, it is desirable to cancel ESD and repeat evaluation after some period.

References

1. Shimizu Y, et al. Endoscopic diagnosis of early squamous neoplasia of the esophagus with iodine staining: high-grade intra-epithelial neoplasia turns pink within a few minutes. J Gastroenterol Hepatol. 2008;23:546–50.
2. Maselli R, et al. The metallic silver sign with narrow-band imaging: a new endoscopic predictor for pharyngeal and esophageal neoplasia. Gastrointest Endosc. 2013;78:551–2.
3. Oyama T, et al. Local recurrences after esophageal endoscopic mucosal resection. Stomach Intestine. 1996;31:1217–22.

4 Diagnosis of Invasion Depths

Tsuneo Oyama and Shigetaka Yoshinaga

4.1 Endoscopic Diagnosis

Since invasion depth and lymphatic metastases are strongly associated, preoperative diagnosis of invasion depth is important in therapeutic decision-making. Invasion depth diagnosis of superficial cancer is performed mainly with endoscopy, magnification endoscopy, and endoscopic ultrasound (EUS). In this section, invasion depth diagnosis is explained for endoscopy and magnification endoscopy.

Invasion Depth Diagnosis Under White Light Imaging

Since invasion depth and disease form types are strongly correlated, disease form typing is useful in invasion depth diagnosis. 0-I and 0-III are mostly T1b. 0-Ip is sometimes T1a. 0IIb is either T1a-EP or T1a-LPM and is indicated for endoscopic treatments. On the other hand, 0-IIa and 0-IIc include wide range of lesions from T1a-EP to T1b, necessitating careful assessments of invasion depths.

Evaluation of Thickness

When a T1a-MM or T1b lesion becomes invasive, local thickness develops within a lesion. It is important to adjust air volume to assess thickness. T1a-EP~LPM lesions may show local thickness when air volume is reduced, but when inflated with enough air, such temporary thickness disappears. Therefore, adequate adjustment of air volume is essential for evaluation of thickness. If thickness and deformed shape remain with sufficient air inflation, greater invasion depth of T1a-MM or more is suspected.

The case below is a 0-IIc + IIa lesion located in the mid-thoracic (Mt) esophagus spreading from the posterior wall to the right wall. With small amount of air, some thickness is noted in 0-IIa portion at 5 o'clock (Fig. 4.1a). With large amount of air, the esophageal lumen expanded, but the thick area had poor

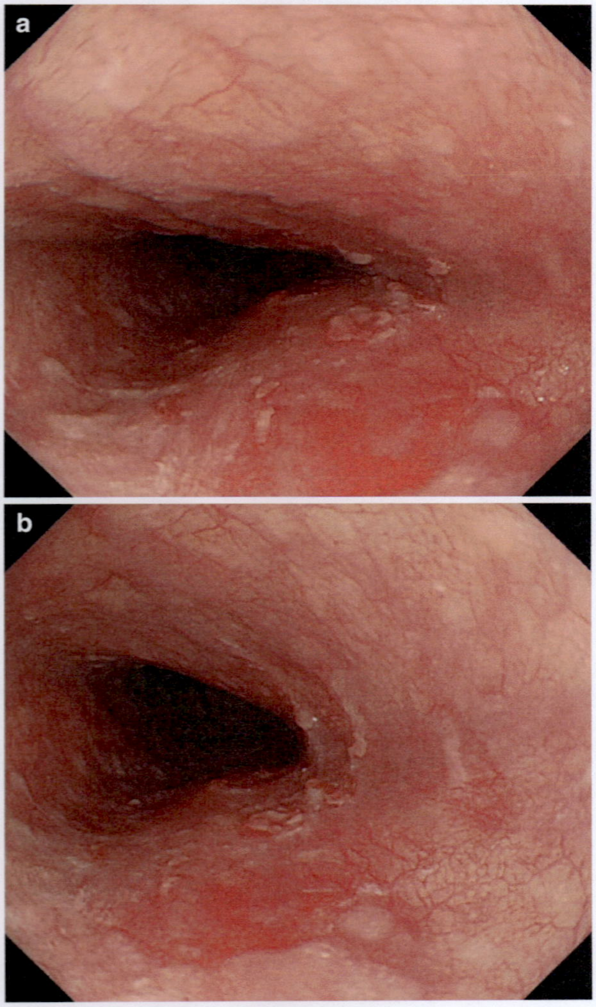

Fig. 4.1 Evaluation of thickness

T. Oyama (✉)
Department of Endoscopy, Saku Central Hospital Advanced Care Center, Nagano, Japan
e-mail: oyama@coral.ocn.ne.jp

S. Yoshinaga
Department of Endoscopy, Saku Central Hospital Advanced Care Center, Nagano, Japan

T. Oyama (ed.), *Endoscopic Diagnosis of Esophageal Carcinoma for ESD*, https://doi.org/10.1007/978-981-32-9030-3_4

expansion with persistent thickness (Fig. 4.1b). Invasion depth of the thick area was T1a-MM. It is important to observe dynamically with varying volume of air to evaluate thickness of lesions.

"Tatami (Japanese Woven Straw) Mat" Pattern

Iodine dye staining stimulates the muscularis mucosal layer to shrink, resulting in a characteristic appearance resembling "tatami" pattern. When cancer remains within T1a-LPM, the pattern is observed. When cancer invades into T1a-MM and deeper, shrinkage of the muscularis mucosa is hindered, resulting in disappearance of the "tatami mat" pattern.

The case below is 0-IIb squamous cell carcinoma and revealed a clearly demarcated unstained area (Fig. 4.2a). Although "tatami mat" pattern was not seen immediately after iodine dye staining, very clear "tatami mat" pattern appeared after waiting for a while (Fig. 4.2b). Invasion depth of a lesion can be diagnosed as T1a-EP~LPM, when "tatami mat" pattern traverses through the lesion.

On the other hand, once invasion depth reaches T1a-MM and deeper, this pattern disappears. Figure 4.3 shows iodine dye staining of the lesion shown in Fig. 4.1. Although "tatami mat" pattern is observed in the posterior wall side of

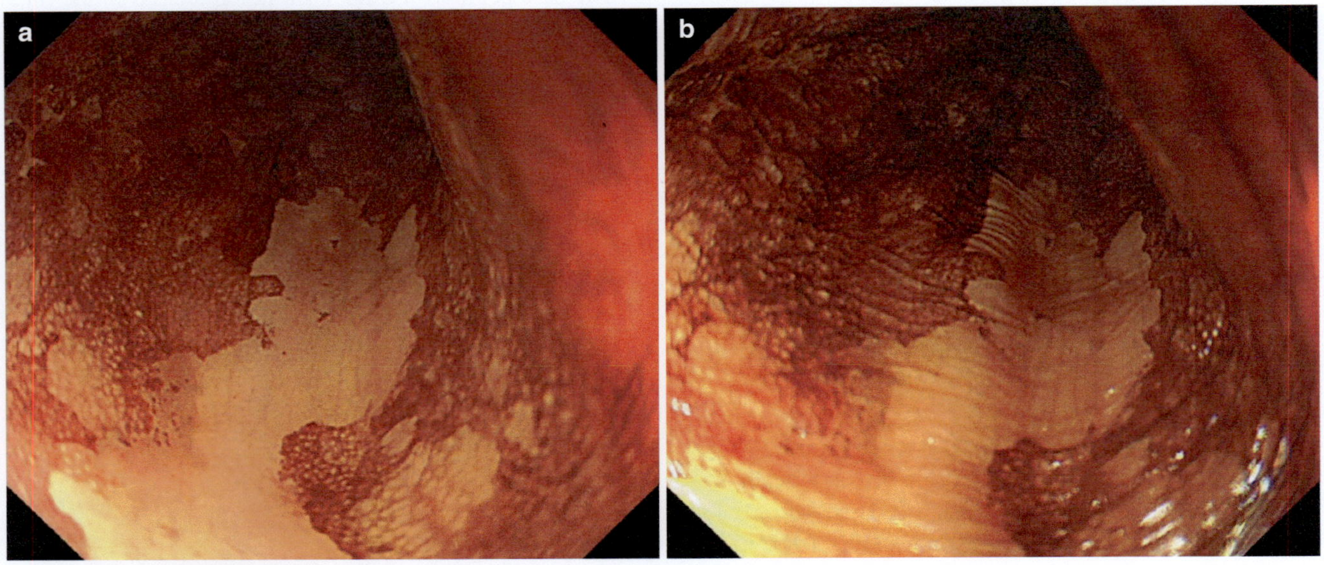

Fig. 4.2 "Tatami (Japanese woven straw) mat" pattern

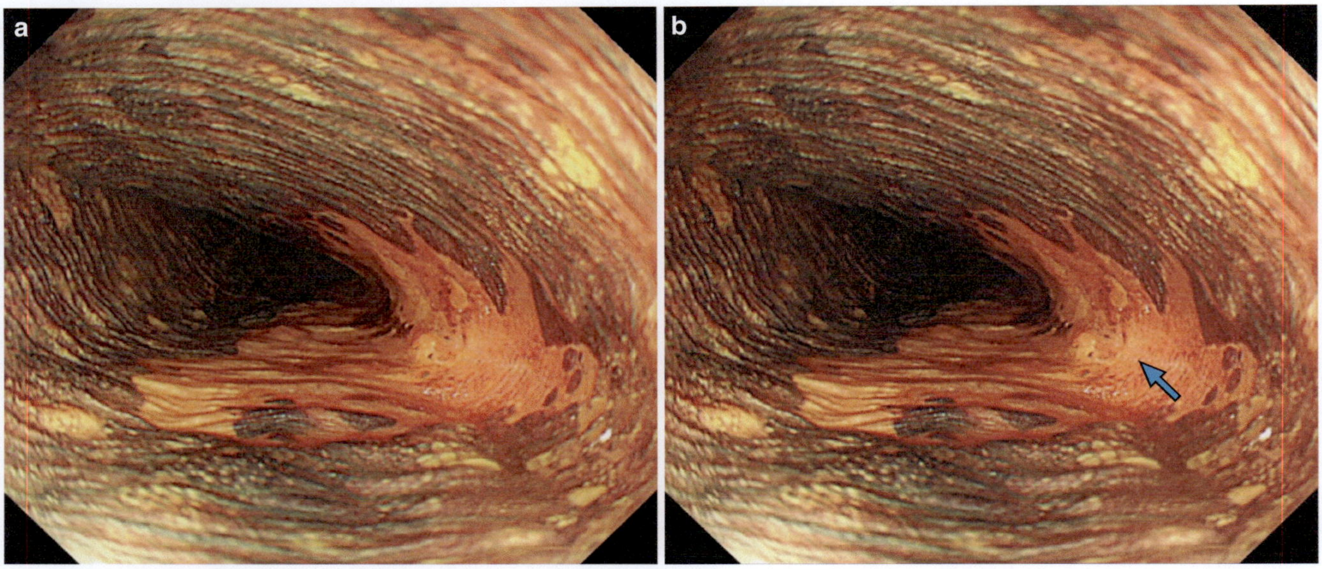

Fig. 4.3 Disappearance of the "tatami mat" pattern

the lesion, it is lost in the 5 o'clock direction where the lesion is noted with localized thickness as shown by the blue arrow (Fig. 4.3).

Invasion Depth Diagnosis with Magnifying Endoscopy

On usual endoscopic observation, the mucosal surface, the lamina propria, and down to the shallow portion of the submucosa are observed, and on magnifying endoscopy, the mucosal surface and the shallow lamina propria are mainly observed. The normal squamous cell layer contains papillary structures, and on magnifying endoscopy, looplike blood vessels running inside the papillae (IPCL) are observed (Fig. 4.4).

Tricks for Performing Magnifying Observation [1]

When performing with magnification, the scope is brought very close to the mucosal surface, nearing to approximately 2 mm in distance. However, this results in very narrow visual field with a very limited area in focus. When a 2 mm transparent attachment hood is placed, the lesion of interest may be observed face on and in clear focus. However, the esophagus moves constantly by respiratory motion and cardiac pulsations, and contacts with the attachment hood may result in bleeding, making a clear observation difficult at times. It is important to utilize respiratory motion as to avoid contacts and frictions while observing.

The Japan Esophageal Society Classification of Findings in Esophageal Cancer Observed with Magnifying Endoscopy [2, 3]

The Japan Esophageal Society utilized intrapapillary capillary loops (IPCL) to classify endoscopic findings using magnifying endoscopy of esophageal cancer.

- **Type A Blood Vessels**

The most representative of the esophageal lesions with brownish area (BA) on NBI is squamous cell carcinoma, but inflammation and thinning of the surface layer may present as BA as well. Sometimes, intraepithelial tumors with little atypia may also present as BA. In such lesions, very slight elongation of the IPCL is observed. These are classified as Type A blood vessels (Fig. 4.5).

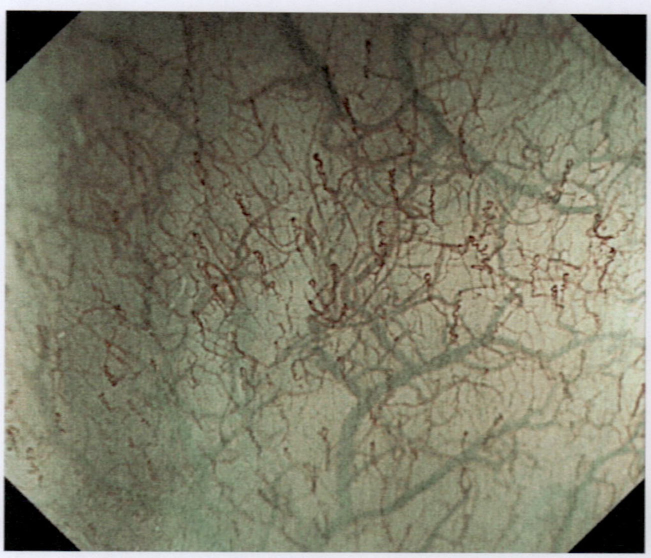

Fig. 4.4 Looplike blood vessels. Same picture as Fig. 1.4 in Chap. 1

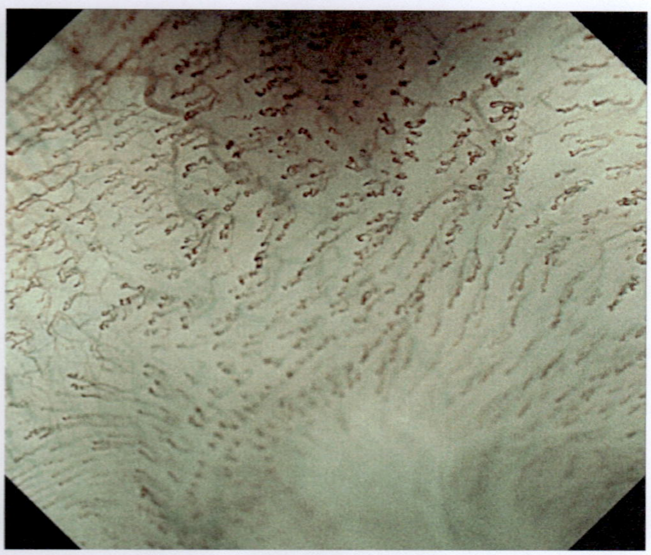

Fig. 4.5 Type A blood vessels

• Type B1 Blood Vessels

When squamous cell cancer with invasion depths of T1a-EP is diagnosed, the cancer grows along the basement membrane replacing the normal cells with neoplastic cells, and papillary structures remain within the cancerous lesion (Fig. 4.6a). Therefore, on magnifying endoscopy, looplike blood vessels are noted running inside these papillae. However, unlike the usual IPCL, irregular looplike vessels characterized with dilation, tortuosity, irregularly traversing patterns, and uneven shapes are noted. These are Type B1 blood vessels (Fig. 4.6b).

On the other hand, once the cancer invades into the LPM, papillary structures become destroyed, and the blood vessels extend horizontally (Fig. 4.6c). Naturally, the intrapapillary blood vessels run within the papillae which extend from their bases in oblique angles and appear as irregular elongated looplike vessels on magnifying endoscopy (Fig. 4.6d). These blood vessels are classified as Type B1, if their looplike structures are kept intact with elongated appearance.

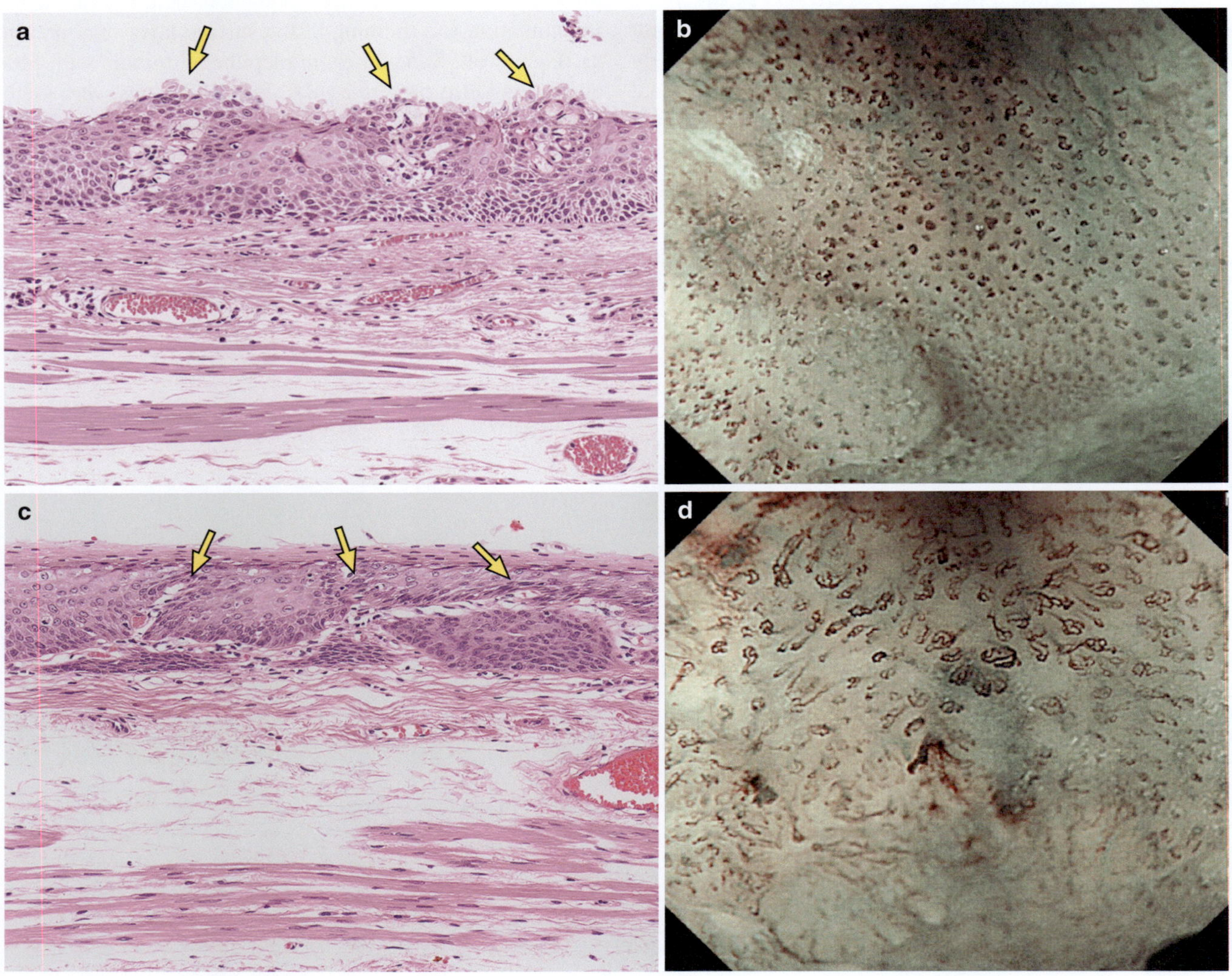

Fig. 4.6 Type B1 blood vessels. (**a**, **b**) Papillary structures (a, yellow arrows) noted within EP cancers, and looplike blood vessels (b) on NBI magnifying endoscopy (Type 1 blood vessels). (**c**, **d**) Papillary structures (c, yellow arrows) noted with LPM cancers, and looplike blood vessels (B1 with elongated vessels)

- **Type B2 Blood Vessels**

When cancer invades further into the muscularis mucosae, the papillary structures are destroyed, and neoplastic blood vessels with looplike formation appear (Fig. 4.7a). Thus appearing non-loop blood vessels are classified as Type B2 (Fig. 4.7b). Therefore, a lesion with Type B2 blood vessels is diagnosed as invasive cancer with destruction of papillary structures, with invasion depth of T1a-MM or T1b-SM1.

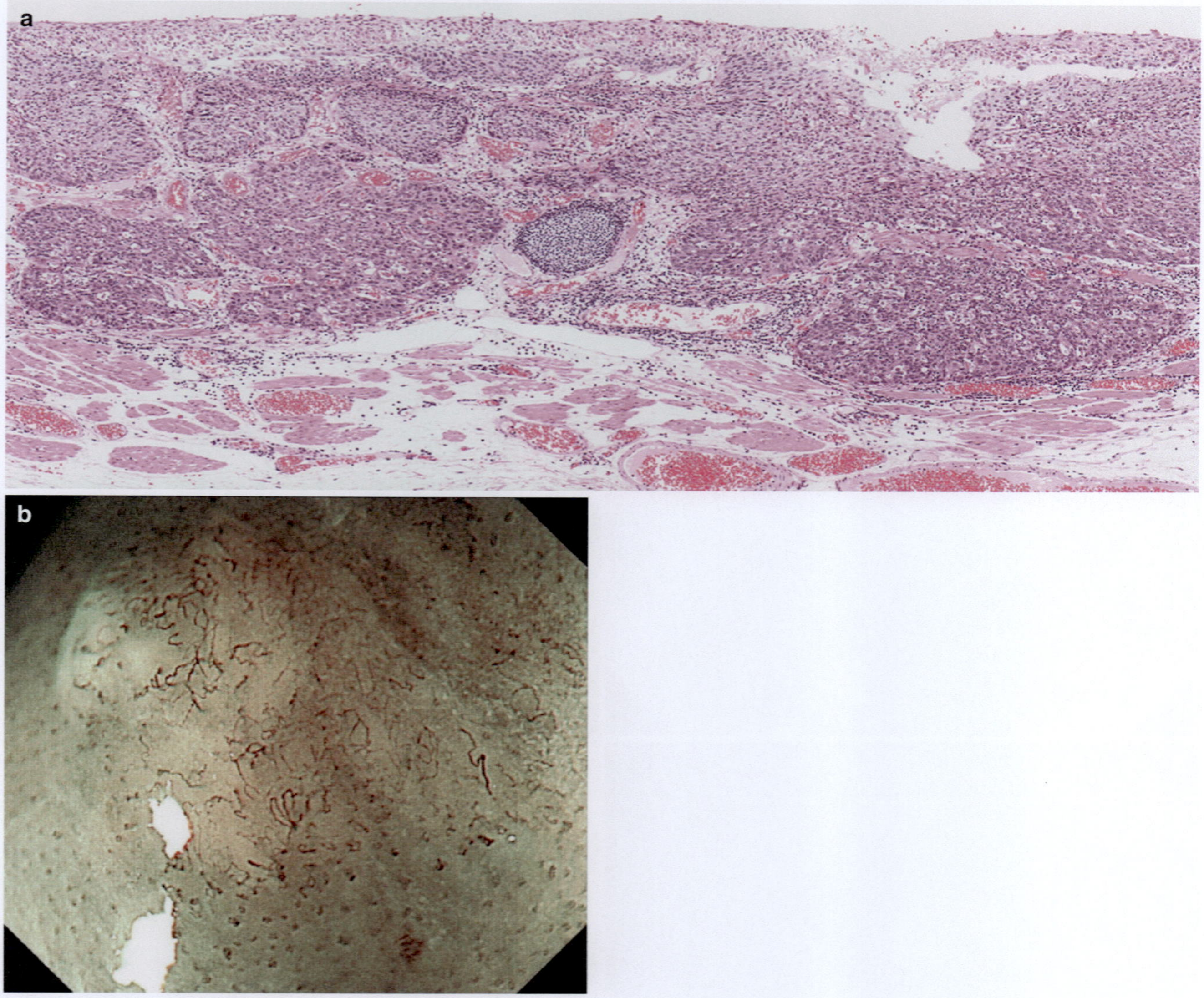

Fig. 4.7 Type B2 blood vessels

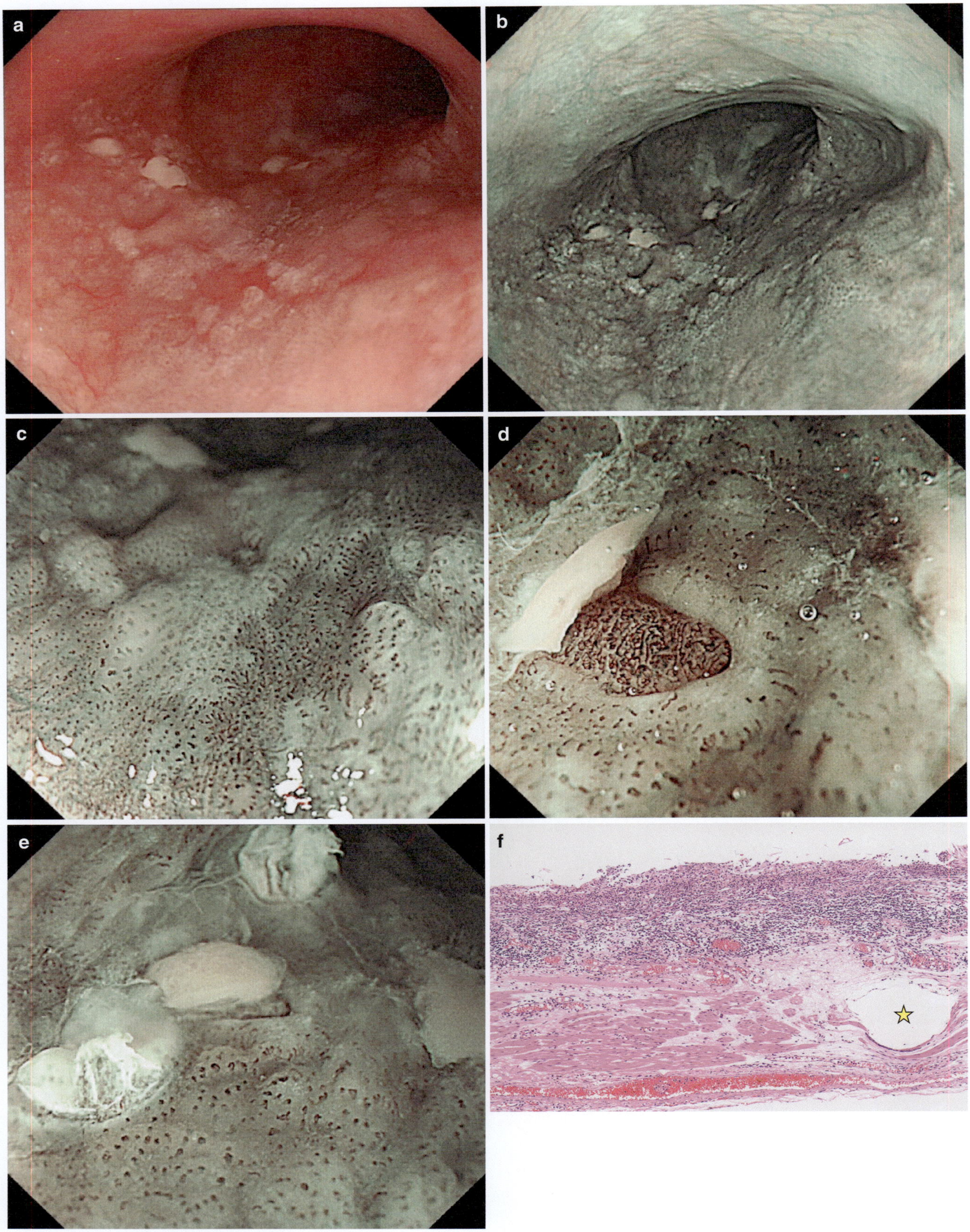

Fig. 4.8 Type B2i blood vessels

• Type B2i Blood Vessels

Often erosions are noted within cancerous lesions, and sometimes non-loop blood vessels without caliber variations are observed.

The case below is a widely spreading posterior wall 0-IIc lesion in the mid-thorax (Mt) (Fig. 4.8b). Blood vessels consist mostly of Type B1 (Fig. 4.8c), but there was an area with densely gathered non-loop blood vessels. Comparing with usual Type B2 blood vessels, these vessels are highly dense and without caliber variations and are diagnosed as B2 like blood vessels seen in granulomas (Fig. 4.8d).

To compare the endoscopic image with the corresponding histological image, two markings (using hook knife) were placed interposing this area (Fig. 4.8). The resected specimen was fixed placing pins in the two markings, and the histological image shows a pinhole marked with yellow star (Fig. 4.8f) next to the area of interest with no cancerous cells, but with infiltrating inflammatory cells with regenerating blood vessels associated with erosive changes.

Since erosions contain no papillary structures, non-loop blood vessels are formed as a natural sequence. Thus formed non-loop vessels associated with erosions are characterized by high density and lack of caliber variations. These characteristic non-loop blood vessels are designated as inflammation-related Type B2i blood vessels.

• Type B3 Blood Vessels

When cancer invades further into the T1b-SM2, tumor-associated blood vessels of larger caliber appear (Fig. 4.9). According to the Japan Esophageal Society classification, Type B3 blood vessels are irregular blood vessels with three times the caliber of usual Type B2 blood vessels (about 60 μm or more).

According to the Japan Esophageal Society's classification, abnormal blood vessels observed by NBI magnifying endoscopy are divided into loop-forming Type B1, non-loop-forming Type B2, and large caliber Type B3, and these types are applied to estimate invasion depth of observed lesions (Table 4.1).

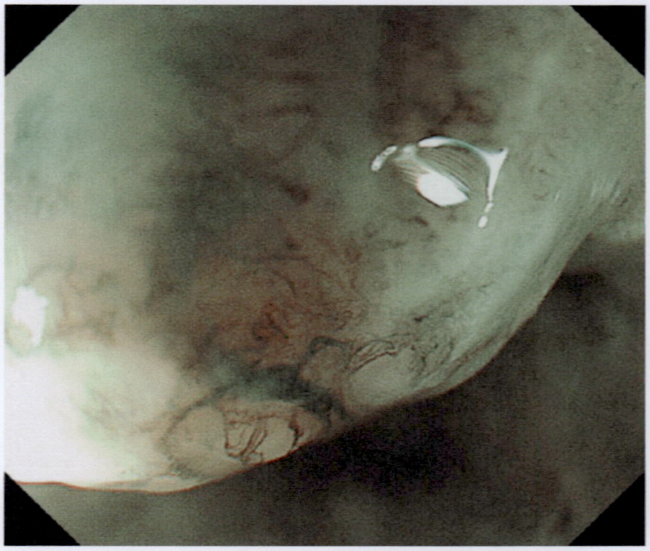

Fig. 4.9 Type B3 blood vessels

Table 4.1 Japan Esophageal Society's classification and invasion depth estimation

B1	T1a-EP, T1a-LPM
B2	T1a-MM, T1b-SM1
B3	T1b-SM2

- **AVA (Avascular Area)**

When squamous cell carcinoma grows expansively forcing blood vessels outside the tumor mass, tumors become surrounded by blood vessels (Fig. 4.10a). When this area is observed with magnified NBI, there appears to be areas of no blood vessels surrounded by Type B2 blood vessels (Fig. 4.10b). The Japan Esophageal Society has classified this finding as avascular areas (AVA). Although described as "avascular area," in actuality, small pieces of blood vessels may be seen scattered within.

AVA were subclassified by size, AVA-small (AVA-S) of less than 0.5 mm, AVA-middle (AVA-M) of 0.5 mm to less than 3 mm, and AVA-large (AVA-L) of greater than 3 mm. It is difficult to accurately measure with endoscopy, but maximum magnification with Olympus H260Z shows on monitor a horizontal width of approximately 3 mm in full zoom, and the size of AVA can be estimated reasonably on full zoom observation.

When Type B2 blood vessels are observed, invasion depth can be diagnosed as T1a-MM~SM1. But if AVA-S is observed, invasion depth may be diagnosed as one level less as T1a-EP~LPM, and if AVA-L is observed, invasion depth may be diagnosed one level above as T1b-SM2 (Table 4.2).

Table 4.2 Japan Esophageal Society's AVA classification and invasion depth estimation

AVA-small	T1a-EP, T1a-LPM
AVA-middle	T1a-MM, T1b-SM1
AVA-large	T1b-SM2

Summary Points

- AVA is an avascular or scantly vascular area surrounded by Type B2 blood vessels.
- Even when Type B2 blood vessels are seen, AVA-S is diagnosed one level less and AVA-L one level above.

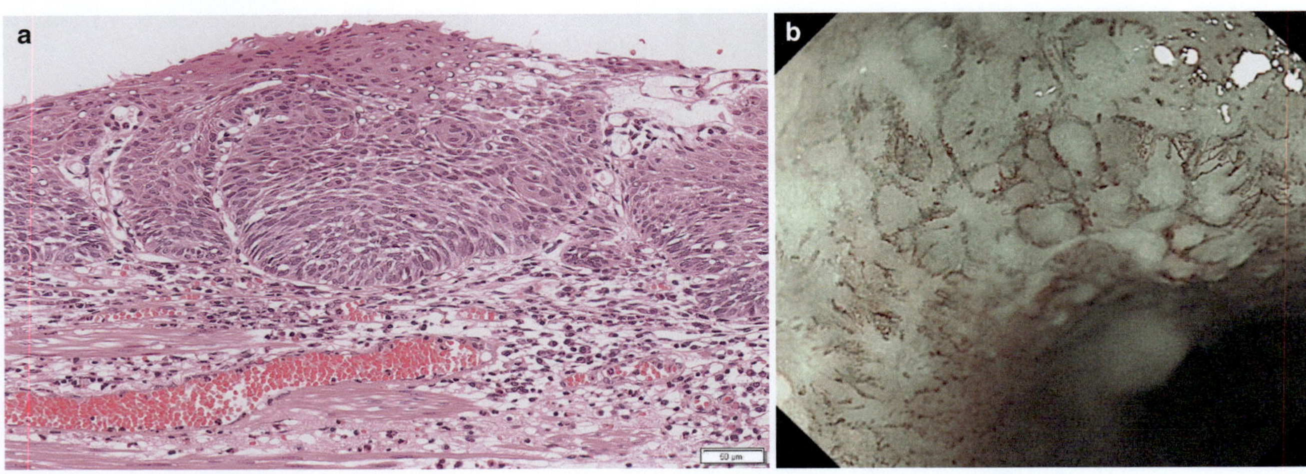

Fig. 4.10 AVA (avascular area)

- **Type R Blood Vessels** [4]

Although squamous cell cancers usually infiltrate expansively, when adhesive factors are lost, they may spread diffusely without forming cancer nests. In such cases, finely branching reticular blood vessels are observed. These blood vessels are designated as reticular (Type R) blood vessels (Fig. 4.11). Type R blood vessels are often seen with undifferentiated- or special-type cancers, and therefore, this classification is useful for histological diagnosis. It should be noted that before-mentioned Type B2i and Type R blood vessels are both non-loop forming, and distinguishing them apart is important. Inflammation-associated Type B2i blood vessels have no caliber variations and highly dense, which are useful points in differentiating from Type R blood vessels.

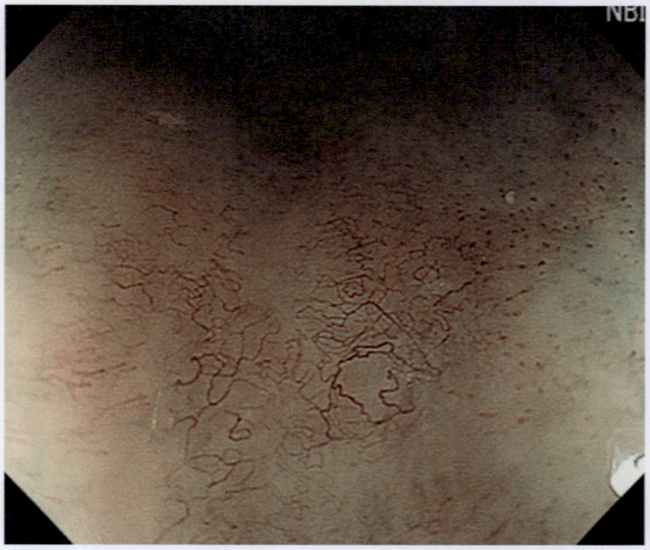

Fig. 4.11 Type R blood vessels. Same picture as Fig. 23.3e in Chap. 23

Limitations of Diagnosis with Magnifying Endoscopy

Magnifying endoscopy allows us to observe merely the top surface of the cancer, and we are not directly visualizing the infiltrating portion. Therefore, information obtained from magnifying endoscopy does not necessarily reflect invasion depths of the lesion observed. Several reasons why magnifying endoscopy findings do not match invasion depth estimations are explained below.

• Case of Type B1 Blood Vessels, but with Invasion Depth of T1a-MM or More

When cancer invades into T1a-MM or T1b level, papillary structures are destroyed, and non-looping blood vessels appear. Therefore, if cancer infiltrates and is exposed to the surface, findings of magnifying endoscopy and invasion depth estimation correlate well. On the other hand, sometimes the surface of deeply invasive cancer is covered over with T1a-EP or T1a-LPM cancer. In such case, white light imaging shows localized thickness, but magnifying endoscopy only shows the lesion surface with Type B1 blood vessels. This is the limit of invasion depth diagnosis with magnifying endoscopy. To arrive at more accurate invasion depth estimation, the use of other modalities such as white light imaging and EUS must be combined with magnifying endoscopy to collectively assess diagnosis.

• Case of Type B2 Blood Vessels, but with Invasion Depth of T1b-SM2

Since magnifying endoscopy can only detect the blood vessels in the topmost surface, it is difficult to diagnose invasion depth. It is possible to make correct diagnosis when findings of high positive predictive value (PPV) such as Type 3 blood vessels or AVA-L are seen. But these findings occur infrequently, and their sensitivities are low. "Detection of Type B2 blood vessels" is not necessarily equal to "T1a-MM or T1b-SM1," but "Type B2 blood vessels" are "destructions of papillary structures," and this should be interpreted as suspicious of invasion depth of T1a-MM or greater. If the area of Type B2 blood vessels is very small, limited to 1 mm, invasion depth should be rated one level below as T1a-LPM, but if the area of Type B2 blood vessels is a wide area over 10 mm in size, T1b-SM2 should be suspected, and other modalities should be used for evaluation.

• Case of Type B1 Blood Vessels, but with Invasion Depth of T1b-SM2

A reddish flat lesion is noted in the mid-thoracic esophagus (Mt), with a slightly raised area within (marked with a yellow arrow) (Fig. 4.12a). On NBI, BA with dot-like blood vessels are noted within (Fig. 4.12b). When the scope is advanced further, a slight localized thickness is noted (Fig. 4.12c). With NBI magnification observation, Type B1 blood vessels are noted full view, with elongated Type B1 blood vessels in part (Fig. 4.12d,e). Iodine dye staining reveals a clearly demarcated unstained area of over 8 cm long and a large superficially spreading-type cancer (Fig. 4.12f).

Based on these findings of mostly flat superficially spreading large cancer, with only a small area of localized thickness, consisting only of Type B1 blood vessels, and with estimated invasion depth of T1a-LPM, a large superficially spreading esophageal cancer was diagnosed, and ESD was performed.

With a clearly demarcated unstained area of a large superficially spreading-type esophageal cancer (Fig. 4.12g), the resected specimen was prepared and sliced for full evaluation. Histological images of the dotted black line (Fig. 4.12g) are shown. Cancer had invaded the muscularis mucosa down widely to the submucosal area (Fig. 4.12h). The topmost surface was covered with T1a-EP cancer, and the deeply invasive cancer was not exposed to the surface (Fig. 4.12i). Since magnifying endoscopy visualizes the blood vessels in the topmost layer, deeply invasive cancer, if covered over by T1a-EP cancer, only Type B1 blood vessels will be observed. In this case, it is important to diagnose by thickness. The final diagnosis was SCC, T1b-SM2 (invasion distance of 360 μm, invasion width of 3600 μm), ly(+), v(−), HMO0, VM0, 0-IIc + IIb, 85 × 50 mm (Fig. 4.12j).

This case was T1b-SM2, but the invasion width was only 3600 μm and covered with T1a-EP cancer, and preoperative diagnosis was difficult. Retrospectively analyzed, the invasion was confirmed at the point marked by the yellow arrow (Fig. 4.12a–c).

> **Summary Points**
> - Magnifying endoscopy merely observes the topmost layer; the final diagnosis needs to be made together with white light imaging.

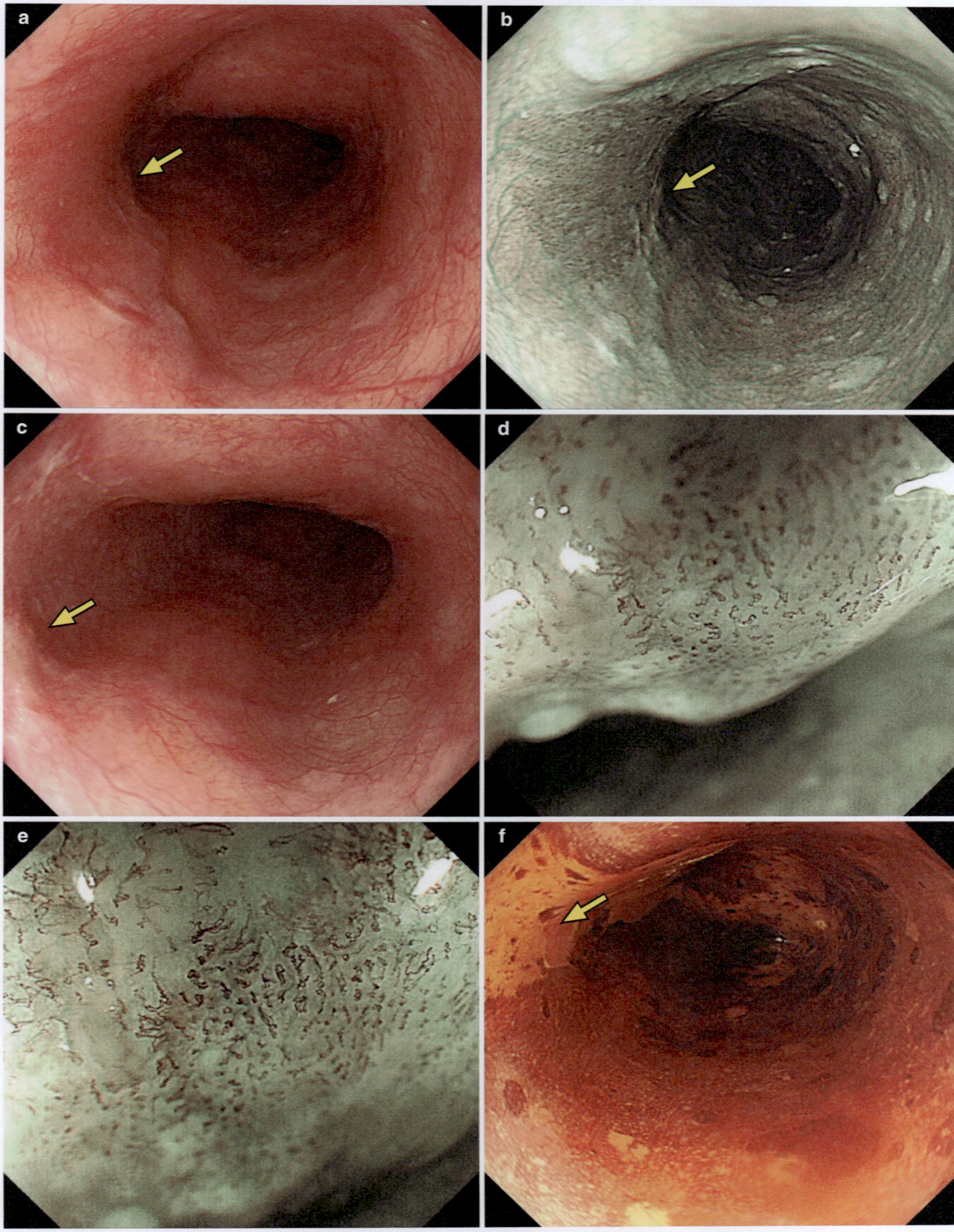

Fig. 4.12 Case of Type B1 blood vessels but with invasion depth of T1b-SM2

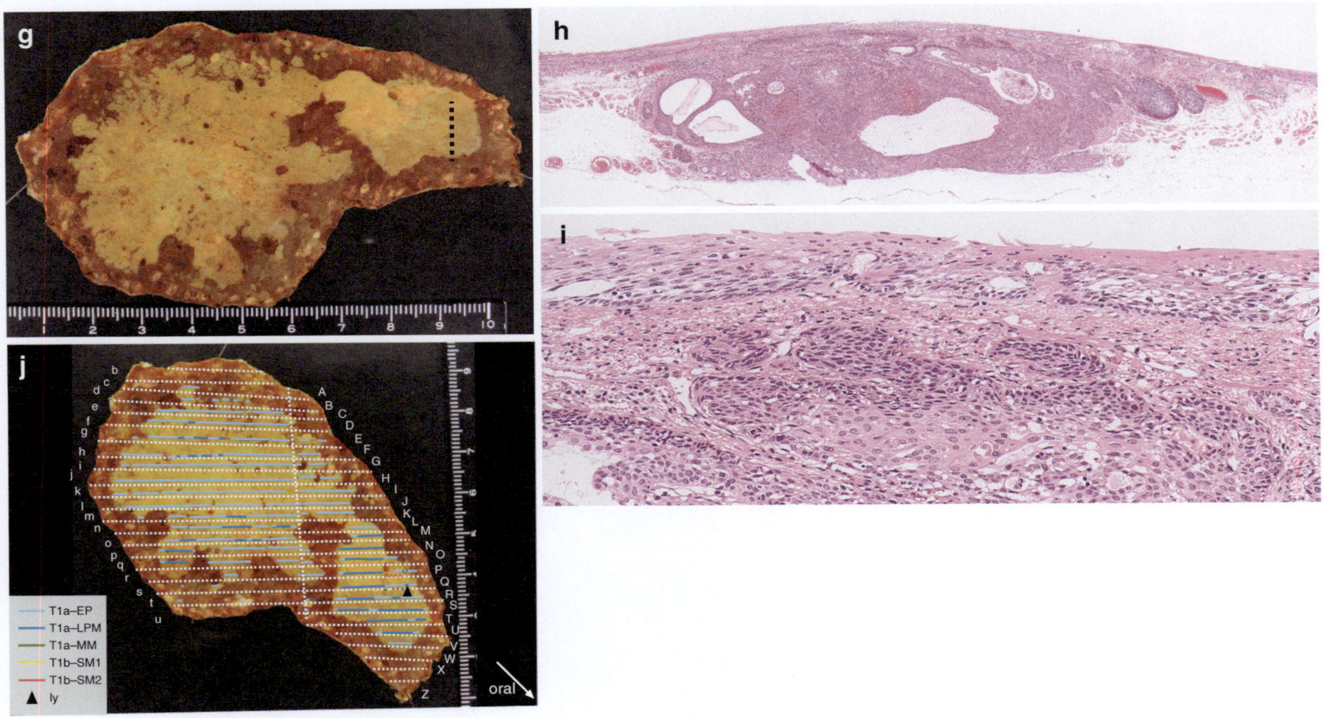

Fig. 4.12 (continued)

4.2 EUS

State of Invasion Depth Diagnosis by EUS

State of Diagnosing Capability

There are various reports concerning invasion depth diagnosis of superficial esophageal cancer by EUS (Table 4.3). Correct diagnosis rates of invasion depth diagnosis by EUS range from 59% to 92% but mostly in 70% ranges. Most of these studies are performed by small-diameter probes inserted through usual endoscope channels rather than dedicated endosonographic scopes. Currently, invasion depth is often classified as either M(T1) or SM(T2) in the USA and Europe, but not standardized. On the other hand, recent studies from Japan used three groups to evaluate based on estimated differences in lymphatic metastases, M1(T1a-EP)-M2(T1a-LPM), M3(T1a-MM)-SM1(T1b-SM1), and SM2(T1b-SM2)-SM3(T1b-SM3). When divided into M and SM cancers, correct diagnosis rate for M is 70–86% and for SM 75–94%, and they are about the same for both M and SM cancers.

When divided into three invasion depth groups, correct diagnosis rate for M1-M2 is 50–100%, M3-SM1 40–75%, and SM2-SM3 76–100%. Correct diagnosis rate of invasion depth for M3-SM1 cancer is lower compared with the other two groups. These are reflecting the current mechanical limitations of sonographic imaging, as well as effects of fibrosis, lymphatic growth, and difficulties in differentiating esophageal glands, retention cysts, and cancer. Diagnostic capabilities may improve with technological advancements.

Comparison of Diagnostic Capability of EUS with Diagnostic Capabilities of Usual Endoscopy and NBI Magnifying Endoscopy

There are many reports on diagnostic capabilities of each modality from various institutions. However, there are very few studies directly comparing these modalities. Goda and colleagues prospectively evaluated correct diagnosis rates of invasion depth with usual endoscopy, NBI magnifying endoscopy, and EUS, and correct diagnosis rates were 92%, 88%, and 85%, respectively, but with no statistically significant differences. Lee and colleagues retrospectively evaluated correct diagnostic rates of NBI magnifying endoscopy and EUS and were 76.1% and 84.8%, again without statistically significant differences, and correct diagnosis rate by both modalities is 94%.

Factors Influencing Diagnostic Capabilities of EUS

There were factors generally thought to affect diagnostic capabilities of EUS, such as nodular components, inflamma-

Table 4.3 Invasion depth diagnosis of superficial esophageal cancers by EUS

Author	Year	Device used	Invasion depth criteria	Correct diagnosis rate
Morita et al. [5]	1996	Probes (15 MHz, 20 MHz)	M1, M2, M3, SM	73.5%[a]
Hasegawa et al. [6]	1996	Probe (15 MHz) EUS scope (12 MHz)	M, SM	92% (probe) 76% (scope)
Fukuda et al. [7]	2000	Probes (12 MHz, 20 MHz)	M1, M2 + M3, SM	80.8%[a]
Murata et al. [8]	2003	Probes (12 MHz, 15 MHz, 20 MHz)	M1 + M2, M3 + SM1, SM2 + SM3	87%
Esaki et al. [9]	2006	Probe (20 MHz)	M1 + M2, M3 + SM1, SM2 + SM3	77.8% (with echo jelly) 59.1% (with soft balloon)
Chemaly et al. [10]	2008	Probes (20 MHz, 30 MHz)	M, SM	74.5%
Goda et al. [11]	2008	Probes (20 MHz)	M, SM	85%
He et al. [12]	2014	EUS scope (7.5 MHz, 12 MHz)	M, SM	70.8%
Jung et al. [13]	2014	Probe (20 MHz)	M, SM	78.9%
Lee et al. [14]	2014	Probe (20 MHz)	M, SM	84.8%
Kawada et al. [15]	2014	Probe (20 MHz)	M1 + M2, M3 + SM1, SM2 + SM3	71.4%
Arima et al. [16]	2015	Probe (20 MHz)	M1 + M2, M3 + SM1, SM2 + SM3	88%

M lesion limited to mucosa, *SM* lesion limited to submucosa, *M1* lesion limited to mucosal surface (T1a-EP), *M2* lesion limited to lamina propria (T1a-LPM), *M3* lesion including muscularis mucosa, *SM1* lesion reaching top 1/3 of submucosa, *SM2* lesion reaching mid 1/3 of submucosa, *SM3* lesion reaching lower 1/3 of submucosa

[a]Only superficial cancer cases are quoted

tion, and scarring, but no clear evidences were found. There were two papers considering factors influencing diagnostic capabilities of EUS in recent years, but only large lesion size (2–3 cm or more) alone was found as a significant factor influencing diagnostic capability by multivariate analysis, and lesion location, histological degree of differentiation, and morphological type were no significant factors. It was thought that longer lesions require frequent scanning movements of the probe, making it rather difficult to detect small invasions relative to the size of the lesion.

Invasion Depth Diagnosis by EUS: Practical Applications

Scanning Methods

There are two main scanning methods in EUS, performed using either an EUS endoscope or a small-diameter probe inserted through an endoscope channel. To use a small-diameter probe, the esophageal lumen must be filled with water first, and it is sometimes difficult to perform scanning. A dedicated EUS scope uses a balloon attachment to the scanner portion, and scanning can be performed with a relative ease by filling of the balloon with water. However, the scope is forward slant viewing and makes viewing of the lesion with a proper orientation somewhat difficult. Because of the pressure applied against target lesions by water-filled balloon, EUS imaging may appear to have deeper invasion depth than the actual, and EUS scopes are reported to have lower correct diagnosis rates than small-diameter probes, although not at statistically significant level [2].

Therefore, EUS by small-diameter probes is thought to have better diagnostic accuracy than EUS by dedicated endoscopes for invasion depth diagnosis of superficial esophageal cancers.

But the use of small-diameter probes require filling of the esophageal lumen with water, and unlike stomach, esophagus does not hold water well, and soft balloon method or echo jelly method is sometimes used.

Soft balloon method utilizes a soft balloon attached to the scope end which then is filled with water allowing observation without leakage of water. Even esophagogastric junction can be observed with this method, but the pressure applied by the balloon may make diagnosis of M1–M2 cancers difficult. Echo jelly method utilizes echo jelly, a highly viscous material used instead of water, to fill the esophageal lumen for observation. Compared with soft balloon method, echo jelly method was reported to have better diagnostic accuracy, though without statistically significant difference.

In our endoscopy unit, we use degassed water with other arrangements to overcome leakage and allow quality imaging. We use an endoscope with water-jet function and have an assistant manually infuse degassed water via the water-jet channel, allowing us to obtain quality scanning images. While manual water infusion minimizes air bubbles, as much air as possible is aspirated from the esophagus before and during scanning. To avoid gastric air reflux, we thoroughly wash the stomach beforehand and fill it with degassed water while completely aspirating air. When possible, antimotility medication is used to minimize esophageal contractions during scanning.

EUS Imaging of Normal Esophageal Wall

EUS imaging of normal esophageal wall show divisions to 5 layers, 7 layers, 9 layers, and 11 layers depending on scanning frequencies. A consensus meeting was held in 2000 to clarify how each of these layers corresponds to actual histology at the 60th meeting of the Japanese Society of Gastrointestinal Endoscopy (Fig. 4.13). Clinically, EUS imaging shows divisions consisting mainly of five layers, seven layers, and nine layers. When divided into nine layers (Fig. 4.14), the third layer (3rd/9 layer) corresponds to muscularis mucosa, the fourth layer (4th/9 layer) to submucosa, and the fifth layer (5th/9 layer) to the border of submucosa and muscularis propria. For seven layer divisions, the third (3rd/7) layer, and for five layer divisions, the third (3rd/5) layer corresponds to submucosa, important in invasion depth diagnosis of superficial cancers.

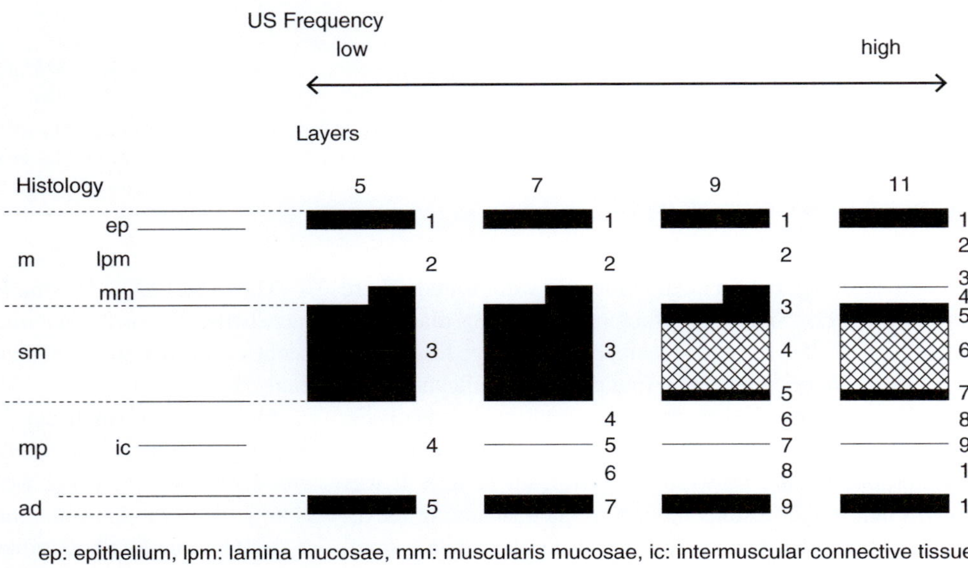

Fig. 4.13 Endosonographic correlation with histology in a layered structure of the gastrointestinal wall (adapted from [17])

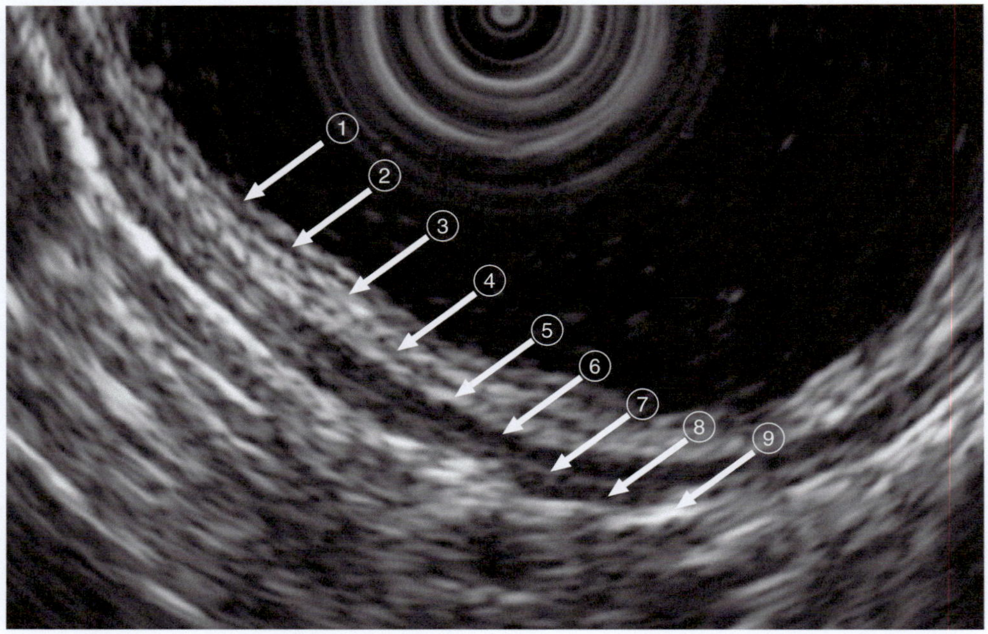

Fig. 4.14 Endosonographic image of a normal esophageal wall in nine layers

Cases: Invasion Depth Evaluation by EUS

Case 1

A male in his 60s was noted to have a reddish depressed lesion of approximately 20 mm in diameter, in the anterior wall of the lower thoracic esophagus (a). The anal side of the depression was clearly demarcated, but the oral side was somewhat unclear. And a partially depressed elevation was noted on the oral side (white arrow), and a possibility of deeper invasion could not be denied (b). By scanning the elevated lesion with EUS, the 3rd/9 layer (white arrow) was pressed downward, but the 4th/9 layer (yellow arrow) remained intact, and invasion depth of T1a-MM was diagnosed (c), leading to resection by ESD. Histologically, the lesion was mostly intraepithelial to the lamina propria, but the lesion at locally elevated point invaded further down to the muscularis propria (T1a-MM) (d) (Fig. 4.15).

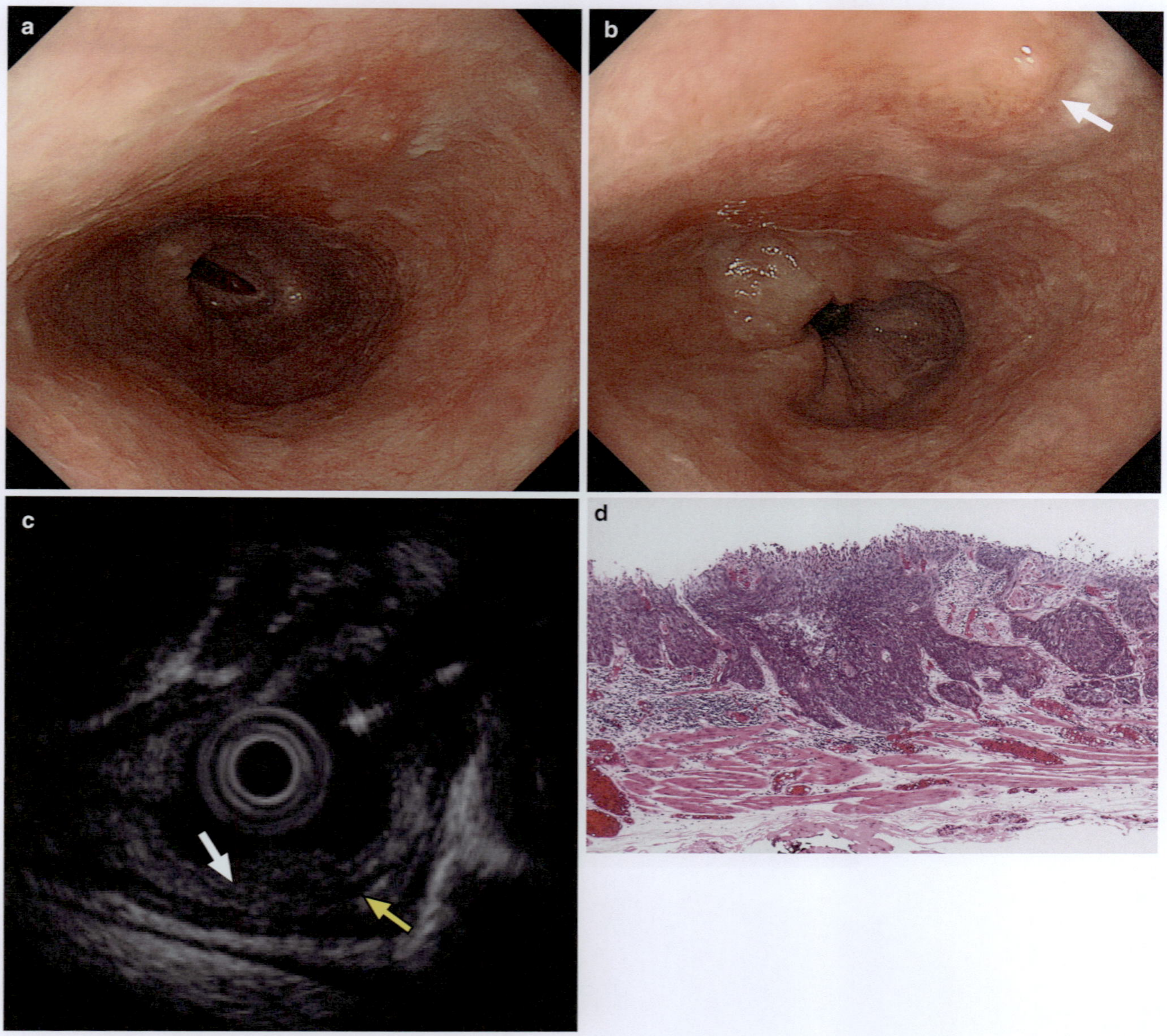

Fig. 4.15 Case 1

Case 2

A female in 70s was noted to have a reddish coarse appearing, approximately 20 mm diameter and one-third the circumferential lesion (a). At the center, a 4 mm elevation was noted. It appeared to be somewhat hard with small air volume. EUS scanning of the raised area showed top 3/9 layer pressed downward by the lesion, but remained intact without obvious invasion, and invasion depth was diagnosed as T1a-MM (c). ESD was performed. Histologically, the lesion was limited down to the lamina propria, and invasion depth was T1a-LPM (d) (Fig. 4.16).

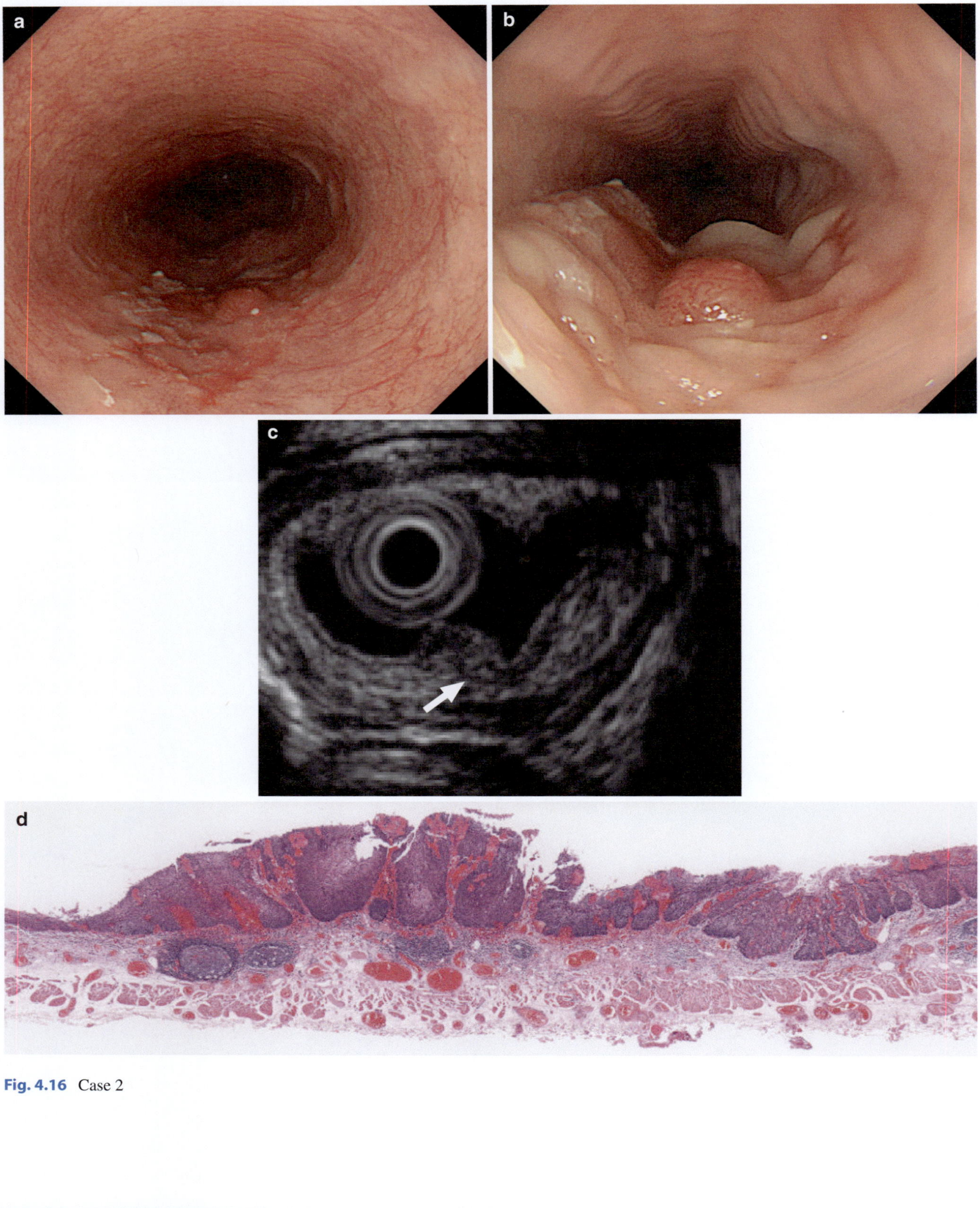

Fig. 4.16 Case 2

Case 3

A male in 70s was found to have a reddish semi-circumferential depressed lesion in the left wall of the mid-thoracic esophagus (a). A depressed lesion was clearly demarcated with nodularities within suggestive of deeper invasion (b). On EUS scanning, the top 2/7 layers showed thickening and the 3rd/7 layer was markedly narrowed (white arrow), and the lesion was diagnosed as invading the deeper SM (c). Although chemoradiation or surgery was recommended, the patient strongly insisted on endoscopic therapy, and ESD was performed. Histologically, the lesion was invading the deeper SM with invasion depth of T1b-SM2(1000 μm) (d) (Fig. 4.17).

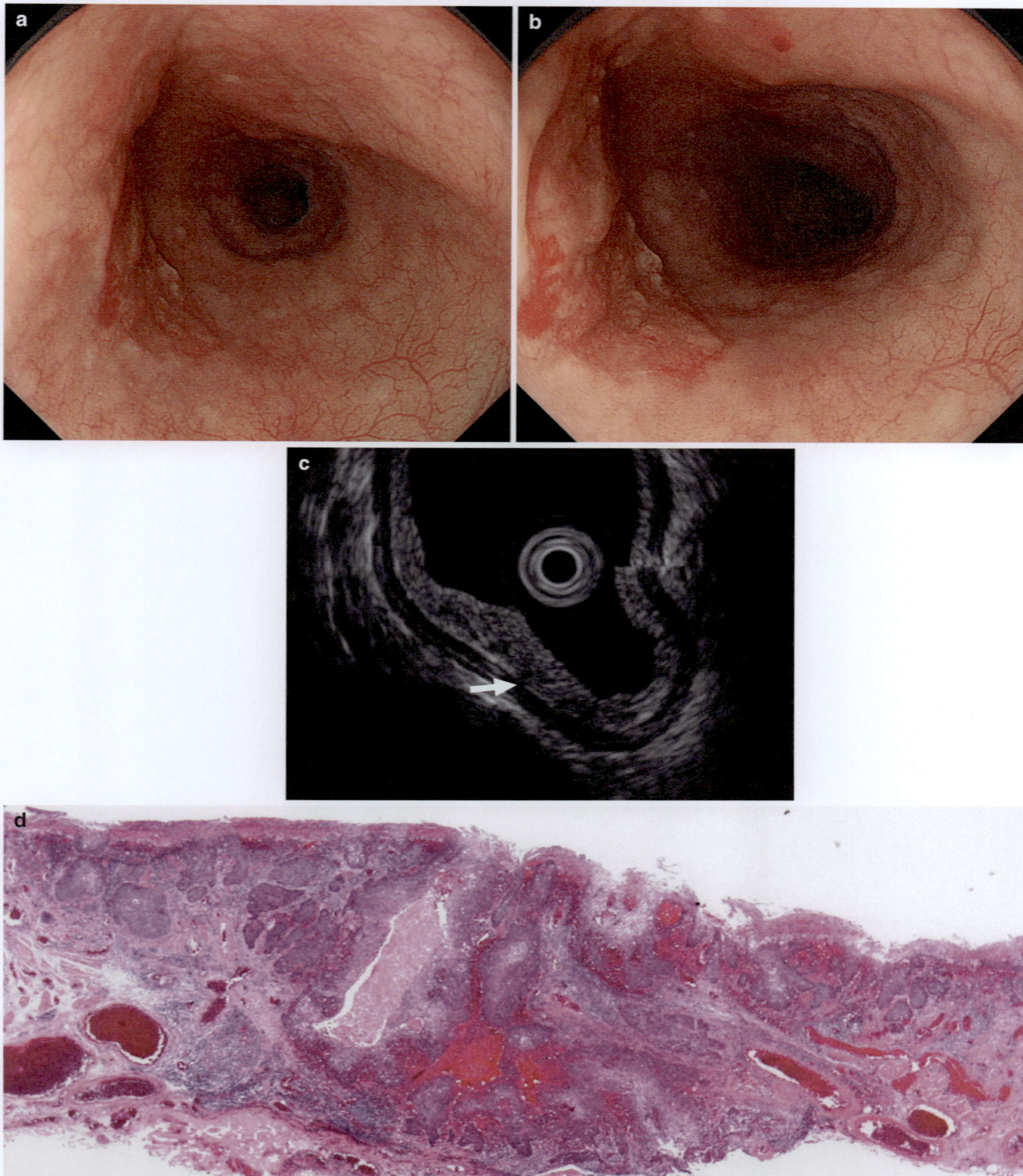

Fig. 4.17 Case 3

Case 4

A male in 70s was noted to have a 10 mm slightly elevated lesion in the posterior wall of the lower thoracic esophagus (a). The top was somewhat depressed, and reddish mucosa spreads within the depression and on oral and anal sides, but with SMT like smooth rise at the base (b). On EUS scanning, disruption of the 3rd/9 and 4th/9 layers (white arrow), as well as narrowing of the 5th/9 layer (yellow arrow), was noted, and invasion depth of the deeper SM was diagnosed (c). Although recommended to undergo surgery, the patient strongly desired endoscopic treatment, and ESD was performed. Histologically, the tumor showed invasion into the deeper submucosa, and invasion depth was T1b-SM2 (500 μm) (d) (Fig. 4.18).

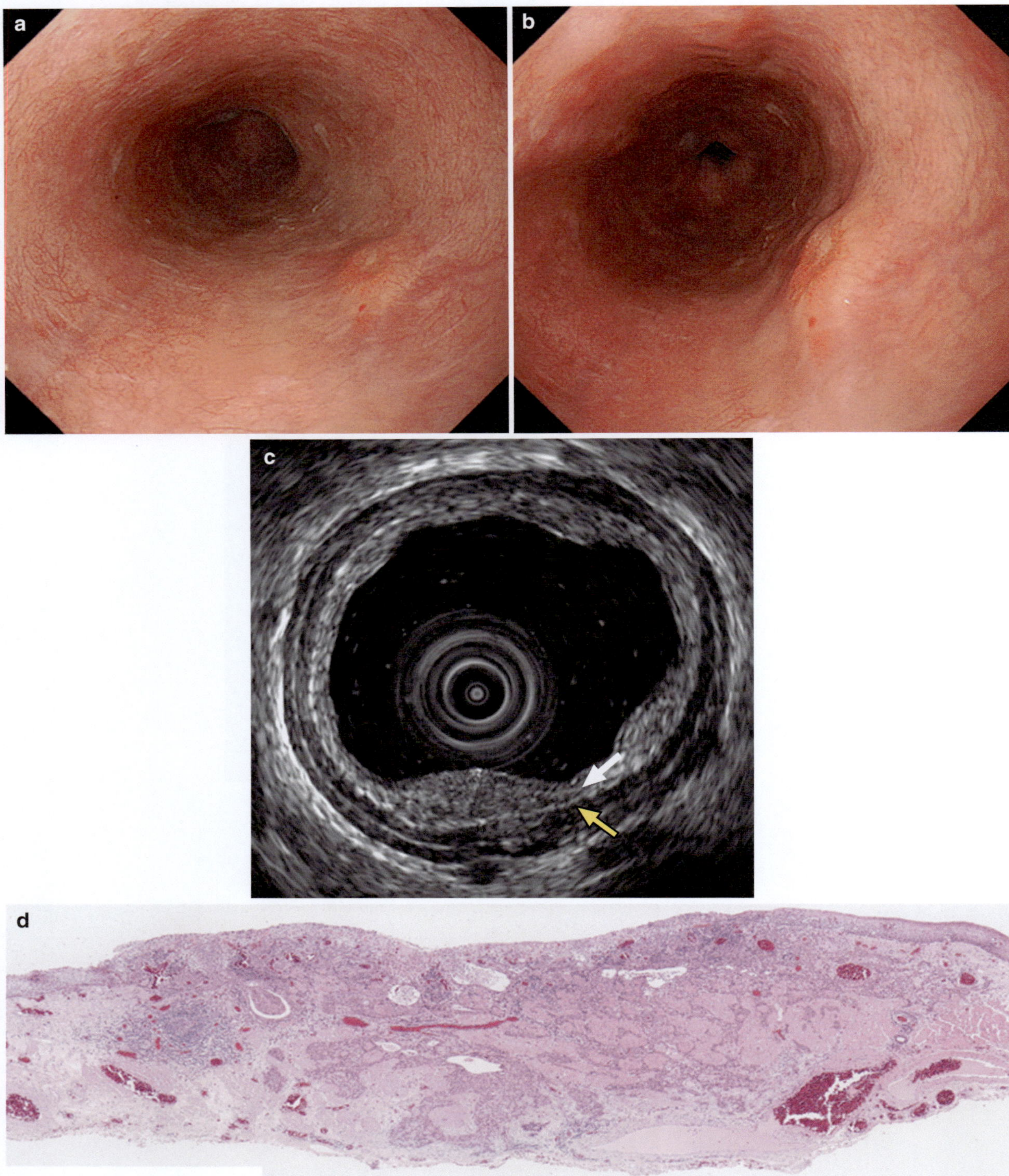

Fig. 4.18 Case 4

4.3 Summary

Current status and practical applications of EUS regarding invasion depth diagnosis were summarized. EUS is an important modality for invasion depth diagnosis, and its characteristics and limitations must be understood when utilizing EUS.

References

1. Oyama T. Procedures of diagnosing small esophageal lesions. Stomach Intestine. 2009;44:1755–8.
2. Oyama T, et al. Prediction of the invasion depth of superficial squamous cell carcinoma based on microvessel morphology: magnifying endoscopic classification of the Japan Esophageal Society. Esophagus. 2017;14:105–12.
3. Oyama T. Japan Esophageal Society's magnifying endoscopic classification. Stomach Intestine. 2014;49:148–52.
4. Arima M, et al. Japan Esophageal Society's magnifying endoscopic classification and invasion depth—Type R blood vessel and histological imaging. Stomach Intestine. 2014;49:213–21.
5. Murata Y, et al. Small ultrasonic probes for determination of the depth of superficial esophageal cancer. Gastrointest Endosc. 1966;44:23–8.
6. Hasegawa N, et al. Prospective staging of superficial esophageal carcinoma: comparison of an ultrasound probe and standard endoscopic ultrasonography. Gastrointest Endosc. 1996;44:388–93.
7. Fukuda M, et al. Endoscopic ultrasonography. Gastrointest Endosc. 1996;44:388–93.
8. Murata Y, et al. High-frequency endoscopic ultrasonography in the evaluation of superficial esophageal cancer. Endoscopy. 2003;35:429–36.
9. Esaki M, et al. Probe EUS for the diagnosis of invasion depth in superficial esophageal cancer: a comparison between a jelly-filled method and water-filled balloon method. Gastrointest Endosc. 2006;63:389–95.
10. Chemaly M, et al. Miniprobe EUS in the pretherapeutic assessment of early esophageal neoplasia. Endoscopy. 2008;40:2–6.
11. Goda K, et al. Magnifying endoscopy with narrow band imaging for predicting the invasion depth of superficial esophageal squamous cell carcinoma. Dis Esophagus. 2009;22:453–60.
12. He LJ, et al. Endoscopic ultrasonography for staging of T1a and T1b esophageal squamous cell carcinoma. World J Gastroenterol. 2014;20:1340–7.
13. Jung JI, et al. Clinicopathologic factors influencing the accuracy of EUS for superficial esophageal carcinoma. World J Gastroenterol. 2014;20:6322–8.
14. Lee MW, et al. Predicting the invasion depth of esophageal squamous cell carcinoma: comparison of endoscopic ultrasonography and magnifying endoscopy. Scand J Gastroenterol. 2014;49:853–61.
15. Kawata K, et al. Invasion depth diagnosis of superficially spreading esophageal cancers. Stomach Intestine. 2014;49:1173–81.
16. Arima M, et al. Invasion depth diagnosis of superficial esophageal cancer with use of high frequency echoprobe. Stomach Intestine. 2014;49:1173–81.
17. Yamanaka T, et al. Interpretation of EUS layer structure. Gastroenterol Endosc. 2001;43:1091–2.

Part II

Diagnosis and Treatment of Each Carcinoma Type

5 Type 0-Is Esophageal Cancer

Manabu Takeuchi

M. Takeuchi (✉)
Department of Gastroenterology, Nagaoka Red Cross Hospital,
Niigata, Japan

T. Oyama (ed.), *Endoscopic Diagnosis of Esophageal Carcinoma for ESD*, https://doi.org/10.1007/978-981-32-9030-3_5

5.1 Let's Try to Diagnose This Lesion

Let's Diagnose with White Light Imaging (Fig. 5.1a)

- At 30 cm from the incisors, on the posterior wall of the mid-thoracic esophagus, an approximately 10 mm diameter elevated lesion was noted with fullness and firmness, sharply and smoothly rising from its base to greater than 1 mm in height with the center of the raised lesion showing clearly demarcated reddish area with irregular bumps.
- Based on above, the sharply rising part is covered by noncancerous squamous epithelium, and squamous cell carcinoma (SCC) with submucosally infiltrating tumor is suspected.

Let's Confirm Hardness of Lesion with Air Volume Adjustment (Fig. 5.1b)

- After full inflation of air to expand the lesion, there was little change in lesion shape, and the lesion was found to be a wide-based hard raised lesion.
- It is important to assess lesion shape change by adjusting air volume in determining invasion depth.

Let's Perform Iodine Dye Staining (Fig. 5.1c)

- After iodine dye staining, the rising part of the lesion was stained like the surrounding area, but the central elevated part was unstained as exposed cancer epithelium, while the rising base was covered by noncancerous epithelium.
- "Tatami mat" pattern was interrupted within the lesion, and the cancer was diagnosed as invading into the muscularis mucosa and below.

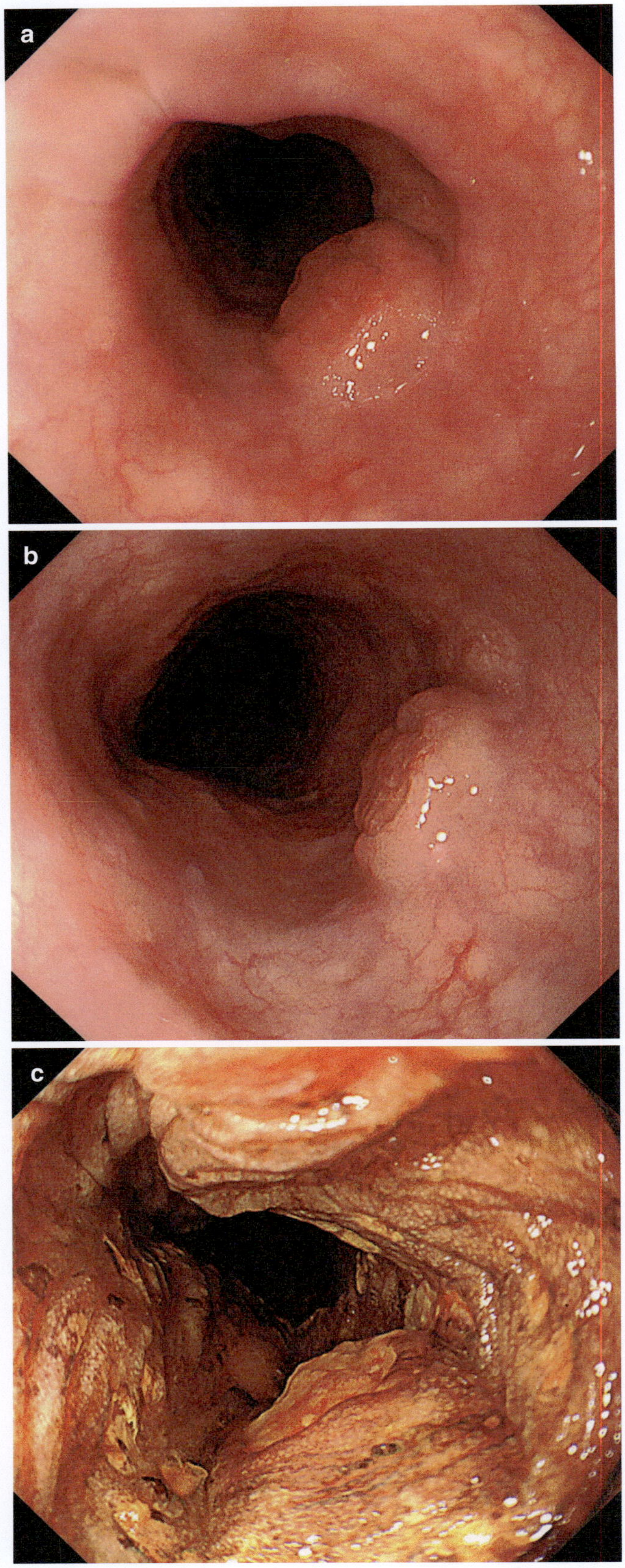

Fig. 5.1 Type 0-Is esophageal cancer. (**a**) White light endoscopic image of the lesion. (**b**) WL white light endoscopic image with decreased the air volume. (**c**) Iodine chromoendoscopic image of the lesion

5.2 From ESD to the Final Diagnosis

Let's Perform Magnifying NBI Observation (Fig. 5.2a)

- The base of the rising part is covered with noncancerous epithelium with non-irregular intrapapillary blood vessels. The center of the raised lesion showed non-loop-forming irregularly traversing Type B2 blood vessels and elongated Type B2 blood vessels and larger caliber cyan-toned Type B3 blood vessels at the periphery.
- Based on above, the lesion can be diagnosed as Type O-Is, SCC, invasion depth of SM massive.

Let's Perform EUS (Fig. 5.2b)

- EUS scanning of the elevated part using a small-diameter probe revealed the lesion as an uniform low echoic area down to the 4th/9 layers. Although without interruptions, high echoic submucosal layer was found to be pressed and thinning, confirming invasion into the submucosa.

Let's Confirm with the Pathological Specimen (Fig. 5.3)

- The fourth pathological section corresponding the elevated lesion showed histopathology of moderately differentiated squamous cell carcinoma penetrating the muscularis mucosa with submucosal invasion (SM2: 2000 μm). The base of the rising lesion is covered with noncancerous squamous cell epithelium with infiltration of cancerous nests beneath.

Conclusive Diagnosis

Esophageal squamous cell carcinoma, 0-Is, T1b-SM2(2000 μm), ly(−), v(−), HM0, VM0, 22 × 20 mm, pCur A, Mt.

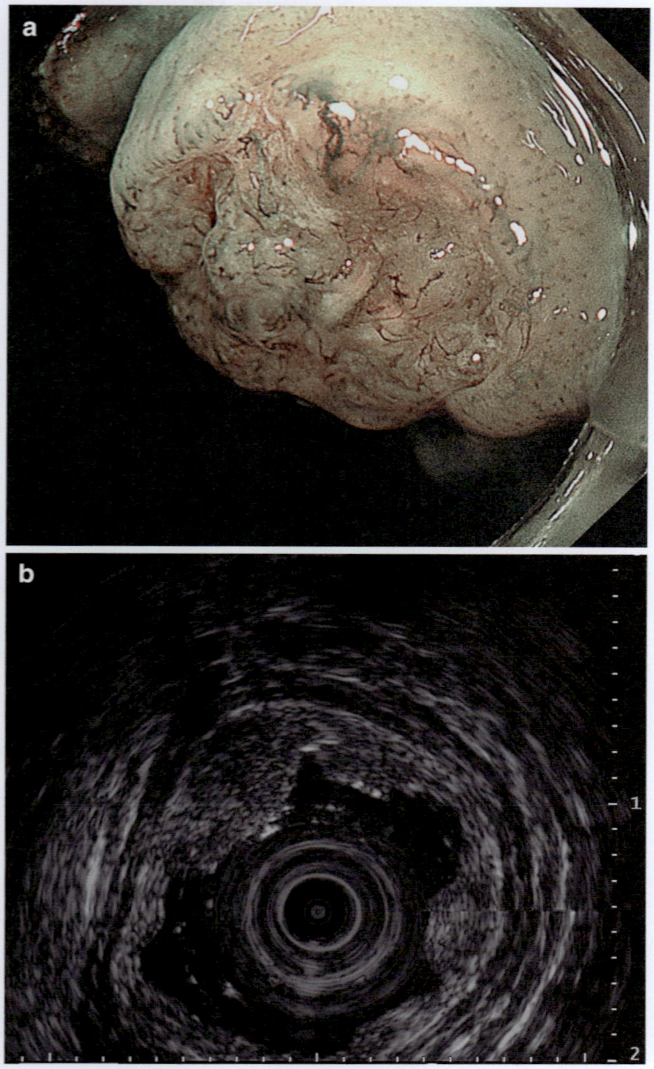

Fig. 5.2 Type 0-Is esophageal cancer. (**a**) NBI magnified endoscopic image. (**b**) EUS scanning image of the elevated part using a small-diameter probe

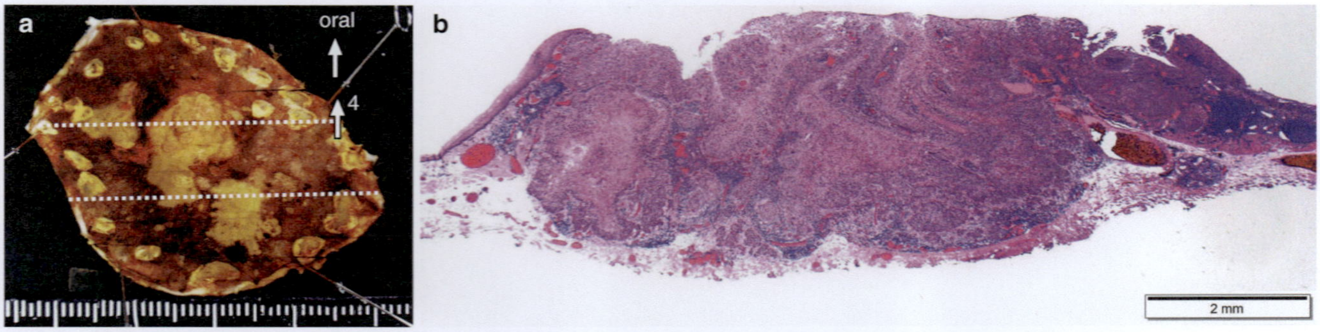

Fig. 5.3 Histopathologic image of the fourth pathological section corresponding the elevated lesion

Type 0-Ip Esophageal Cancer

6

Manabu Takeuchi

M. Takeuchi (✉)
Department of Gastroenterology, Nagaoka Red Cross Hospital,
Niigata, Japan

T. Oyama (ed.), *Endoscopic Diagnosis of Esophageal Carcinoma for ESD*, https://doi.org/10.1007/978-981-32-9030-3_6

6.1 Let's Try to Diagnose This Lesion

Let's Diagnose with White Light Imaging

- On white light imaging, a reddish flat coarse mucosa with longitudinal length of 6 cm extending from the lower thoracic esophagus to the abdominal esophagus was noted, and on its anal side, an approximately 15 mm reddish tall raised lesion was noted on the right wall (Fig. 6.1a).
- On close-up observation, the lesions base was noted with a narrow stalk, and the lesion surface appears papillary and granular (Fig. 6.1b).

Let's Observe the Stalk form Changes with Esophageal Peristalsis

- The stalk portion extended and flattened easily with peristaltic movements, suggesting its soft extensible nature (Fig. 6.1c).

Let's Observe the Surface of the Lesion

- The head of the lesion was observed in the stomach with a retroflexed view, showing granular and papillary surface appearance without firmness. These findings of a tall raised lesion with granular and papillary surface and a very soft extensible stalk suggested invasion depth of T1a-MM, one level shallower than usual O-Is lesions (Fig. 6.1d).

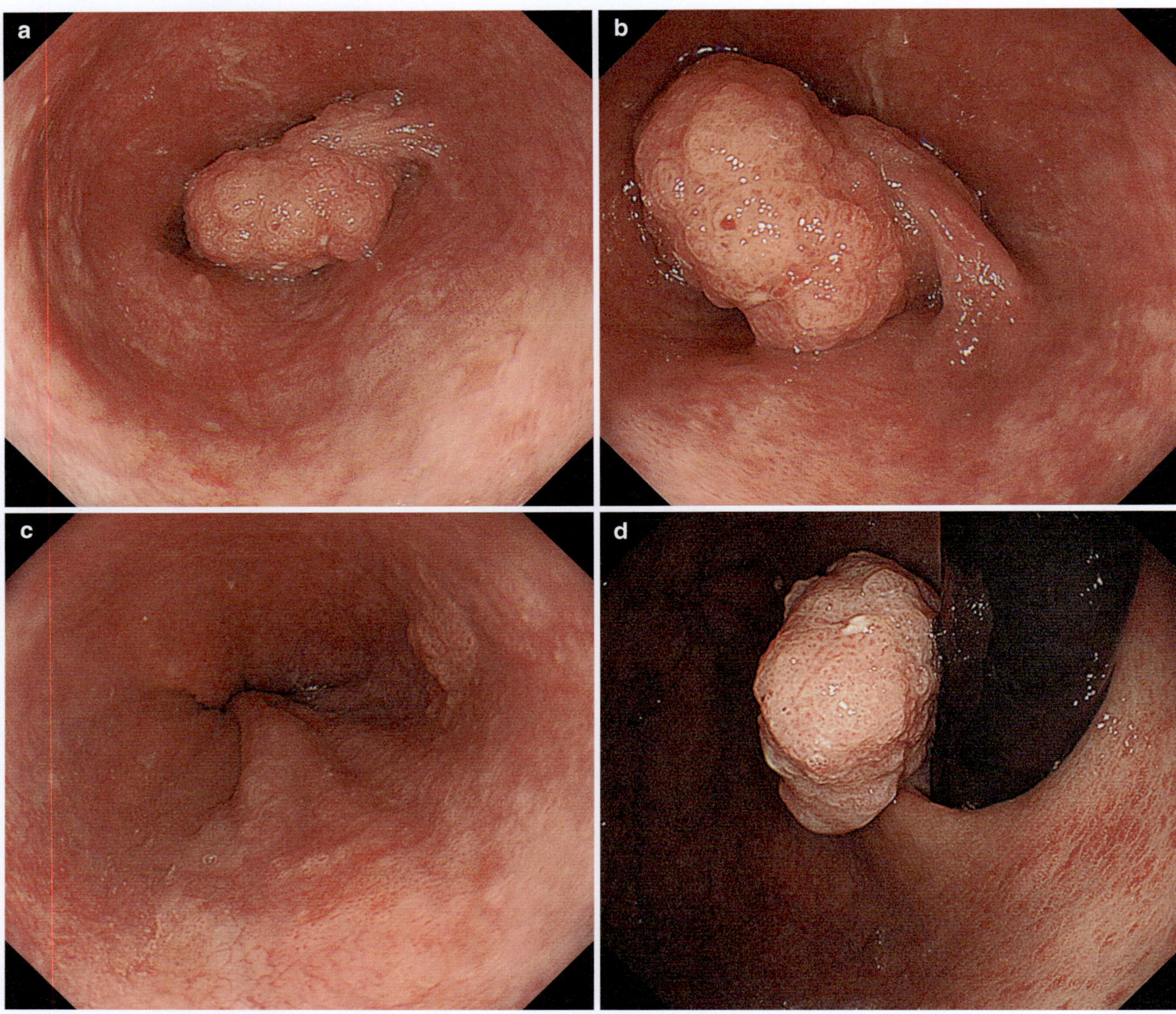

Fig. 6.1 Type 0-Ip esophageal cancer. (**a**–**c**) White light endoscopic images of the lesion

6.2 From ESD to the Final Diagnosis

Let's Observe with Magnifying NBI

- On magnifying NBI observation, the surface was uneven, uniformly papillary and granular, and filled with aggregates of spiral Type B1 blood vessels, showing "salmon roe-like" appearance (Fig. 6.2a).
- The stalk portion showed dot like Type B1 blood vessels similar to the surrounding flat portion, and noncancerous squamous epithelium was noted in part (Fig. 6.2b).

Let's Perform Iodine Dye Staining

- On iodine dye staining, a circumferentially unstained area was noted with the raised portion which was also unstained. With reduced air inflation, the flat area surrounding the raised portion showed "tatami mat" patterns, but not the raised portion. But, it is prudent to remember that tall raised lesions do not necessarily show "tatami mat" patterns because of lesion thickness and not because of invasion of muscularis mucosa (Fig. 6.3).

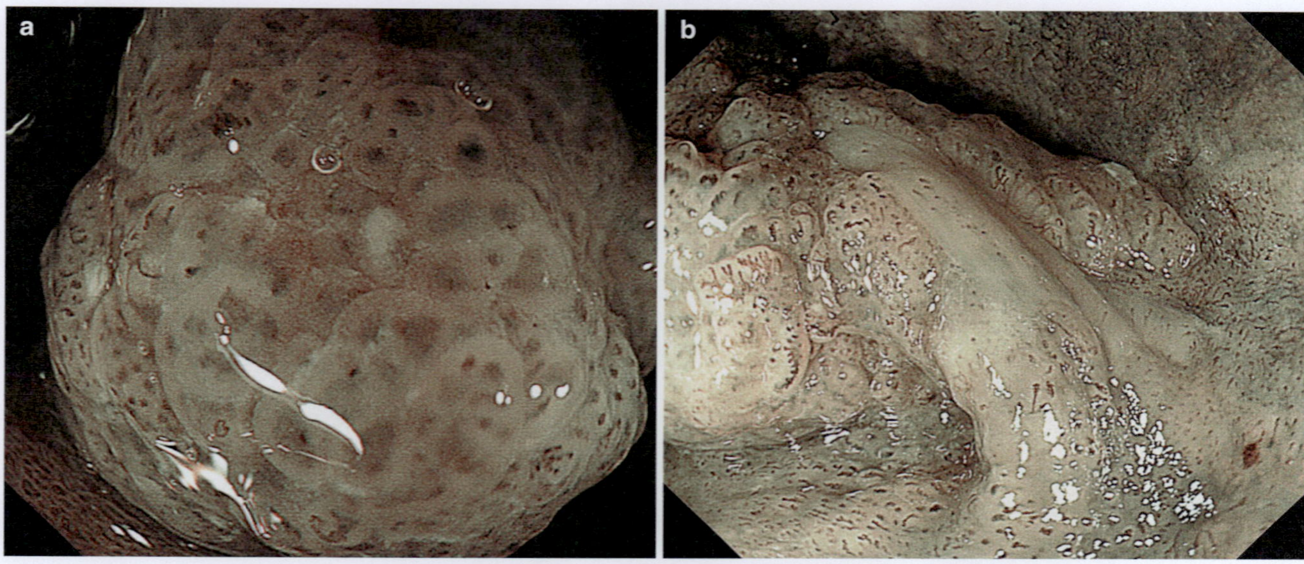

Fig. 6.2 Type 0-Ip esophageal cancer. (**a**, **b**) NBI magnified endoscopic images of the lesion

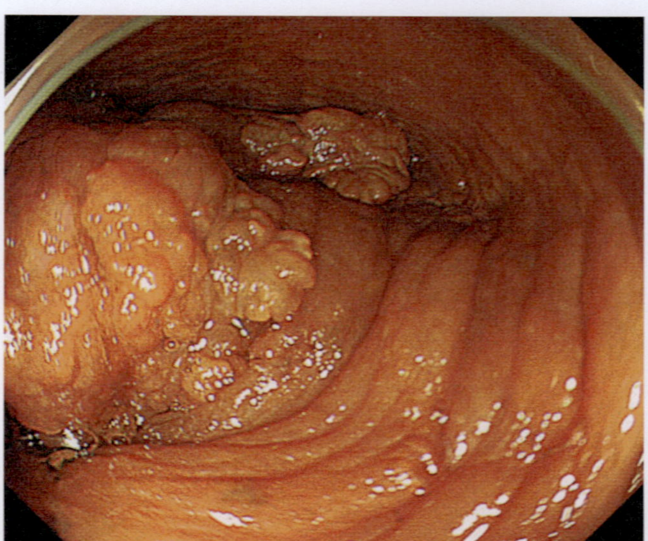

Fig. 6.3 The lesion staining with iodine

Let's Confirm with the Pathological Specimen

- The 13th pathological section corresponding to the raised lesion showed the raised portion to be consisting of the tumor, muscularis mucosa (drawn with dotted line) lifted with the tumor, and the submucosal structures. On magnified viewing of the section marked by white dotted line, well-differentiated to moderately differentiated squamous cell carcinoma.

  Invading the lamina propria, but not into the muscularis mucosa, with invasion depth of T1a-LPM (Fig. 6.4).

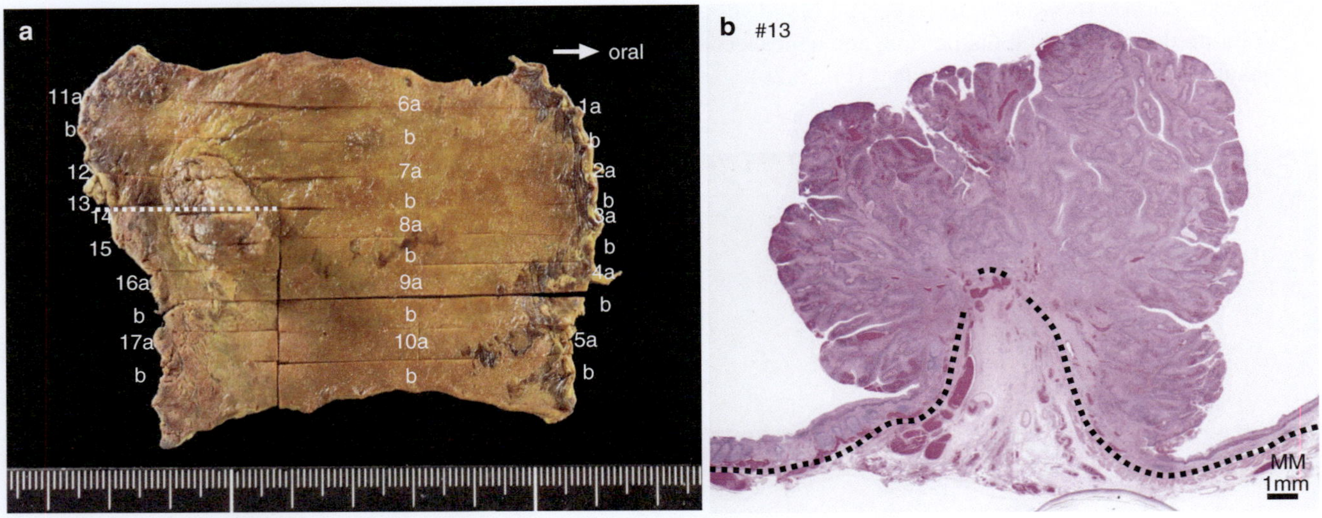

Fig. 6.4 (**a**) The resected specimen of the lesion. (**b**) The 13th pathological section corresponding to the raised lesion

> **Conclusive Diagnosis**
> Esophageal squamous cell carcinoma, 0-"IIc" + Ip + IIb, T1b-SM2, ly(−), v(−), HM0, VM0, 56 × 60 mm, pCurA, Lt, Ae.

7 Type 0-Isp Esophageal Cancer

Manabu Takeuchi

M. Takeuchi (✉)
Department of Gastroenterology, Nagaoka Red Cross Hospital,
Niigata, Japan

T. Oyama (ed.), *Endoscopic Diagnosis of Esophageal Carcinoma for ESD*, https://doi.org/10.1007/978-981-32-9030-3_7

7.1 Let's Try to Diagnose This Lesion

Let's Diagnose with White Light Imaging

- At 42 cm from the incisors in the lower thoracic esophagus on the right wall, approximately 10 mm reddish raised lesion was noted with a surrounding flat reddish area (Fig. 7.1a).

Let's Observe the Surface Mucosa

- On close-up observation, the base of the raised lesion was noted with narrowing, and the surface showed papillary and granular mucosa without tenseness or firmness (Fig. 7.1b).

Let's Confirm Movability of the Raised Portion (Fig. 7.1c)

- With adjustments of air volume and scope movements, the raised portion was found to be movable with clear narrowing at its base.
- Based on these findings of papillary and granular appearance of the raised portion, clear narrowing at its base, with easy movability, invasion depth was determined one level shallower as T1a-MM like the previous Type Ip case.

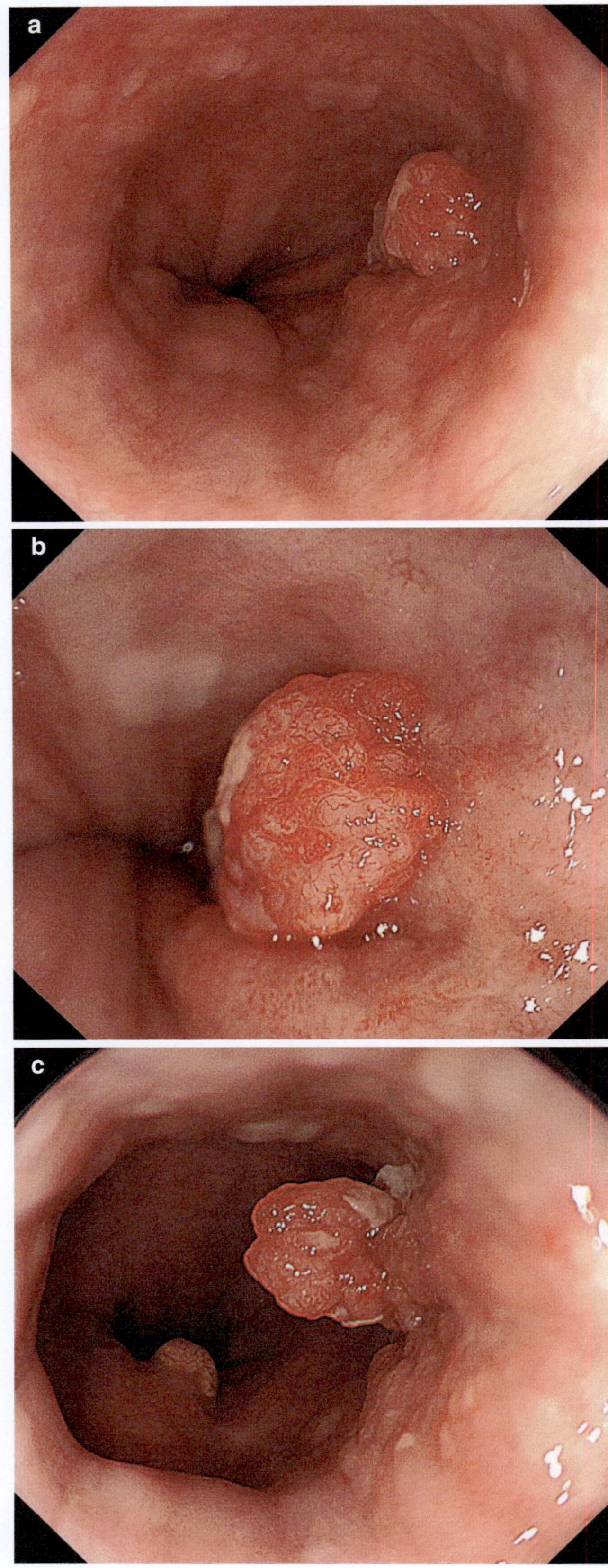

Fig. 7.1 Type 0-Isp esophageal cancer. (**a–c**) White light endoscopic images of the lesion

7.2 From ESD to the Final Diagnosis

Let's Perform Magnifying NBI

- The raised portion was noted on lower magnification NBI as a brownish area, with elongated intrapapillary blood vessels (Fig. 7.2a).

Let's Observe with Higher Magnification

- On full magnifying NBI, elongated non-loop-forming B2 blood vessels inside clearly papillary structures, but loop-forming spiral blood vessels are occasionally noted as well. Like this case, when clearly recognizable papillary and granular surface is noted, upward growing tumor is considered, and invasion depth is diagnosed one level shallower as T1a-LPM even with the presence of Type B2 blood vessels (Fig. 7.2b).

Let's Confirm with the Pathological Specimen

- The seventh pathological section corresponding to the raised portion of the lesion showed upward growing SCC not reaching down to the muscularis mucosa, with invasion depth diagnosis of T1a-LPM (Fig. 7.3).

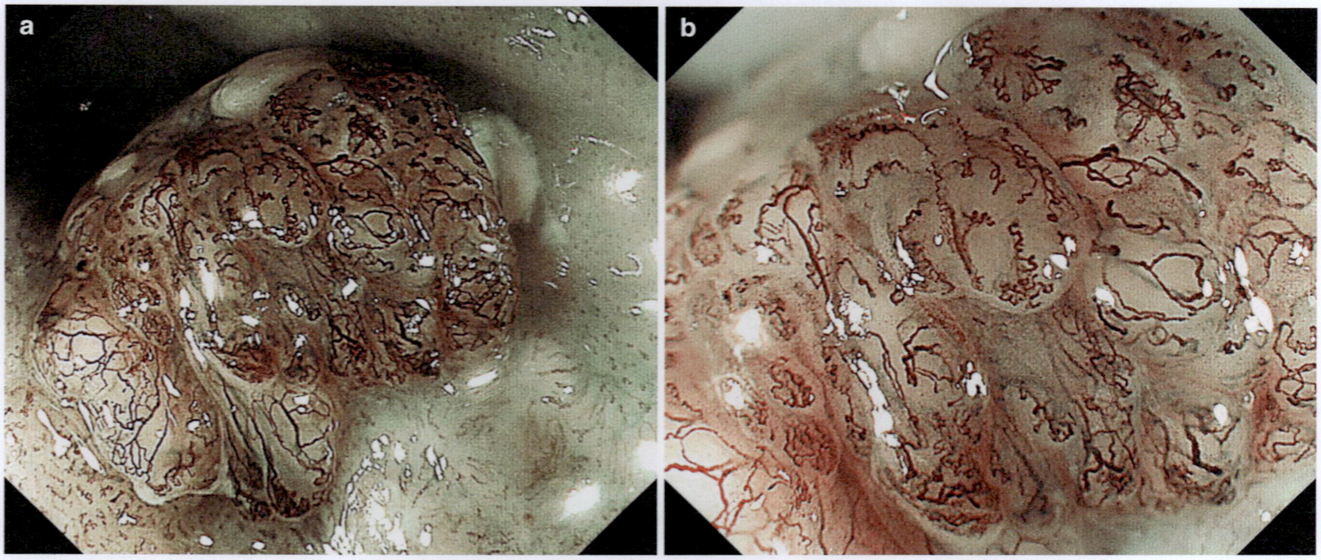

Fig. 7.2 Type 0-Isp esophageal cancer. (**a**, **b**) NBI magnified endoscopic images

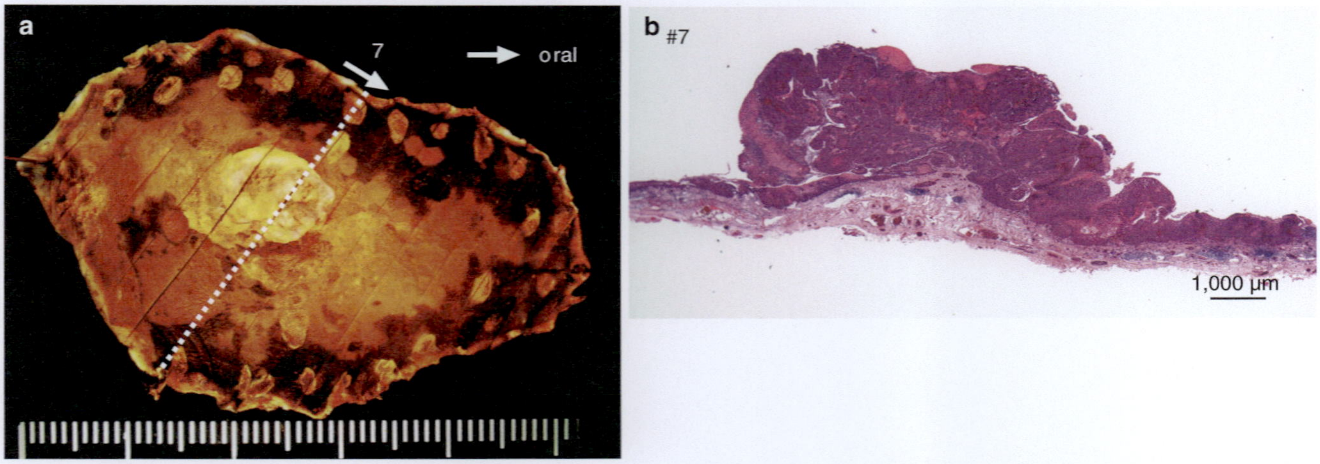

Fig. 7.3 (**a**) The resected specimen of the lesion. (**b**) The seventh pathological section corresponding to the raised portion of the lesion

Conclusive Diagnosis

Esophageal squamous cell carcinoma, O-Isp, T1a-LPM, ly (−), v (−), HM0, VM0, 41 × 26 mm, pCurA, Lt.

Summary

Many of Type 0-I esophageal cancers are deeply invasive lesions infiltrating submucosa. White light imaging is important in invasion depth diagnosis, and it is important to combine findings at bases of raised lesions, surface texture, and firmness of lesions confirmed by air volume adjustments. When findings such as widely based raised lesion, irregularly uneven unclear surface, tense appearance, or firmness are observed, submucosal (SM) invasions are strongly suspected. But in the case of easily movable pedunculated or semi-pedunculated lesions with papillary or granular surface, without tenseness or firmness, invasion depth can be assessed one level shallower. For pedunculated lesions, stalk width also is an important finding as wider stalks increase risks of submucosal invasions. With magnifying NBI observations, Type B3 blood vessels are often associated with deeper submucosal (SM) invasions but infrequently encountered. EUS is also useful in invasion depth diagnosis but often difficult to obtain quality scanning images of lesions with basal narrowing. Although these modalities are of auxiliary help, white light imaging remains the basis of invasion depth diagnosis.

Type 0-IIa Esophageal Cancer: First Case

8

Dai Hirasawa

D. Hirasawa (✉)
Department of Gastroenterology, Sendai Kosei Hospital, Sendai, Miyagi, Japan
e-mail: hirasawa@sendai-kousei-hospital.jp

T. Oyama (ed.), *Endoscopic Diagnosis of Esophageal Carcinoma for ESD*, https://doi.org/10.1007/978-981-32-9030-3_8

8.1 Let's Try to Diagnose This Lesion

Let's Diagnose with White Light Imaging (Fig. 8.1a)

- A whitish flat elevated lesion was noted in the mid-thoracic esophagus on the anterior left wall.
- Whitish color tone changes reflect keratosis of the surface epithelium. A sharply rising rim without a table-like elevation was noted, and it was suspected that the surface epithelium grew upward with strong keratinization.

Let's Consider Causes of an Elevated Lesion Form (Fig. 8.1a)

- There are two types of O-IIa esophageal squamous cell carcinoma: (1) upward growth of epithelium resulting in elevation and (2) thickness of cancer nests resulting in elevation. This case is thought to be caused by keratosis of upward growing epithelium and belongs to the first type.

Invasion Depth Diagnosis Should Be Made by Collective Judgments

Invasion Depth of Whitish Lesions Should Be Made Shallower (Fig. 8.1b)

- Blood vessels cannot be seen by NBI due to keratosis.
- Invasion depth cannot be estimated due to vascular morphologies. But whitish lesions with keratosis tend to be highly differentiated and are often lacking in invasiveness, suggesting shallower invasion depth. Based on size (7–8 mm), softness of the lesion, and color tone, invasion depth was diagnosed as T1a-EP ~ LPM.

Let's Perform EUS (Fig. 8.1c)

- EUS scanning of the elevated part using a 20 MHz small-diameter probe revealed that the 1st–2nd layers are thickened and raised upward.
- Nothing observed in the high echoic 3rd/5 layers, the invasion depth was diagnosed as T1a-EP ~ LPM.

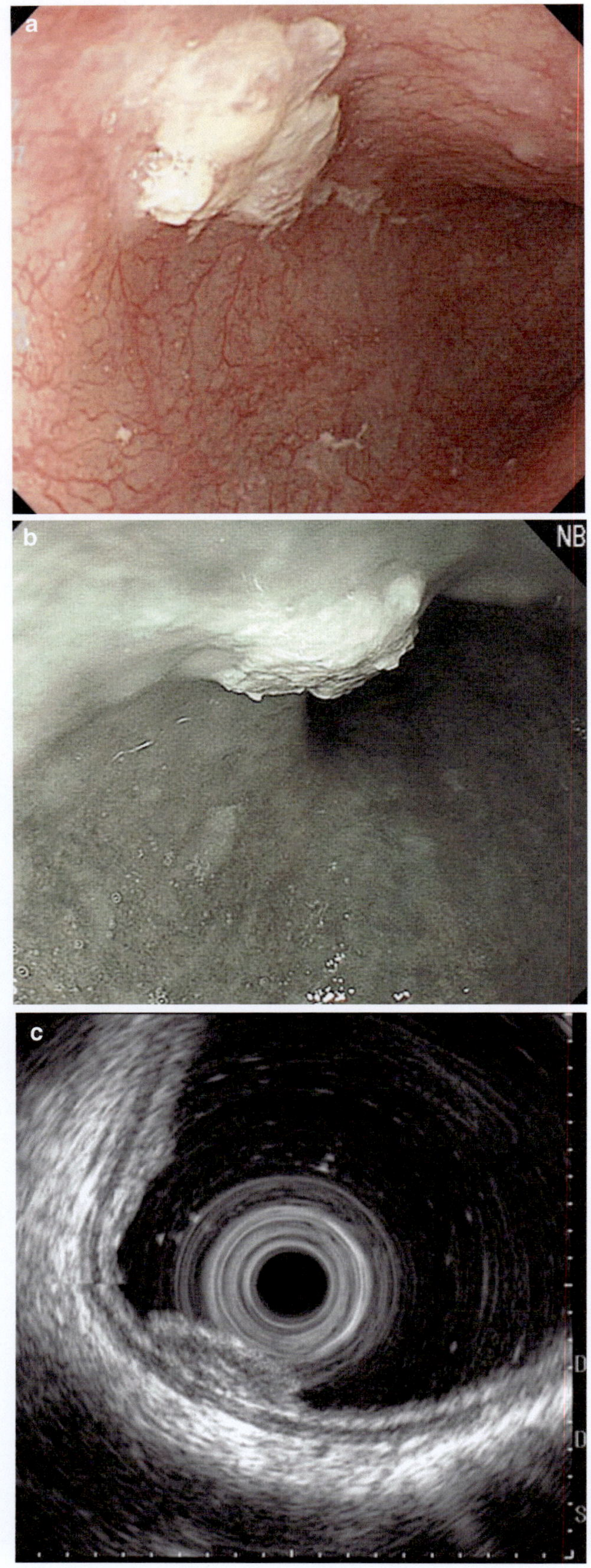

Fig. 8.1 Type 0-IIa esophageal cancer. (**a**) White light endoscopic images of the lesion. (**b**) NBI endoscopic image of the lesion. (**c**) EUS scanning image of the lesion

8.2 From ESD to the Final Diagnosis

Let's Observe the Freshly Resected Specimen (Fig. 8.2a)

- The left side of the image is the oral side, and the whitish flat raised lesion is noted.
- The size of the flat raised lesion was 9 × 6 mm.

Let's Observe the Iodine Dye-Stained Specimen (Fig. 8.2b)

- The raised lesion was unstained by iodine dye.
- There was a linear unstained area extending anally from the raised lesion.

Let's Observe the Histopathological Image

- H&E staining image of the section (yellow dotted line on the left image) through the raised lesion. A thick layer of atypical cells with large nuclei is growing upward replacing the normal epithelial layer. Well-developed squamous cell cancer with invasion depth of T1a-LPM was diagnosed (Fig. 8.3a).
- The anal part of the iodine dye unstained lesion was shown by a H&E section represented by blue dotted line. Squamous cell carcinoma was noted extending in the basal layer of the epithelium (Fig. 8.3b).

Conclusive Diagnosis

Esophageal squamous cell carcinoma, O-IIa, T1a-LPM, INFα, ly(−), v(−), HM0, VM0, 24 × 8 mm, pCurA, Mt.

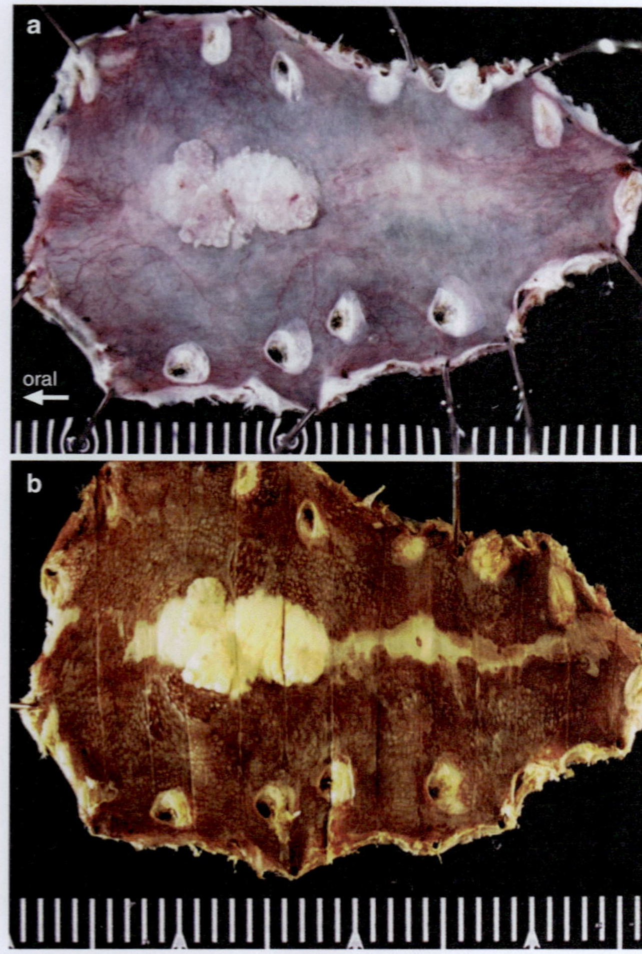

Fig. 8.2 (a) Fleshly resected specimen. (b) The specimen staining with iodine

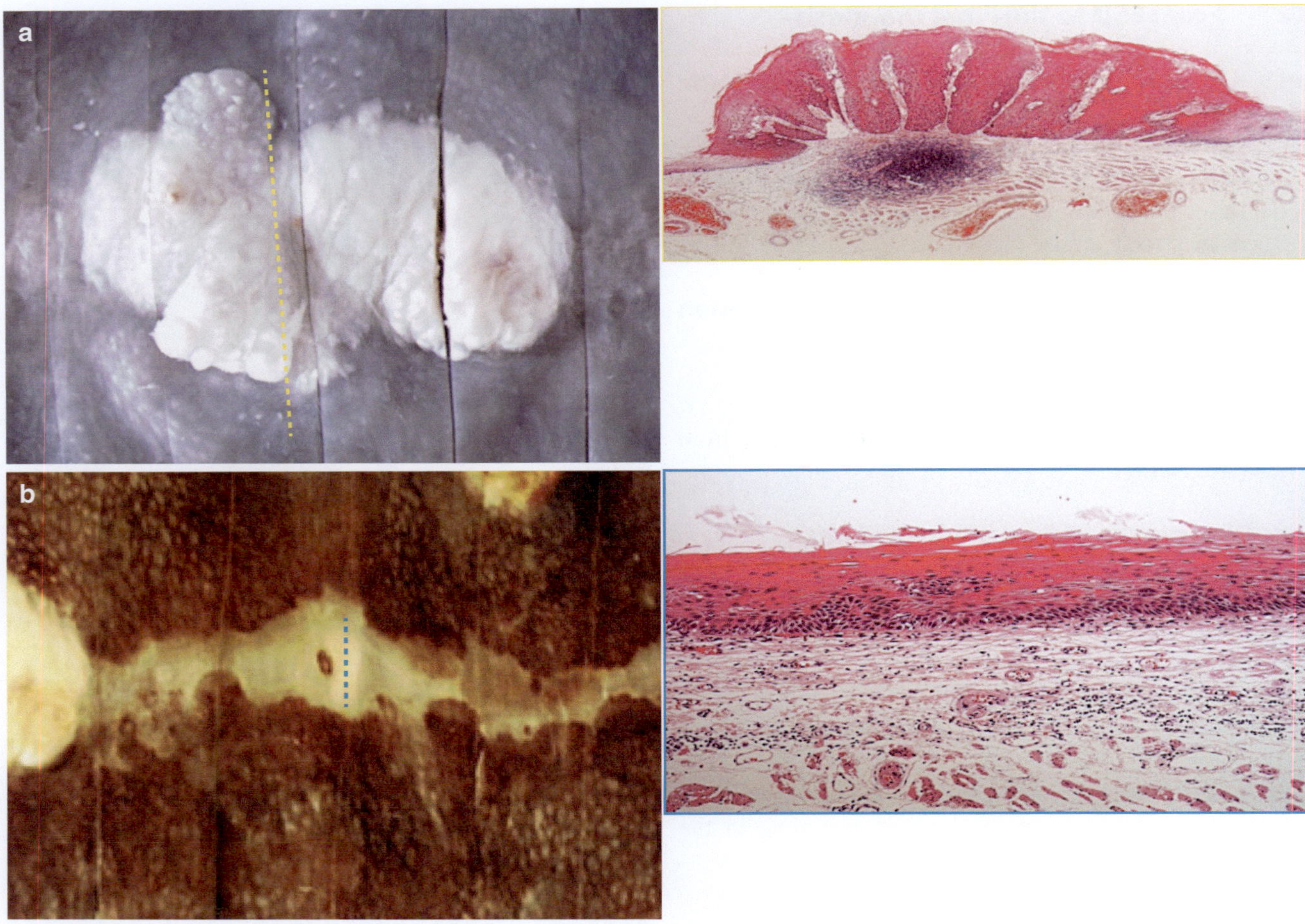

Fig. 8.3 (**a**) H&E staining image of the section (yellow dotted line on the left image) through the raised lesion. (**b**) The anal part of the iodine dye-unstained lesion was shown by a H&E section represented by blue dotted line

9 Type 0-IIa Esophageal Cancer: Second Case

Dai Hirasawa

D. Hirasawa (✉)
Department of Gastroenterology, Sendai Kosei Hospital,
Sendai, Miyagi, Japan
e-mail: hirasawa@sendai-kousei-hospital.jp

T. Oyama (ed.), *Endoscopic Diagnosis of Esophageal Carcinoma for ESD*, https://doi.org/10.1007/978-981-32-9030-3_9

9.1 Let's Try to Diagnose This Lesion

Let's Diagnose with White Light Imaging (Fig. 9.1a)

- A reddish flat raised lesion with 1/3 the circumference was noted on the right wall of the lower thoracic esophagus (black arrows).
- The lesion was clearly demarcated, with loss of vascular visibility compared with the surrounding area.

Let's Observe the Lesion with Air Volume Adjustments (Fig. 9.1b)

- The lesion was noted to change its shape by air volume adjustments, appearing taller with desufflation of air.
- Although being a tall raised lesion, with easily extensible lesion form as noted by the previous image, the lesion seemed unlikely to have submucosal invasions.

Let's Consider Causes of an Elevated Lesion form (Fig. 9.1b)

- The lesion was sparsely keratotic, with visible papillary structures, appeared to have upward growth tendency. Since the lesion height was noted to vary with air volume adjustments, tumor volume appears to be abundant as well. Causes of the elevated lesion form are thought to be due to both upward growth tendency and tumor volume.

Let's Observe with Magnifying NBI (Fig. 9.1c)

- Dot like blood vessels mostly of Type B1 were noted, but there were some non-loop blood vessels of Type B2 in the central portion as noted in the image on the left (pink arrows).
- Based on magnifying NBI, invasion depth of T1a-MM ~ T1b-SM1 were suggested.

Let's Determine Invasion Depth with Comprehensive Diagnosis (Fig. 9.1c)

- On white light imaging, the lesion was noted to be easily extensible.
- On magnifying NBI, Type B2 blood vessels were seen, but within a very limited area where both Type B1 and B2 vessels were seen mixed together. Considering both easy flexibility of the lesion and tumor volume abundancy, the lesion was suspected to be mostly T1a-LPM, with partial T1a-MM-level invasions.

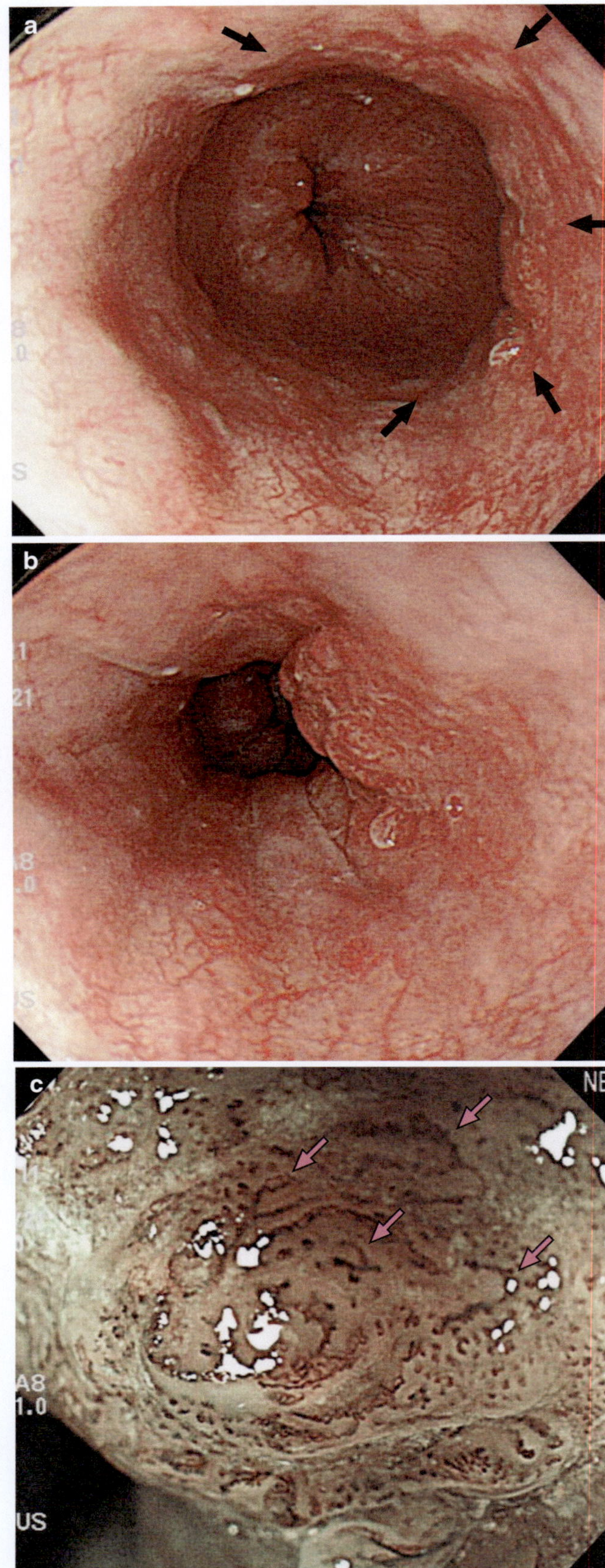

Fig. 9.1 Type 0-IIa esophageal cancer. (**a**) White light endoscopic image of the lesion. (**b**) White light endoscopic image with decreased the air volume. (**c**) NBI magnified endoscopic image of the lesion

9.2 From ESD to the Final Diagnosis

Let's Perform Iodine Dye Staining (Fig. 9.2a)

- There was an unstained area corresponding to the raised lesion.
- The lesion was clearly demarcated.

Let's Observe the Freshly Resected Specimen (Fig. 9.2b)

- The freshly resected specimen was observed.
- The resected specimen measured 35 × 30 mm.
- The lesion was slightly raised as a whole, with nodular elevations at the central part.
- The lesion measured 16 × 20 mm.

Let's Observe the Histopathological Image (Fig. 9.2c)

- H&E-stained histopathology of the lesion showed well-developed squamous cell carcinoma with keratosis.

Summary

There are two types of superficially raised (0-IIa) esophageal cancer: (1) upward growth type, and (2) thickening of cancer nests resulting in lesion lifting type. The first type with strong keratosis shows white color tone with shallower invasion depth. The second type sometimes shows invasion depth of T1a-MM or deeper, and invasion depth must be carefully diagnosed.

Conclusive Diagnosis

Esophageal squamous cell carcinoma, well differentiated, 0-IIa, T1a-LPM, INFα, ly (−), v(−), HM0, VM0, 20 × 16 mm, pCur B, Mt.

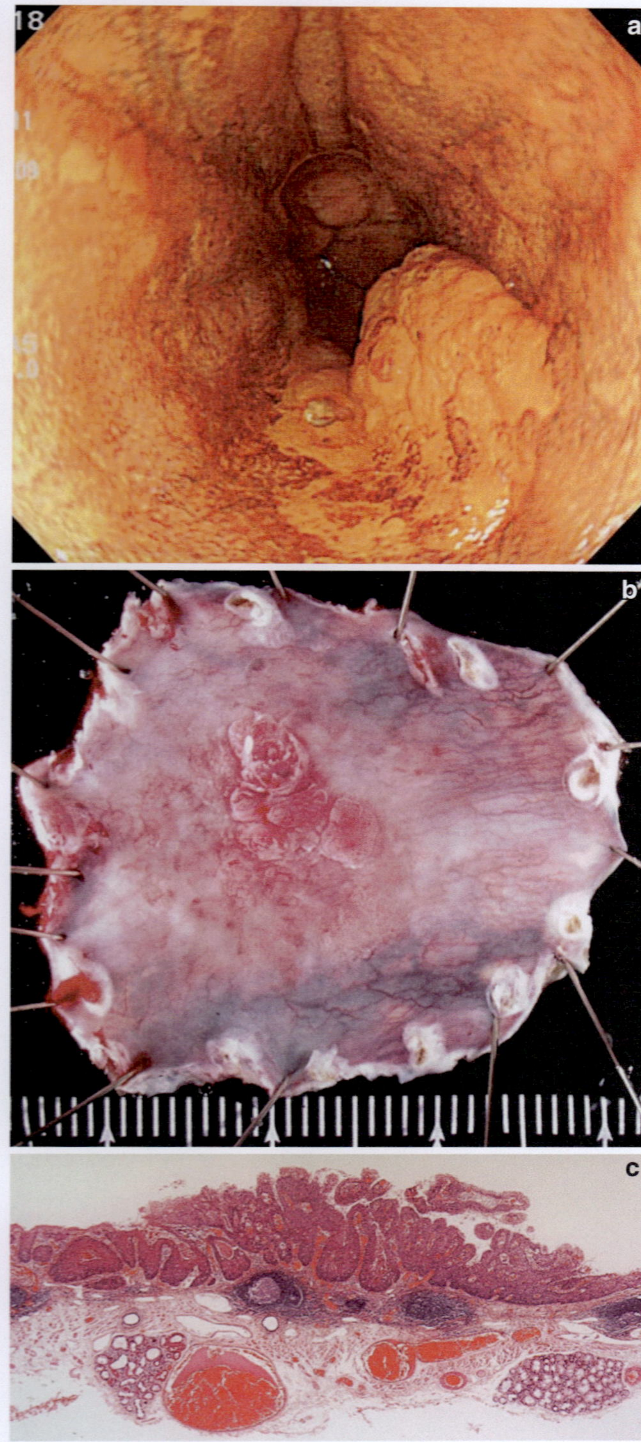

Fig. 9.2 (**a**) The lesion staining with iodine. (**b**) Fleshly resected specimen. (**c**) H&E-stained histopathological image of the area of interest

Type 0-IIb Esophageal Cancer: First Case

10

Nobukazu Yorimitsu

N. Yorimitsu (✉)
Department of Endoscopy, Saku Central Hospital Advanced Care Center, Nagano, Japan
e-mail: 99097ny@jichi.ac.jp

T. Oyama (ed.), *Endoscopic Diagnosis of Esophageal Carcinoma for ESD*, https://doi.org/10.1007/978-981-32-9030-3_10

10.1 Let's Try to Diagnose This Lesion

Let's Diagnose with White Light Imaging (Fig. 10.1a)

- The mid-thoracic esophagus was observed with white light imaging.
- Vascular visibility was good throughout.

Let's Observe with Non-Magnifying NBI (Fig. 10.1b)

- On non-magnifying NBI, the reddish area observed above corresponded to a brownish area (BA).
- A clear demarcation was noted as color difference extending nearly half the circumference.
- The lesion was smooth flat squamous cell carcinoma, O-IIb, with invasion depth of T1a-EP being suspected.

Let's Observe from the Periphery with Low-Magnification NBI (Fig. 10.1c)

- An aggregation of dense dot-like blood vessels were noted with faint intervascular background coloration.
- Cyan-tone veins were less visible within the lesion.
- The lesion was clearly demarcated from its surrounding area by blood vessel density and color tone differences.

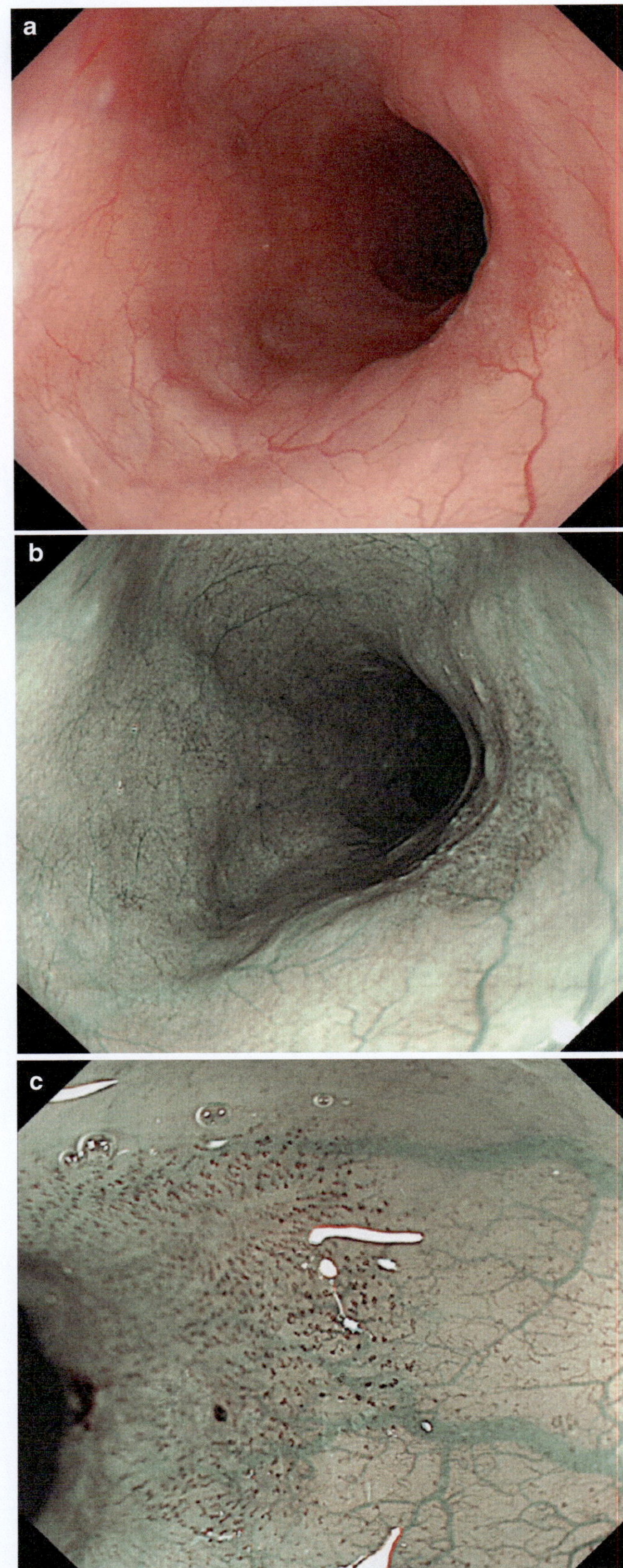

Fig. 10.1 Type 0-IIb esophageal cancer. (**a**) White light endoscopic image of the lesion. (**b–d**) NBI magnified endoscopic image of the lesion. (**e**) Endoscopic image after marking. (**f**) The lesion staining with iodine

Let's Observe with Full-Magnification NBI (Fig. 10.1d)

- On full-magnification NBI, loop-like blood vessels with dilation, tortuosity, caliber differences, and uneven shapes were noted suggestive of Type B1 blood vessels.
- In the area marked by a blue-dotted circle, blood vessels were noted horizontally traversing but with both the beginning and the ending parts in the same place, consistent with elongated loops of Type B1 blood vessels, and squamous cell carcinoma with invasion depth of T1a-LPM was diagnosed.

Let's Place Markings to Evaluate the Area of Interest (Fig. 10.1e)

- The Type B1, elongated loop vessel part marked by the blue-dotted circle was chosen as the area of interest.
- To make comparative assessment possible with histopathological images, the area of interest was designated with two interposing markings (red arrows) placed, one on each side of the elongated loop vessel portion.

Let's Perform Iodine Dye Staining (Fig. 10.1f)

- With application of 0.75% iodine dye, the lesion became an irregularly shaped unstained area, with positive pink color sign.
- Based on this, the lesion was diagnosed as esophageal SCC, 0-IIb, with invasion depth of T1a-LPM, and ESD was performed.

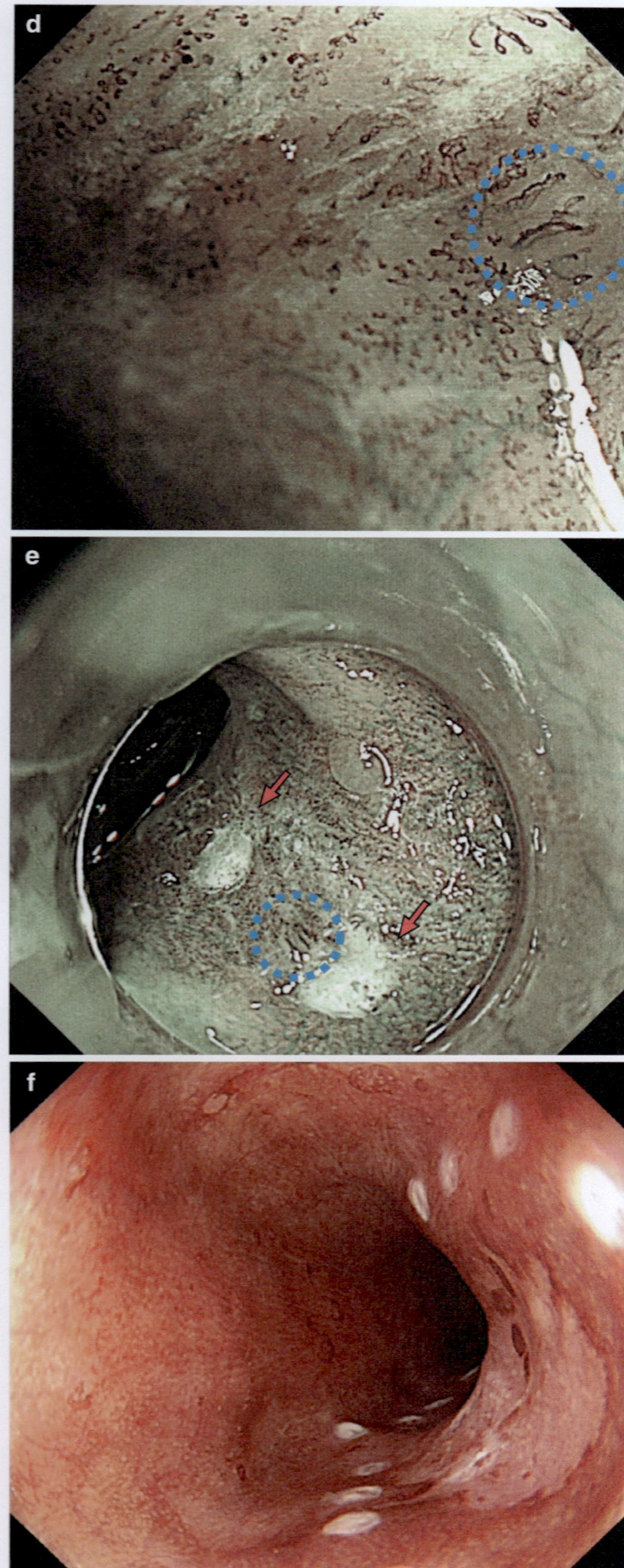

Fig. 10.1 (continued)

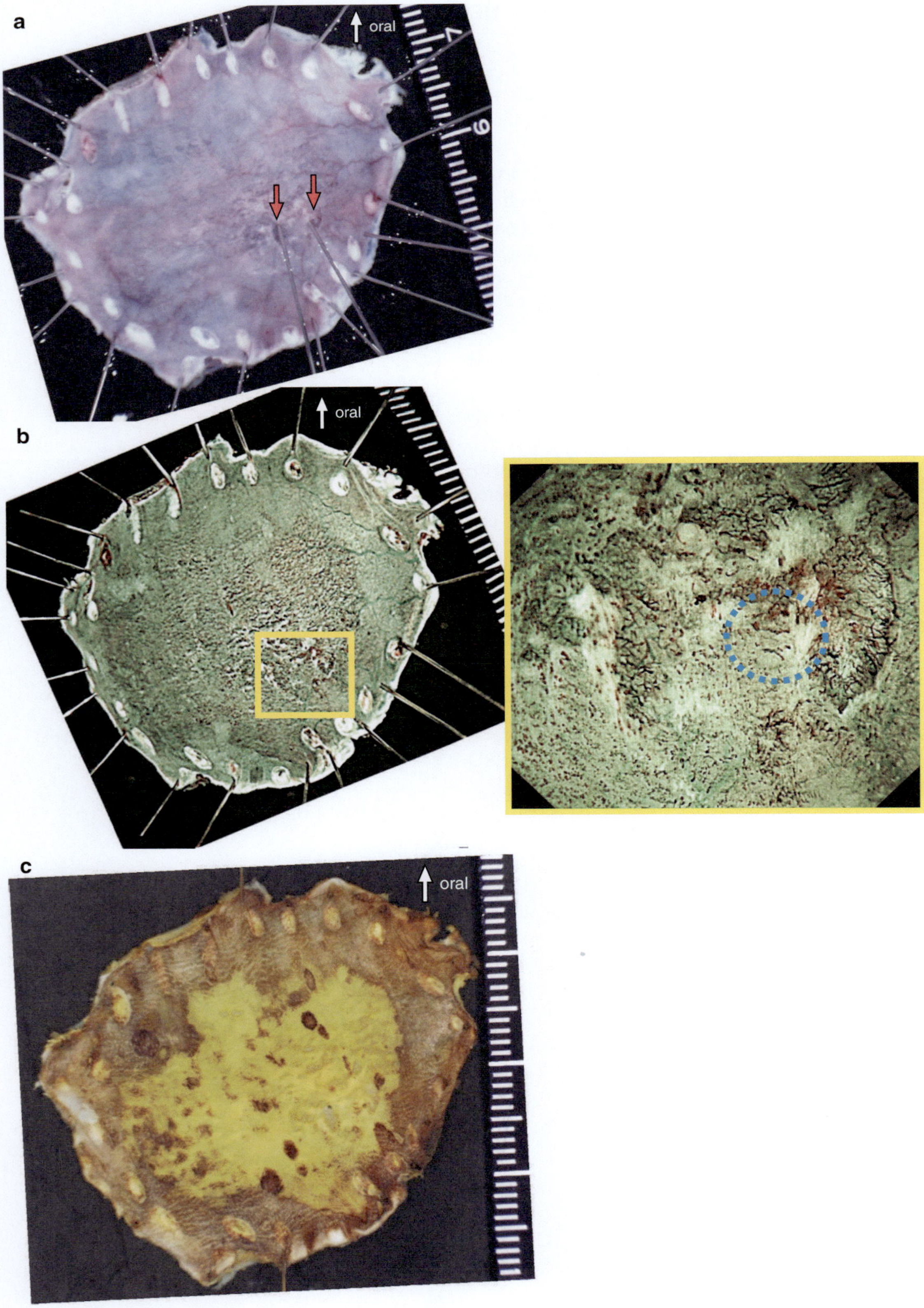

Fig. 10.2 (**a**) Fleshly resected specimen of the lesion. (**b**) NBI-magnified endoscopic image of the resected specimen. (**c**) The specimen staining with iodine

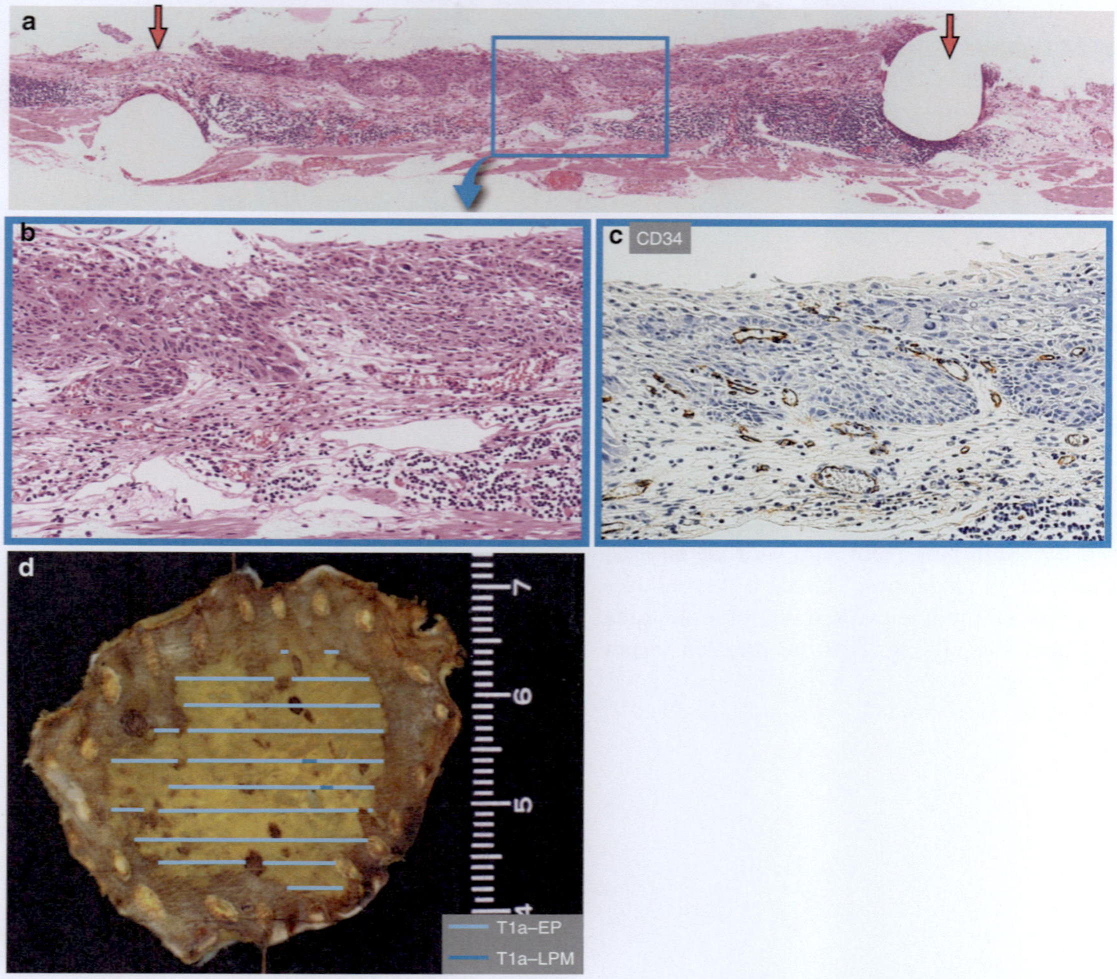

Fig. 10.3 (**a**) H&E-stained histopathological image of the area of interest is shown. The parts marked with red arrows are the two pinholes designating the area of interest. (**b**) The blue square when magnified showed enlarged nuclei of the tumor cells in the full thickness of the epithelium, with partial invasion of the submucosal layer, diagnosing the lesion as SCC, with invasion depth of T1a-LPM. (**c**, **d**) When CD34 is used to stain vascular endothelia, blood vessels traversing within papillary structures were observed. These blood vessels were thought to have been observed as elongated Type B1 blood vessels

10.2 From ESD to the Final diagnosis

Let's Observe the Freshly Resected Specimen (Fig. 10.2a)

- The specimen was oriented with the top right as the oral side.
- There was a faintly reddish area within the resected specimen but with unclear margin.
- For comparative analysis of the area of interest, the two markings placed were pinned (red arrows) before tissue fixation.

Let's Observe the Freshly Resected Specimen with Magnified NBI (Fig. 10.2b)

- A brownish area was noted, corresponding the faintly reddish area of the freshly resected specimen with clear demarcation. The area of interest framed with a yellow square was observed with magnified NBI, showing elongated loop-like Type B1 blood vessels in the area marked by blue-dotted circle.

Let's Observe the Iodine Dye-Stained Specimen (Fig. 10.2c)

- With iodine dye staining, the brownish area noted by NBI observation of the resected specimen was found as an unstained area.
- Iodine dye staining made the demarcation the clearest and confirmed en bloc resection of the lesion.

Conclusive Diagnosis

Esophageal squamous cell carcinoma, 0-IIb, T1a-LPM, INFα, ly(−), v(−), HM0, VM0, 27 × 22 mm, pCurA, Mt., Rt.

Summary

By white light imaging, a reddish flat lesion was noted with unclear demarcation. By NBI, the lesion was recognized as a brownish area (BA) with clear demarcation. Magnifying NBI showed mostly dot-like Type B1 blood vessels, but an area with elongated loop-like Type B1 blood vessels was found to be T1a-LPM. Iodine dye staining showed irregularly shaped unstained area with pink color sign with the clearest demarcation of all modalities. This case showed usefulness of NBI and iodine dye staining in lesion area diagnosis and magnifying NBI in invasion depth diagnosis.

11 Type 0-IIb Esophageal Carcinoma: Second Case

Nobukazu Yorimitsu

N. Yorimitsu (✉)
Department of Endoscopy, Saku Central Hospital Advanced Care Center, Nagano, Japan
e-mail: 99097ny@jichi.ac.jp

T. Oyama (ed.), *Endoscopic Diagnosis of Esophageal Carcinoma for ESD*, https://doi.org/10.1007/978-981-32-9030-3_11

11.1 Let's Try to Diagnose This Lesion

Let's Observe with White Light Imaging (Fig. 11.1a)

- The mid-thoracic esophagus was observed with white light imaging.
- Vascular visibility was good throughout.
- Subtle color tone variations and unevenness of the surface mucosa were noted but with no apparent lesion.

Let's Observe with Non-Magnifying NBI (Fig. 11.1b)

- On non-magnifying NBI observation, a 5 mm brownish area (BA) was noted in the left wall side.
- The lesion had clear demarcation and was suspected to be squamous cell carcinoma (SCC).

Let's Observe with Close-Up Non-Magnifying NBI (Fig. 11.1c)

- On close-up observation, the demarcation became distinctively recognizable by color differences.
- The lesion was flat and was suspected to be SCC, 0-IIb, T1a-EP.

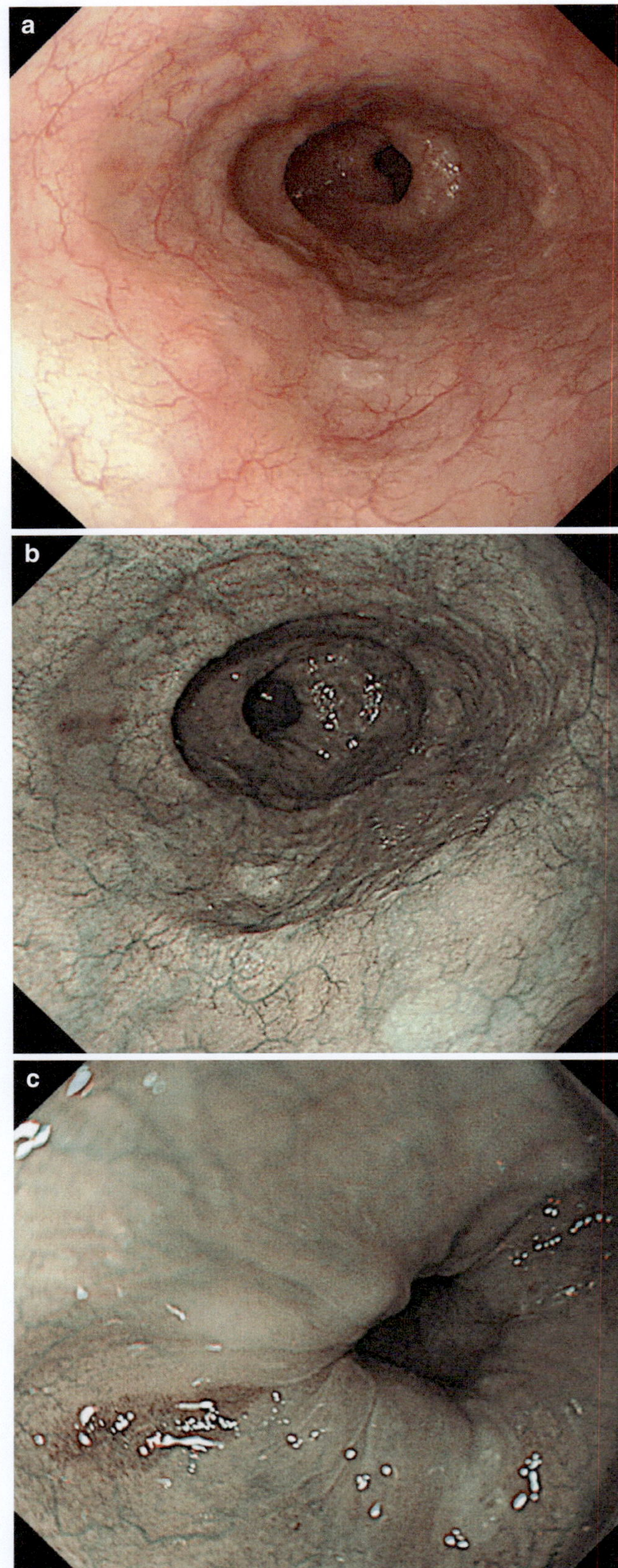

Fig. 11.1 Type 0-IIb esophageal carcinoma. (**a**) White light endoscopic image of the lesion. (**b**, **c**) NBI endoscopic images of the lesion. (**d**, **e**) NBI magnified endoscopic images of the lesion. (**f**) The lesion staining with iodine

Let's Observe with Low-Magnification NBI (Fig. 11.1d)

- The lesion was brought to 12 o'clock position by rotating the scope and observed by low-magnification NBI.
- The entire lesion was densely filled with dot-like blood vessels with intervascular background coloration.
- The demarcation of the lesion from the surrounding mucosa was evident by the differences in color tone and vascular density.

Let's Observe with High-Magnification NBI (Fig. 11.1e)

- On high-magnification NBI, the surrounding mucosa showed normal IPCL without irregularities, clearly branching from the subepithelial capillary network (SECN).
- The lesion revealed aggregations of the irregular loop-like blood vessels with dilation, tortuosity, and irregular calibrations and shapes, consistent with Type B1 blood vessels, supporting the invasion depth diagnosis of T1a-EP.

Let's Perform Iodine Dye Staining (Fig. 11.1f)

- Upon 0.75% iodine dye spraying, the background mucosa showed irregularly staining patchy appearance.
- The lesion had a regularly shaped and clearly demarcated unstained area, supporting the diagnosis of esophageal SCC, 0-IIb, T1a-EP, and ESD was performed.

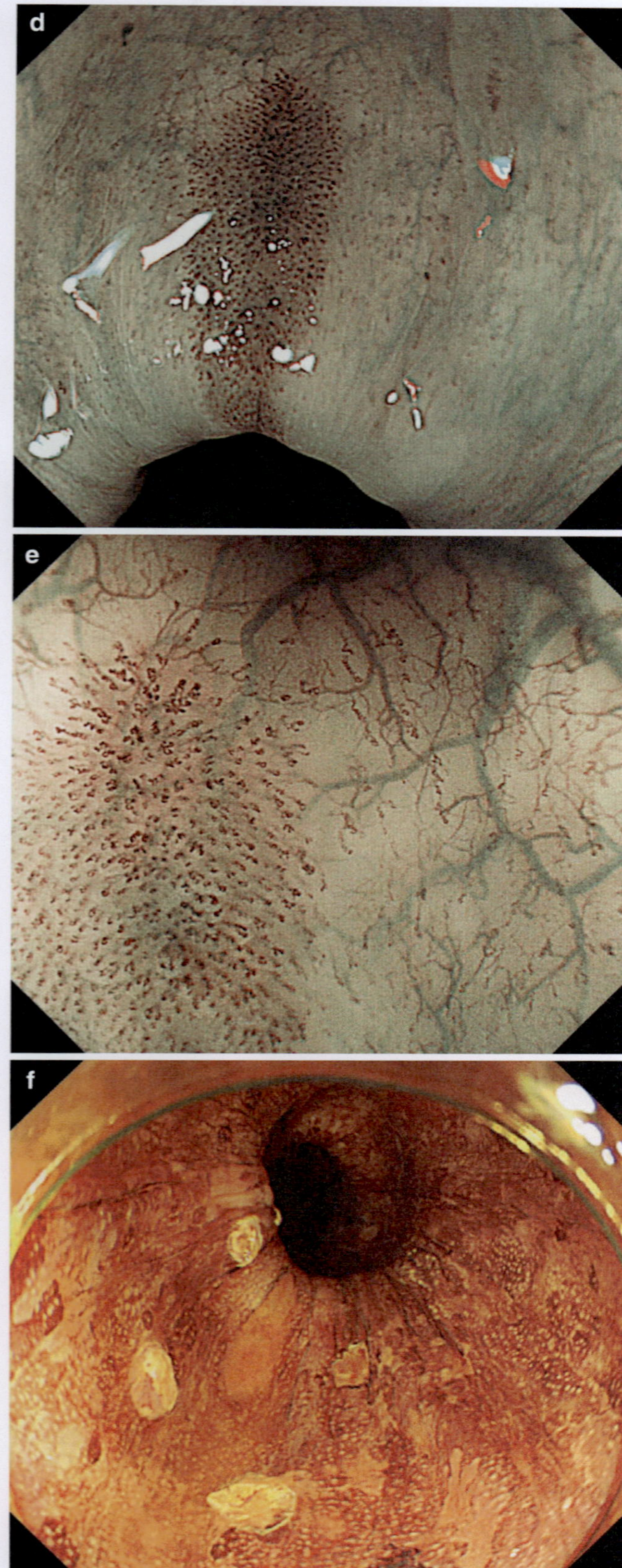

Fig. 11.1 (continued)

11.2 From ESD to the Final Diagnosis

Let's Observe the Freshly Resected Specimen (Fig. 11.2a)

- The resected specimen is shown with the oral side towards the bottom.
- There is a 5 × 3 mm reddish area in the center of the resected specimen.
- The lesion was flat, but clearly demarcated by color tone differences.

Let's Observe the Freshly Resected Specimen with NBI (Fig. 11.2b)

- The reddish area in the resected specimen clearly demarcated as BA.
- The vessels in the specimen revealed dotted-like blood vessels with highly condensed at the center and loop-like blood vessels with dilation and tortuosity at the marginal area. The vessels are determined as Type B1 blood vessels.

Let's Observe the Iodine Dye-Stained Specimen (Fig. 11.2c)

- Upon iodine dye staining, the area corresponding to the reddish flat lesion of the freshly resected specimen was found as an unstained area.
- The lesion was clearly demarcated with somewhat irregular border, suggestive of SCC.

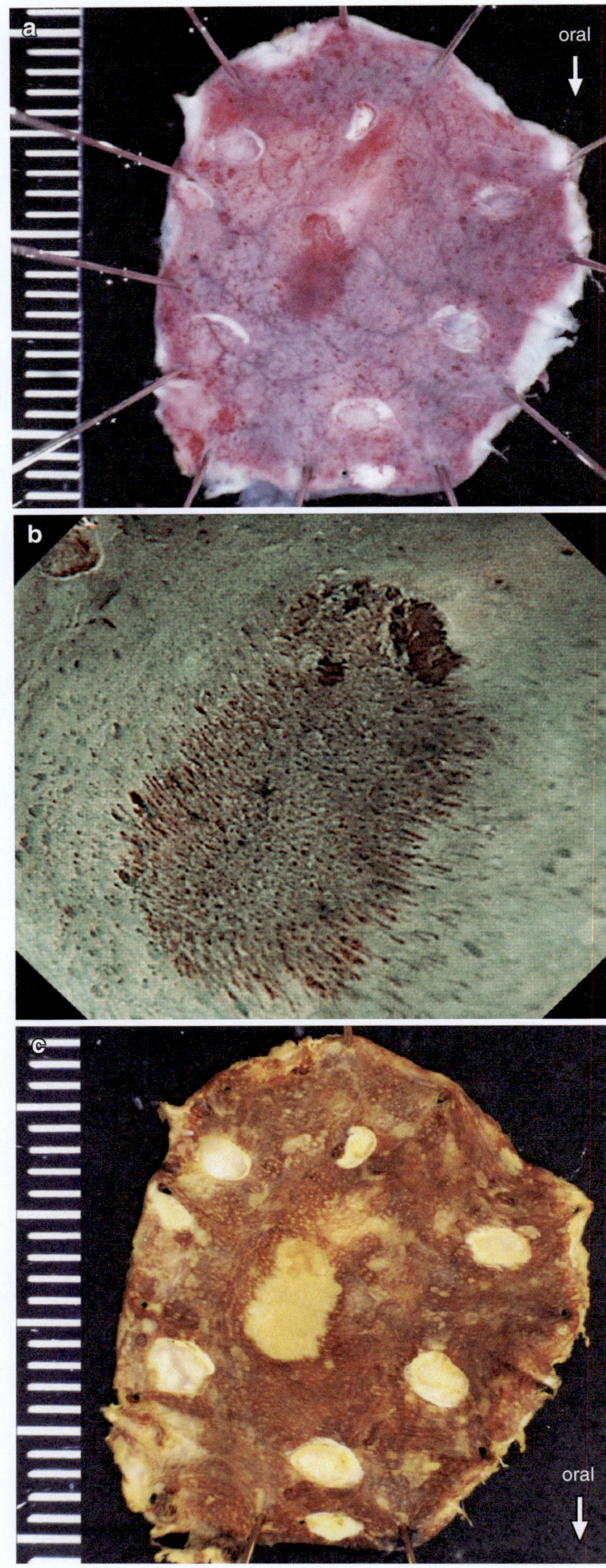

Fig. 11.2 (**a**) Fleshly resected specimen. (**b**) NBI magnified endoscopic images of the resected specimen. (**c**) The resected specimen staining with iodine

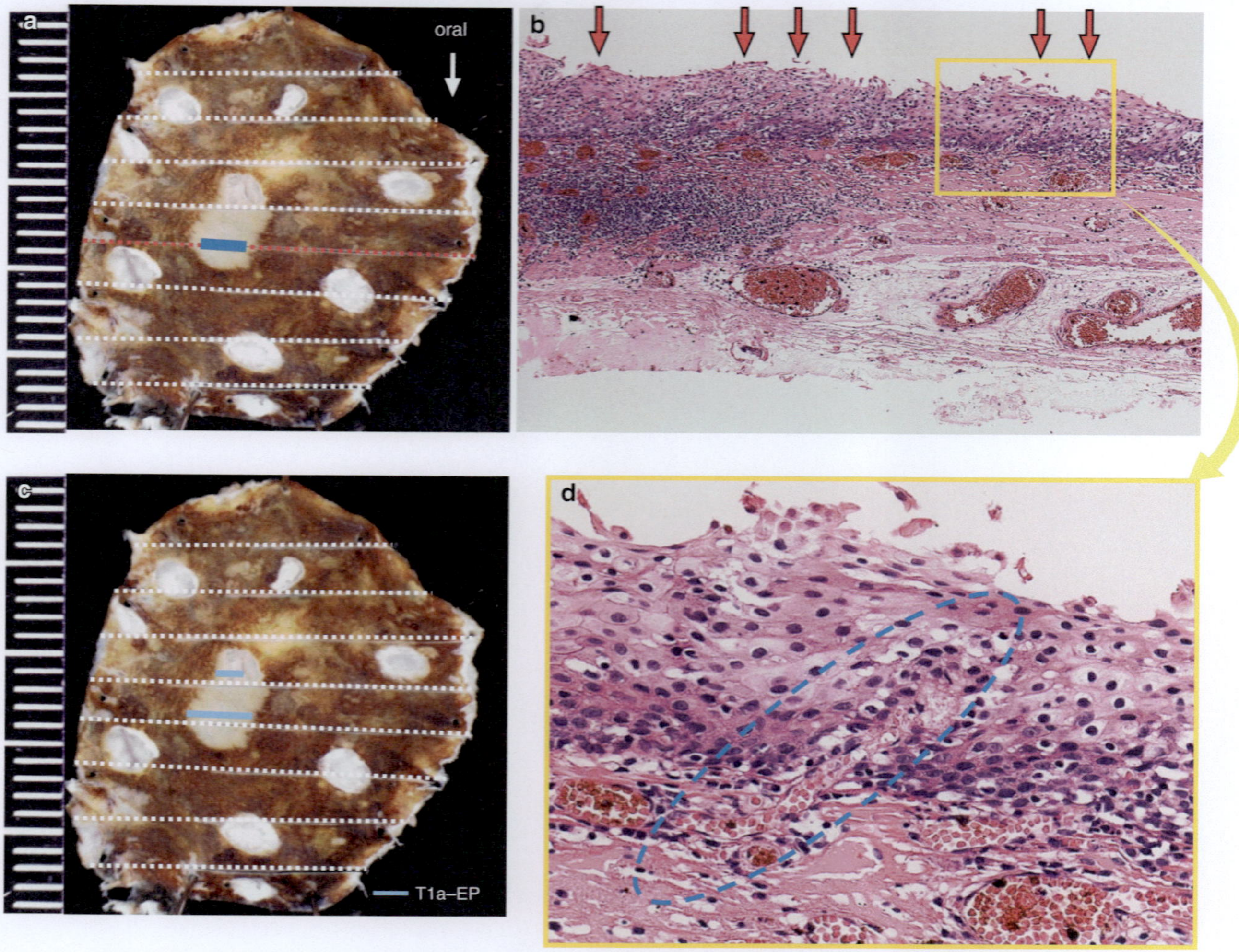

Fig. 11.3 (**a**, **b**) The section noted with the red dotted line in the above left image of this portion was shown in the above right image. Lymphoid follicles were noted within the lamina propria, and atypical cells with large nuclei were noted in the whole layer of the mucosal epithelium. The basal layer was kept intact and SCC with invasion depth of T1a-EP was diagnosed. Vascular structures were noted as marked by the red arrows. (**c**) The portion marked by the yellow square was magnified further. (**d**) A papillary structure was noted in the EP cancer, containing a blood vessel within as circled by the blue-dotted line. This was thought to represent Type B1 blood vessels observed by magnifying NBI. Mapping of the lesion is shown here. SCC with invasion depth diagnosis of T1a-EP is noted corresponding to the unstained area

Conclusive Diagnosis

Esophageal squamous cell carcinoma, 0-IIb, T1a-EP, ly(−), v(−), HM0, VM0, 5 × 3 mm, pCur A, Mt., Lt.

Summary

A small 0-IIb lesion was noted in the left lateral wall of the mid-thoracic esophagus. It was difficult to notice on white light imaging, but became an easily recognizable clearly demarcated BA by NBI. Magnifying NBI revealed Type B1 vessels within the lesion. Iodine dye staining revealed the lesion as a clearly demarcated unstained area, leading to the diagnosis of SCC, T1a-EP. Non-magnifying NBI was useful in detection of this SCC, and magnifying NBI was useful in invasion depth diagnosis.

Type 0-IIc Esophageal Carcinoma: First Case

12

Dai Hirasawa

D. Hirasawa (✉)
Department of Gastroenterology, Sendai Kosei Hospital,
Sendai, Miyagi, Japan
e-mail: hirasawa@sendai-kousei-hospital.jp

T. Oyama (ed.), *Endoscopic Diagnosis of Esophageal Carcinoma for ESD*, https://doi.org/10.1007/978-981-32-9030-3_12

12.1 Let's Try to Diagnose This Lesion

Let's Observe with White Light Imaging (Fig. 12.1a)

- A reddish depressed lesion was noted on the right lateral wall in the mid-thoracic esophagus as marked by the black arrows.
- Corresponding to the depressed area, loss of vascular visibility was noted. The demarcation was evident.
- A whitish mucosal area was noted in the center as marked by the green arrow.

Let's Observe if the Lesion Shape Changes with Air Volume Variation (Fig. 12.1b)

- The lesion was observed with air volume reduction.
- Unevenness became more distinct making the lesion easily recognizable. It is important to use air volume variation when screening for esophageal lesions.
- No stiffness was noted with the lesion and invasion depth diagnosis of T1a-EP~LPM.

Let's Observe with NBI (Fig. 12.1c)

- The lesion was noted as a brownish area with NBI observation.
- NBI is useful for screening evaluations because of its superior lesion detectability compared with WLI.
- An island-like normal mucosa was noted in the center of the lesion as marked by the green arrow.

Let's Observe with Magnifying NBI (Fig. 12.1d)

- Loop-like blood vessels are observed throughout the depressed area.
- Based on the presence of Type B1 blood vessels, invasion depth diagnosis was estimated to be T1a-EP~LPM.

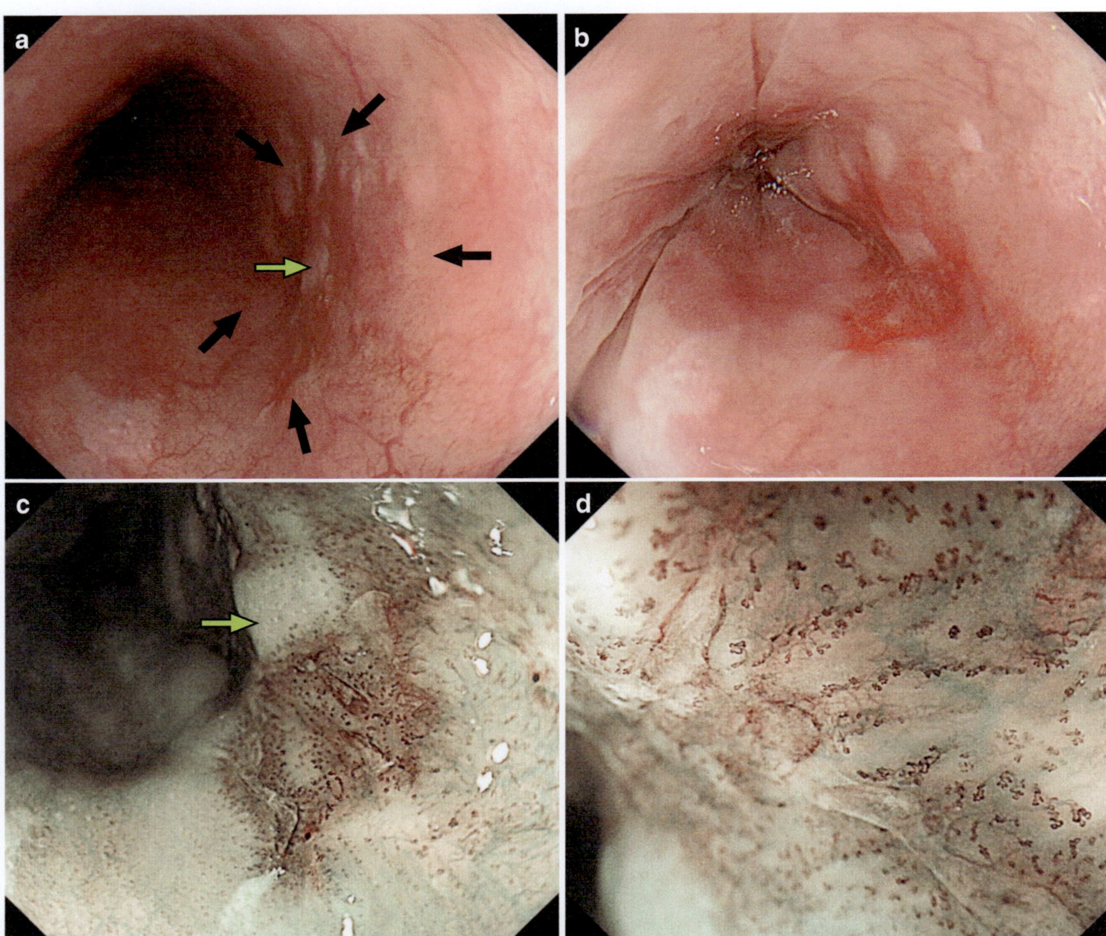

Fig. 12.1 Type 0-IIc esophageal carcinoma. (**a**) White light endoscopic image of the lesion. (**b**) White light endoscopic image with decreased air volume. (**c**) NBI endoscopic image of the lesion. (**d**) NBI magnified endoscopic image of the lesion

Let's Observe with Magnifying NBI (Fig. 13.1d)

- The lesion was rotated to the 12 o'clock for observation. The Olympus-made endoscopes have CCD toward the 12 o'clock direction, making it easier to focus short distance with full-magnification NBI on 12 o'clock direction. On the other hand, for viewing from a distance to capture the entire lesion, the 6 o'clock directional view is better suited.
- Weakly brownish area other than the area marked by the green arrow in the prior image showed loop-like Type B1 blood vessels.

Let's Observe the Areas of Interest in Detail (Fig. 13.1e)

- The stronger brownish area marked by the green arrow in the first NBI image of this case was observed by magnifying NBI.
- Non-loop-forming Type B2 blood vessels were observed as shown.
- Most of the lesion in the prior image is Type B1 blood vessels suggestive of invasion depth diagnosis of T1a-EP~LPM. On the other hand, this area was suspected to have invasion depth diagnosis of T1a-MM~T1b-SM1.

Let's Perform Iodine Dye Staining (Fig. 13.1f)

- This image was obtained after spraying of 1% iodine dye solution.
- There was a semi-circumferential unstained area in the right lateral wall.
- The lesion was clearly demarcated.

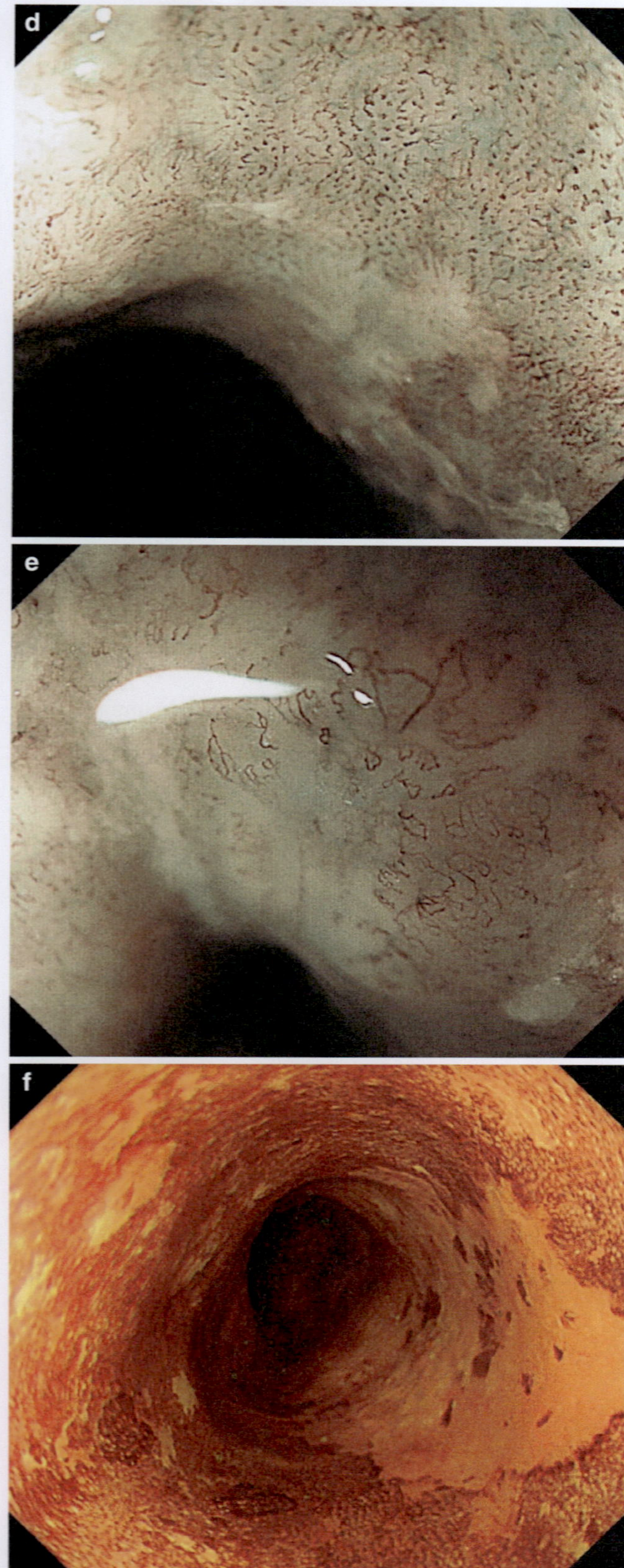

Fig. 13.1 (continued)

13.2 From ESD to the Final Diagnosis

Let's Place Markings Around the Lesion (Fig. 13.2a)

- The lesion occupies more than half of the luminal circumference towards its anal side; the resected area was about three-quarters of the luminal circumference.
- With iodine dye spraying, lesion areas sometimes are found to differ from those observed by NBI. Therefore, it is essential to confirm the lesion area with iodine dye spraying before resection by ESD.
- Because of the caustic nature of iodine dye, mucosal surface damages may result in staining by the second spraying of iodine dye on the regenerated epithelia. It is desirable to wait at least 1 month before the second iodine dye spraying, or it is also important to plan only on the treatment day to spray iodine dye.

Let's Perform ESD (Fig. 13.2b)

- This image shows an endoscopic view after the resection of the lesion.
- The resection was seven-eighth of the circumference at the end.
- Triamcinolone was submucosally injected to prevent stenosis.

Let's Observe the Freshly Resected Specimen (Fig. 13.3a, b)

- The resected specimen was immediately pinned to be spread and immersed under saline water to perform stereoscopic observation and capturing of images.
- The resected specimen measured 60 × 40 mm.
- The lesion was resected with a minimal margin around the markings to prevent stenosis.
- The area surrounded by the green square corresponds to the strongly brownish area marked by the green arrow with NBI observation.
- This magnified image corresponds to the area surrounded by the green square of the resected specimen.
- While the surrounding areas marked by blue-dotted circles showed Type B1 blood vessels, the central area showed non-loop-forming Type B2 blood vessels as marked by the yellow arrows.
- These findings were consistent with magnified NBI observation.

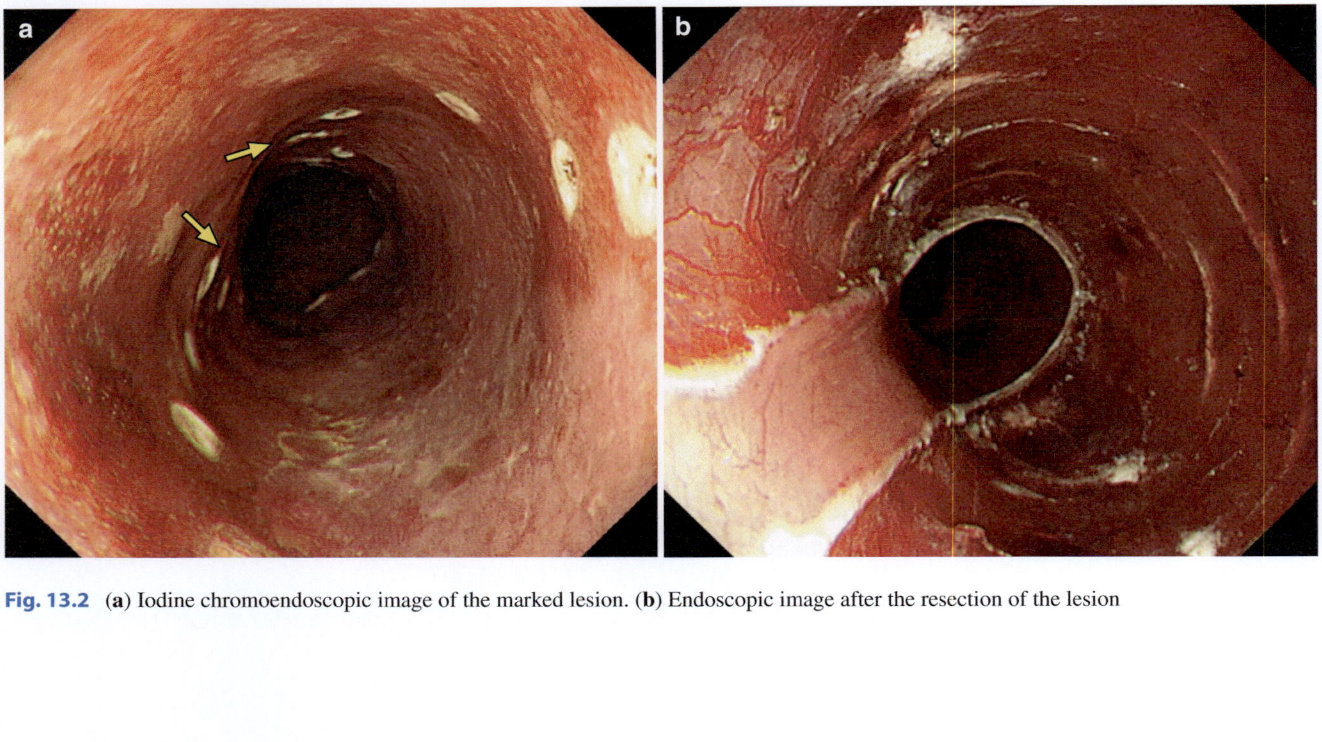

Fig. 13.2 (**a**) Iodine chromoendoscopic image of the marked lesion. (**b**) Endoscopic image after the resection of the lesion

Let's Observe the Iodine Dye-Stained Resected Specimen After Fixation with Formalin (Fig. 13.4a, b)

- After formalin fixation, the fixed specimen was immerse in water for 6 h, sliced for preparation of histopathological sections, and stained by iodine to obtain this image under stereomicroscopy.
- The unstained area representing the lesion measured 50 × 30 mm.
- The surrounding area was circumferentially stained, suggesting no involvement of tumor at the resection margin by stereomicroscopic observation.

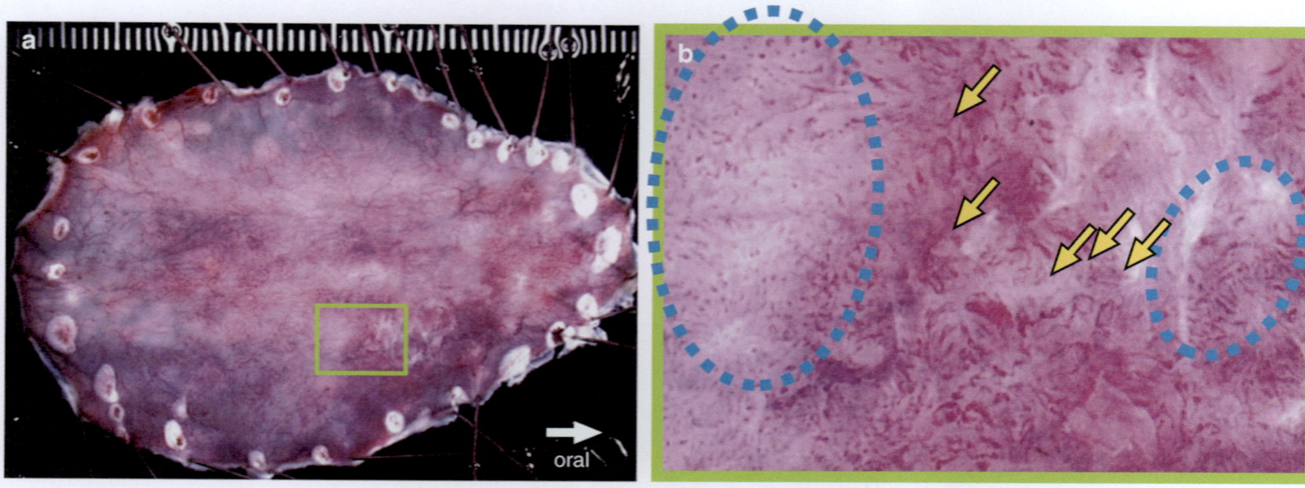

Fig. 13.3 (**a**) Fleshly resected specimen of the lesion. (**b**) Magnified image of the surrounded by the green square

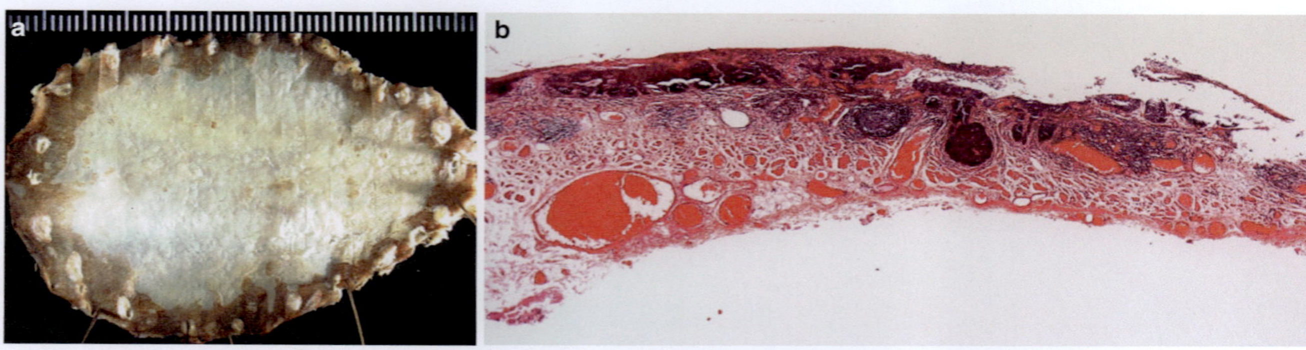

Fig. 13.4 (**a**) Fixed specimen of the lesion. (**b**) Histopathological image of the resected specimen (HE stain) showed moderately differentiated squamous cell carcinoma with obvious interstitial infiltration. Invasion of the muscularis mucosa by carcinoma was noted in the area in which Type B2 blood vessels were observed

Conclusive Diagnosis

Esophageal squamous cell carcinoma, moderately differentiated, 0-IIc, T1a-MM, INFb, ly(−), v(−), HM0, VM0, 50 × 30 mm, pCurB, Mt.

Summary

Among superficial esophageal carcinoma, flat depressed disease form (Type 0-IIc) is the most frequently observed disease form, accompanied with a wide range of invasion depths from T1a-EP~T1b-SM3.

Type 0-III Esophageal Carcinoma

14

Shinichi Furutachi

S. Furutachi (✉)
Department of Gastroenterology, Okayama Medical Center,
National Hospital Organization, Okayama, Japan

T. Oyama (ed.), *Endoscopic Diagnosis of Esophageal Carcinoma for ESD*, https://doi.org/10.1007/978-981-32-9030-3_14

14.1 Let's Try to Diagnose This Lesion

Let's Observe to Diagnose with White Light Imaging (Fig. 14.1a)

- A depressed lesion with surrounding SMT-like elevation was noted on the right wall of the mid-thoracic esophagus. The difference in height of the lesion was very distinct. The surface of the depression appeared shiny. The depression appeared one level deeper suggesting submucosal invasion.

Let's Observe with Reduced Air Volume (Fig. 14.1b)

- With reduced air volume, the shape of the depressed area did not change, and submucosal invasion was suspected endoscopically.

Let's Perform Iodine Dye Staining (Fig. 14.1c)

- The depressed area was unstained with iodine dye staining, and the area surrounding the depressed area showed partially dark staining.

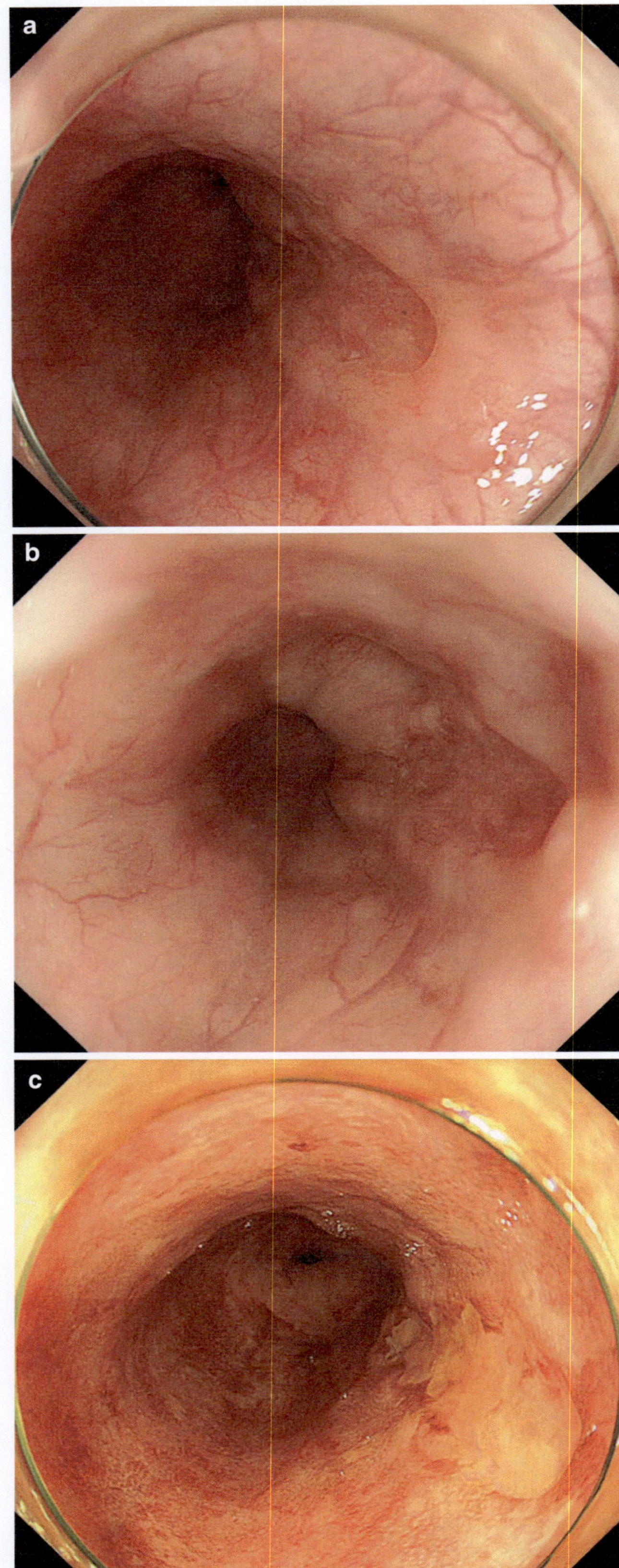

Fig. 14.1 Type 0-III esophageal carcinoma. (**a**) White light endoscopic image. (**b**) White light endoscopic image with decreased air volume. (**c**) Iodine chromoendoscopic image of the lesion. (**d–f**) NBI magnified endoscopic image of the lesion

Let's Observe with NBI (Fig. 14.1d)

- Non-magnifying NBI observation revealed the depressed area and the surrounding area as a faintly brownish area (background coloration).

Let's Observe the Oral Side of the Lesion with Magnification View (Fig. 14.1e)

- The area marked by the yellow square in the left image was observed with the scope turned counterclockwise 90° and with magnification.
- The blood vessels within the depression were thin and non-loop forming, different from Type B2 blood vessels.

Let's Observe the Central Part of the Lesion with Magnification View (Fig. 14.1f)

- The area marked by the red square in the left image was observed with the scope turned counterclockwise 90° and with magnification view.
- The central part of the lesion was covered with squamous cell epithelium with lower vascular densities.

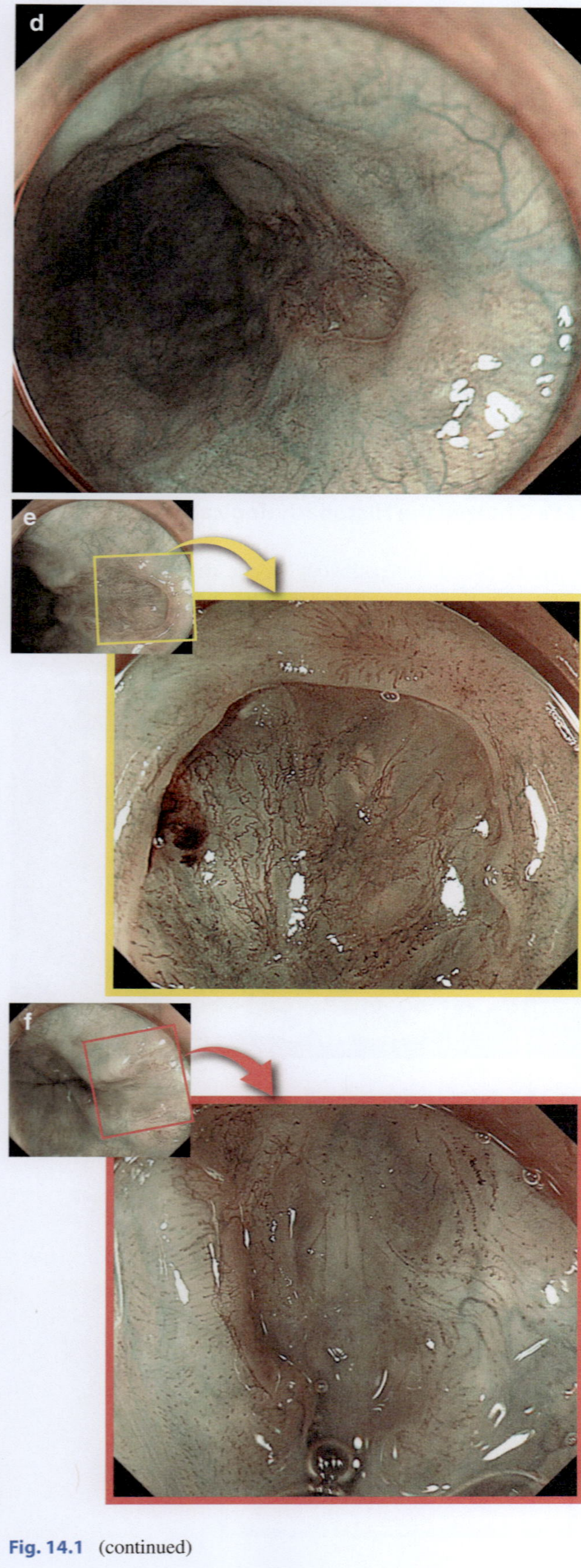

Fig. 14.1 (continued)

14.2 From ESD to the Final Diagnosis

Let's Observe the Fixed Specimen (Fig.14.2)

- The right side the image is the oral side.
- The lesion clearly showed difference in height of the depressed lesion except for a part of the lower side.
- Demarcation of the depression was clear.

Let's Observe the Pathological Specimen (Fig.14.3)

- The section through the central part of the lesion was stained for desmin, and magnified image from three parts marked by color squares were shown below. Muscularis mucosa rises towards the depressed area and appears to be torn apart within the depressed area.

Let's Observe the Histopathological Images

- H&E-stained histopathology of the depressed area of the lesion is shown. Tumor components had infiltrated into the submucosal area. The magnified view of the red squared area shows a squamous epithelium over the carcinoma (Fig. 14.4).
- Dotted color lines represent lesion covered with nontumor epithelium (Fig. 14.5).

Let's Compare the Mapping Image with the Endoscopic Image (Fig. 14.6)

- The stereomicroscopic image of iodine dye staining on the right side was rotated to align with the endoscopic image of iodine dye staining on the left side. Each of the areas marked by colored arrows and circles corresponded one on one. Invasion depth diagnosis of the depressed area was T1a-MM~T1b-SM2.
- Since this person firmly refused surgery, ESD was performed followed by chemoradiation treatment. As of 2 years after treatment, no recurrence was noted.

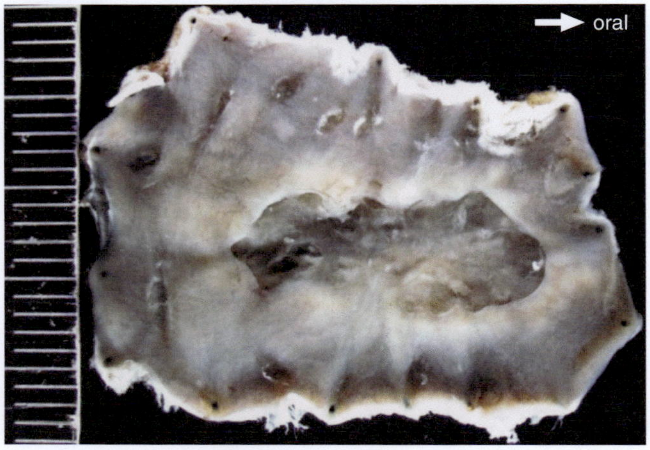

Fig. 14.2 Fixed specimen of the lesion

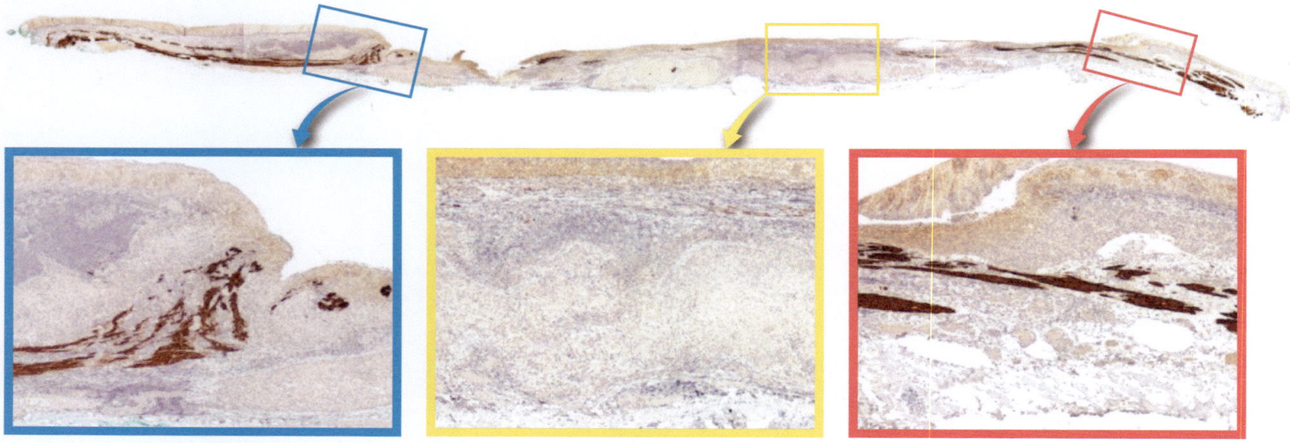

Fig. 14.3 Histopathological image of the resected specimen

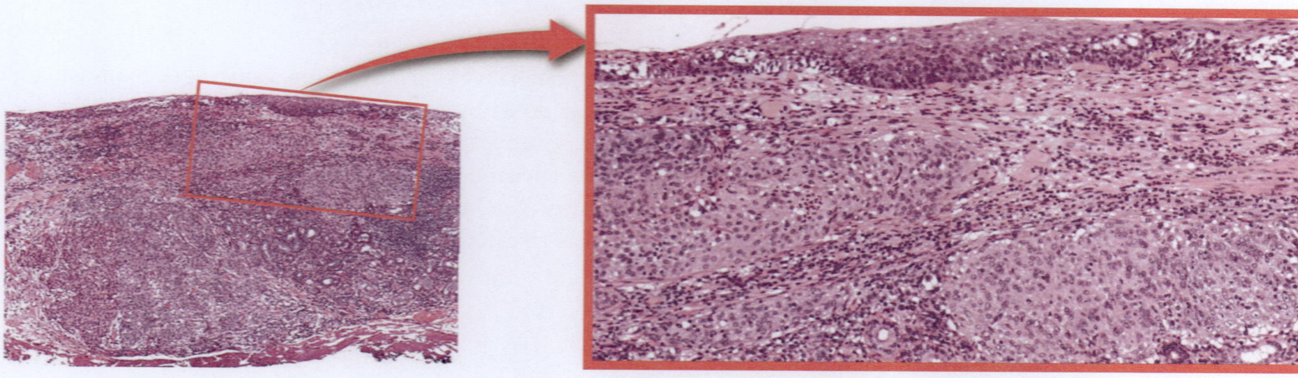

Fig. 14.4 H&E-stained histopathological image of the resected specimen

Fig. 14.5 The resected specimen stained with iodine

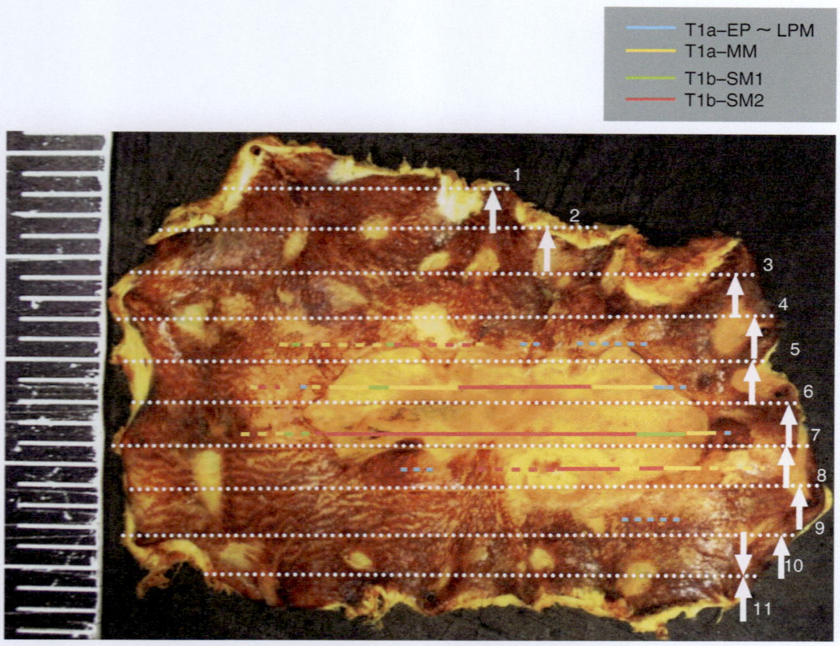

Fig. 14.6 Comparison to the mapping image with the endoscopic image

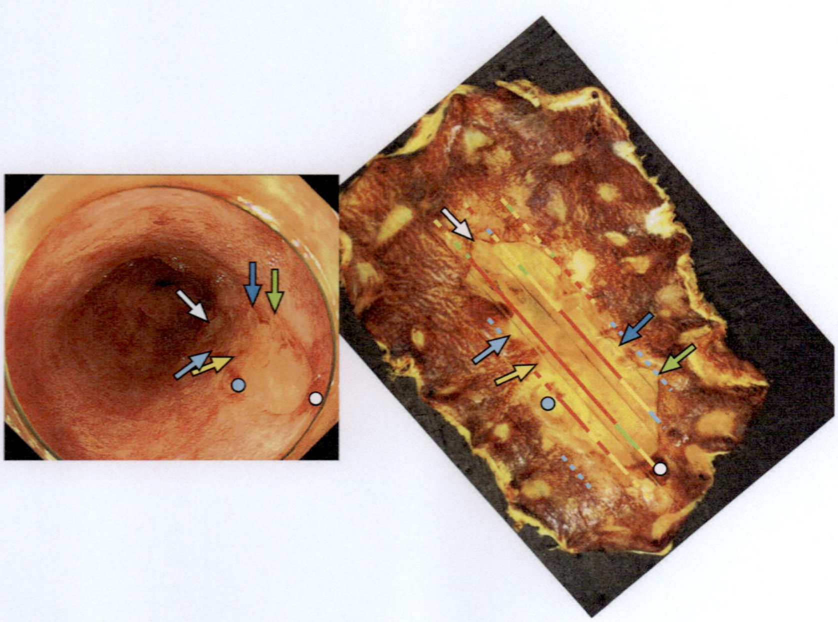

Conclusive Diagnosis

Esophageal squamous cell carcinoma, 0-III, T1b-SM2 (1200 μm), INFb, ly(+), v(+), HM0, VM0, 21 × 9 mm, pCurA, Lt.

Summary

Although no blood vessels suggestive of deep invasion were noted by magnification NBI, based on one-step deeper appearance of the depressed lesion as well as firm appearance with reduced air volume, white light endoscopic imaging was suggestive of deeper submucosal invasion.

Large Superficially Spreading Esophageal Carcinoma

15

Manabu Takeuchi

M. Takeuchi (✉)
Department of Gastroenterology, Nagaoka Red Cross Hospital,
Niigata, Japan

T. Oyama (ed.), *Endoscopic Diagnosis of Esophageal Carcinoma for ESD*, https://doi.org/10.1007/978-981-32-9030-3_15

15.1 Let's Try to Diagnose This Lesion

Let's Find the Definition of Large Superficially Spreading Esophageal Carcinoma (Fig. 15.1a)

- According to the 11th edition of the Japanese Classification of Esophageal Cancer, large superficially spreading esophageal carcinoma is defined as Type 0-II superficial lesion with the largest diameter of 5 cm or greater. This lesion type requires particularly careful assessment of invasion depths because of wide lesion area.

Let's Observe with White Light Imaging (Fig. 15.1a)

- A reddish slightly uneven circumferential lesion was noted with white light imaging extending from 35 to 40 cm from the incisors with its largest diameter of greater than 50 mm, fulfilling the diagnostic criteria of large superficially spreading esophageal carcinoma.

Let's Perform Iodine Dye Staining (Fig. 15.1b)

- Iodine dye staining revealed a large unstained area matching the noted reddish area of unevenness surface.

Let's Observe with White Light Imaging the Area of Uneven Surface (Fig. 15.1c)

- While the anal side revealed circumferential reddish uneven area like the oral side, the anterior wall was noted to have somewhat hardened appearance.

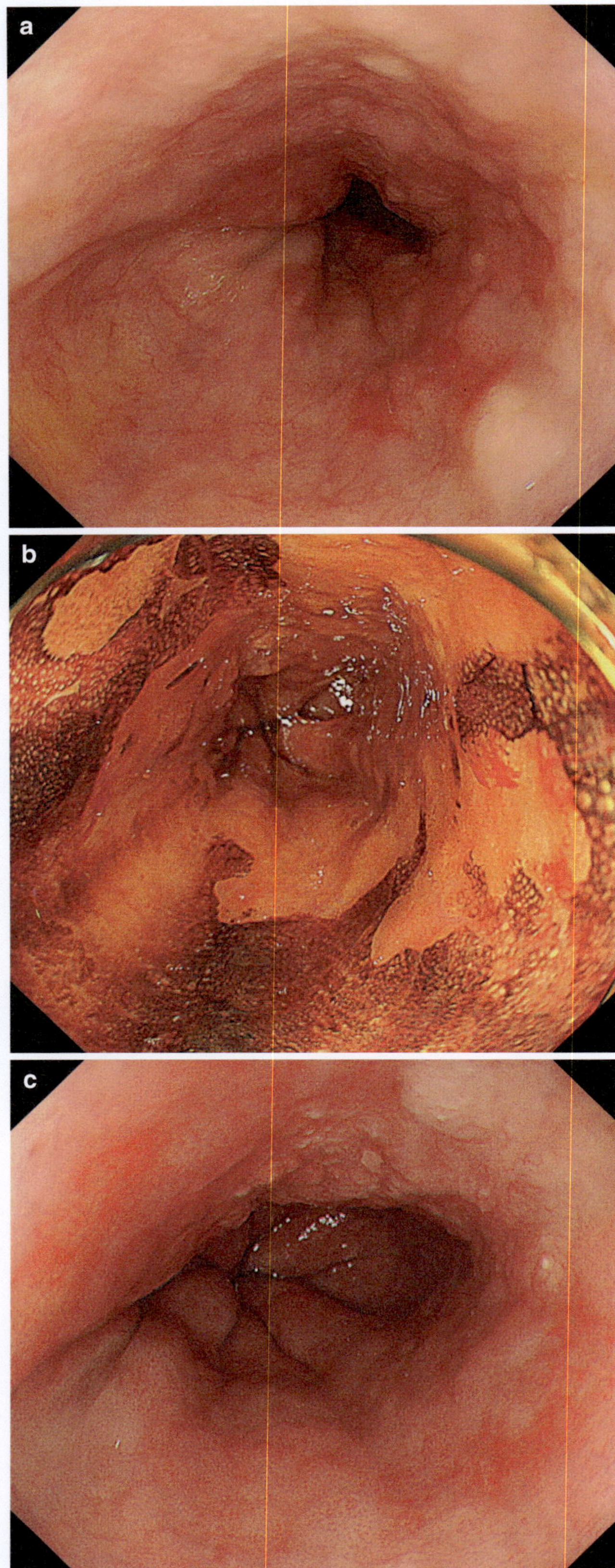

Fig. 15.1 Large superficially spreading esophageal carcinoma, (**a**–**f**) white light endoscopic images

Let's Insert Further and Observe (Fig. 15.1d)

- With further insertion of the scope, the anterior wall was noted with a slightly elevated area compared with its surrounding mucosa.

Let's Observe Closely (Fig. 15.1e)

- On closer observation, a relatively clear flat elevated area of approximately 10 mm was noted with little surface unevenness.

Let's Get Even Closer and Observe (Fig. 15.1f)

- Approaching very closely to the elevated portion, dot-like Type B1 blood vessels were observed even with white light imaging, as well as mild tenseness of the elevation.

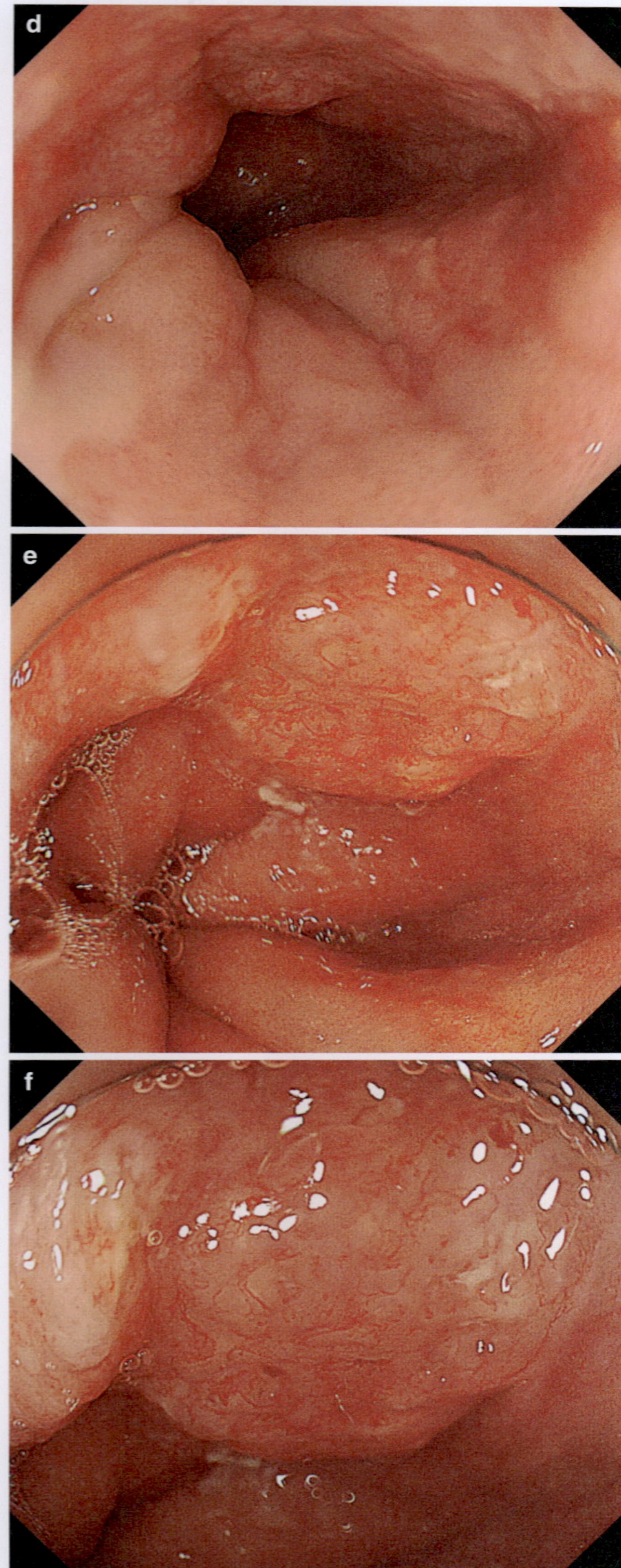

Fig. 15.1 (continued)

Let's Observe the Whole Lesion with NBI, Gradually Increasing Magnification

- With low-magnification NBI observation of the whole lesion, the reddish unevenness was noted to be with Type B1 blood vessels (Fig. 15.2a).
- But with low-magnification NBI of the elevated part, traversing blood vessels of a different type from the surrounding Type B1 blood vessels were noted (Fig. 15.2b).
- On full-magnification NBI of the elevated part, non-loop-forming Type B2 blood vessels were noted in the elevated part with elongated Type B2 blood vessels in the periphery (Fig. 15.2c).

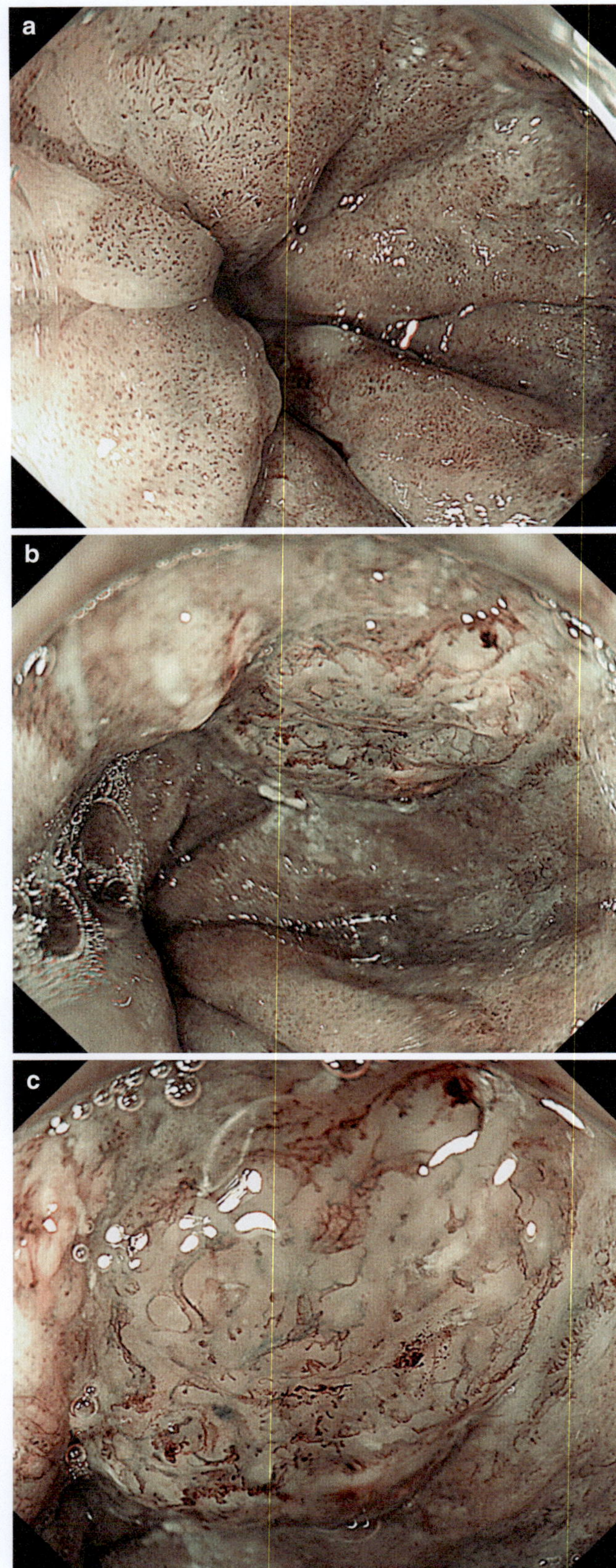

Fig. 15.2 (**a–f**) NBI magnified endoscopic images of the lesion

- On full-magnification NBI of the oral and the anal sides of the elevated lesion, the blood vessels were mainly Type B2 with Type B1 blood vessels mixed in part. There were also areas with very sparse blood vessels (Fig. 15.2d,e).
- Based on observations with white light imaging and NBI, the elevated part can be diagnosed as having the deepest depth of invasion (Fig. 15.2d,e).
- Invasion depth of T1a-MM~T1b-SM1 can be diagnosed based on Type B2 blood vessels, but based on white light imaging showing relatively smooth, flat surface with some hardness and relatively large size of the area of 10 mm diameter, T1b-SM2 may be possible (Fig. 15.2d,e).

Let's Place Two-Point Markings on Both Sides of the Area of Interest (Fig. 15.2f)

- For superficially spreading lesions which will be hard to compare before and after resection like this case, two-point markings interposing the raised area of interest like A and B are useful.

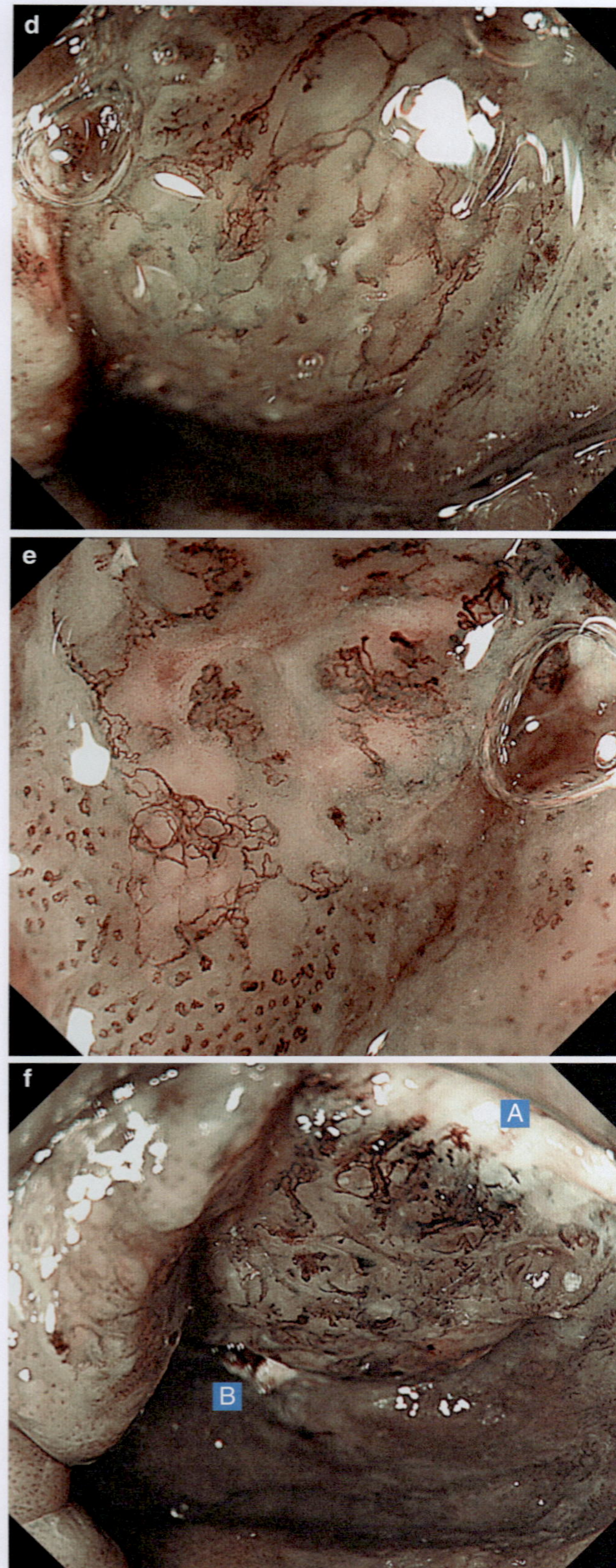

Fig. 15.2 (continued)

15.2 From ESD to Final Diagnosis

Let's Compare the Resected Specimen with Histopathology (Fig. 15.3)

- Two-point markings can be recognized in this iodine dye-stained resected specimen (Fig. 15.3a). The slicing line can be placed near the markings so that the markings can be recognized on the histopathological microslide (Fig. 15.3b).
- The sixth section showed both markings A and B, with raised area in between. Most of the raised area showed well- to moderately differentiated squamous cell carcinoma with invasion depth of T1a-MM contacting the muscularis mucosa. The area marked by the red square showed cancer with invasion depth of T1b-SM2, measuring invasion depth of 1050 μm into the submucosa.

Prognoses Post-ESD of Superficially Spreading Esophageal Cancers

- According to the paper [1], treatment outcomes of superficially spreading esophageal cancers are about the same as superficial esophageal carcinomas. On the other hand, it was also noted that 40% of the cases were found to have invasion depth greater than T1a-MM, requiring careful preoperative evaluation of invasion depth diagnoses. Therefore, prognoses post-ESD are influenced more by invasion depth with more dose correlation with lymphatic metastases than tumor diameters. It is therefore important to improve the accuracy of preoperative invasion depth diagnosis for superficially spreading esophageal carcinomas.

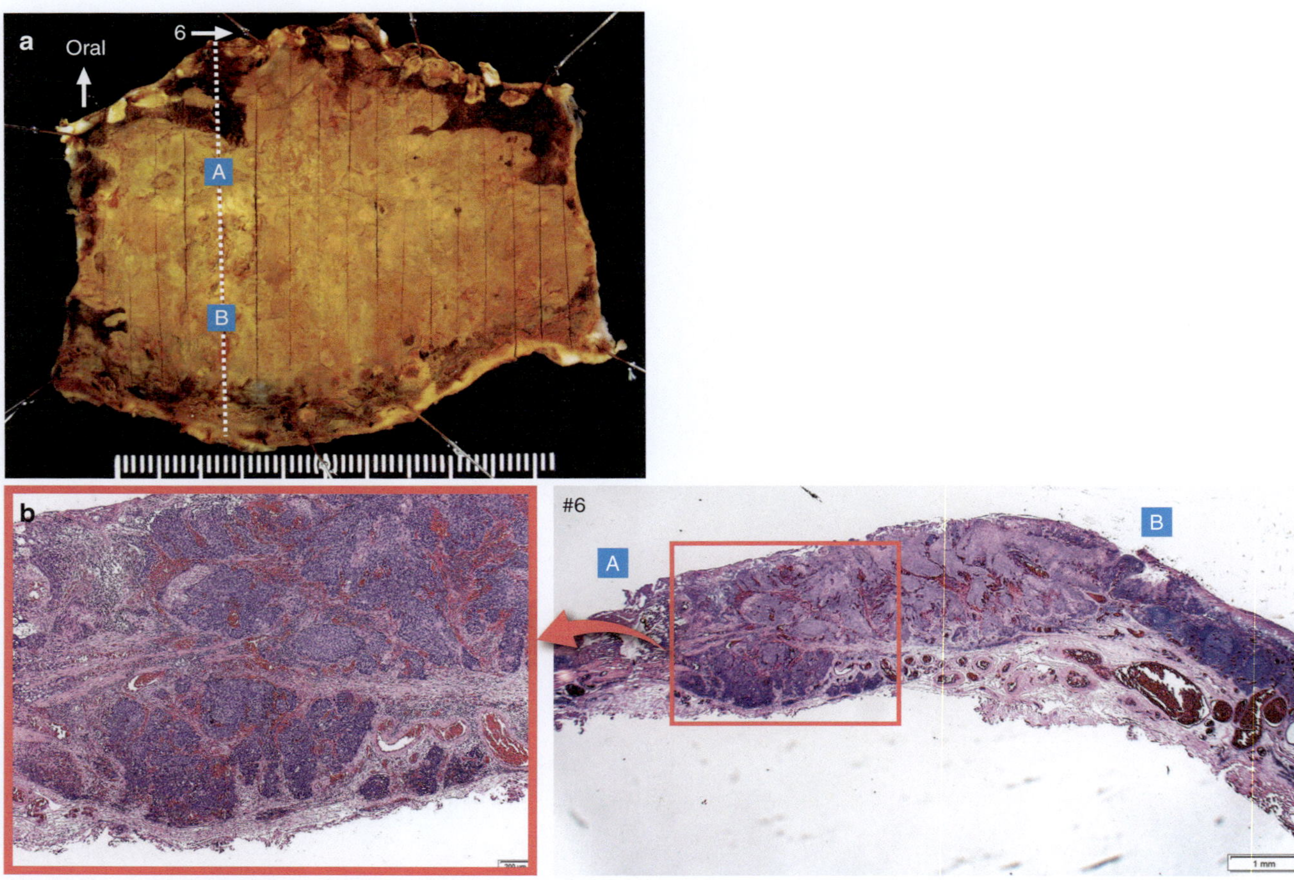

Fig. 15.3 Comparison of the resected specimen with the histopathological image

Conclusive Diagnosis

Esophageal squamous cell carcinoma, 0-IIc + "0-IIa", T1b-SM2 (1050 μm), ly(−), v(−), HM0, VM0, 60 × 45 mm, pCurA, Lt, Ae.

Summary

Invasion depth diagnostic strategy for superficially spreading carcinoma involves first to observe the entire lesion with white light imaging adjusting air volume to confirm degrees of elevations or depressions, firmness, and tenseness. Next, the entire lesion is to be observed by low-magnification NBI and then the area of vascular irregularities with full-magnification NBI. If this area matches with the area of firmness and tenseness, invasion depths diagnosis is made based on combined findings. However, if the findings don't correspond with each other as in a case of a superficially covering T1a-EP~LPM cancer over a deeper lesion, other modalities such as EUS should be used to confirm the diagnosis.

Reference

1. Oyama T, et al. Outcomes of ESD for superficial spreading esophageal cancers, multiple facilities collaborative study. Stomach Intestine. 2014;49:1182–9.

Part III

Practices

Question 1: What Is the Invasion Depth?

16

Kotaro Shibagaki

K. Shibagaki (✉)
Department of Endoscopic Diagnosis and Therapeutics, Shimane University School of Medicine Hospital, Matsue, Shimane, Japan
e-mail: shibagaki@zb.wakwak.com

T. Oyama (ed.), *Endoscopic Diagnosis of Esophageal Carcinoma for ESD*, https://doi.org/10.1007/978-981-32-9030-3_16

Which Is the Correct Invasion Depth? (Fig. 16.1)

1. T1a-EP~LPM
2. T1a-MM~T1b-SM1
3. T1b-SM2

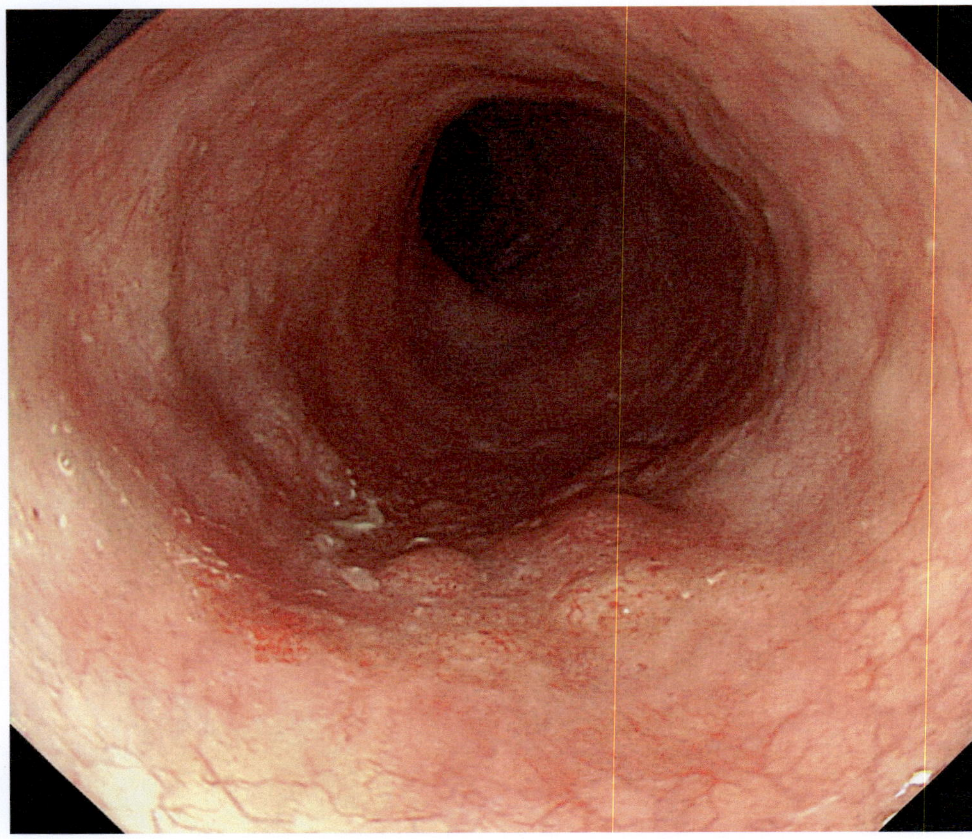

Fig. 16.1 Which is the correct invasion depth?

16.1 Let's Look at These Six Images and Think (Fig. 16.2)

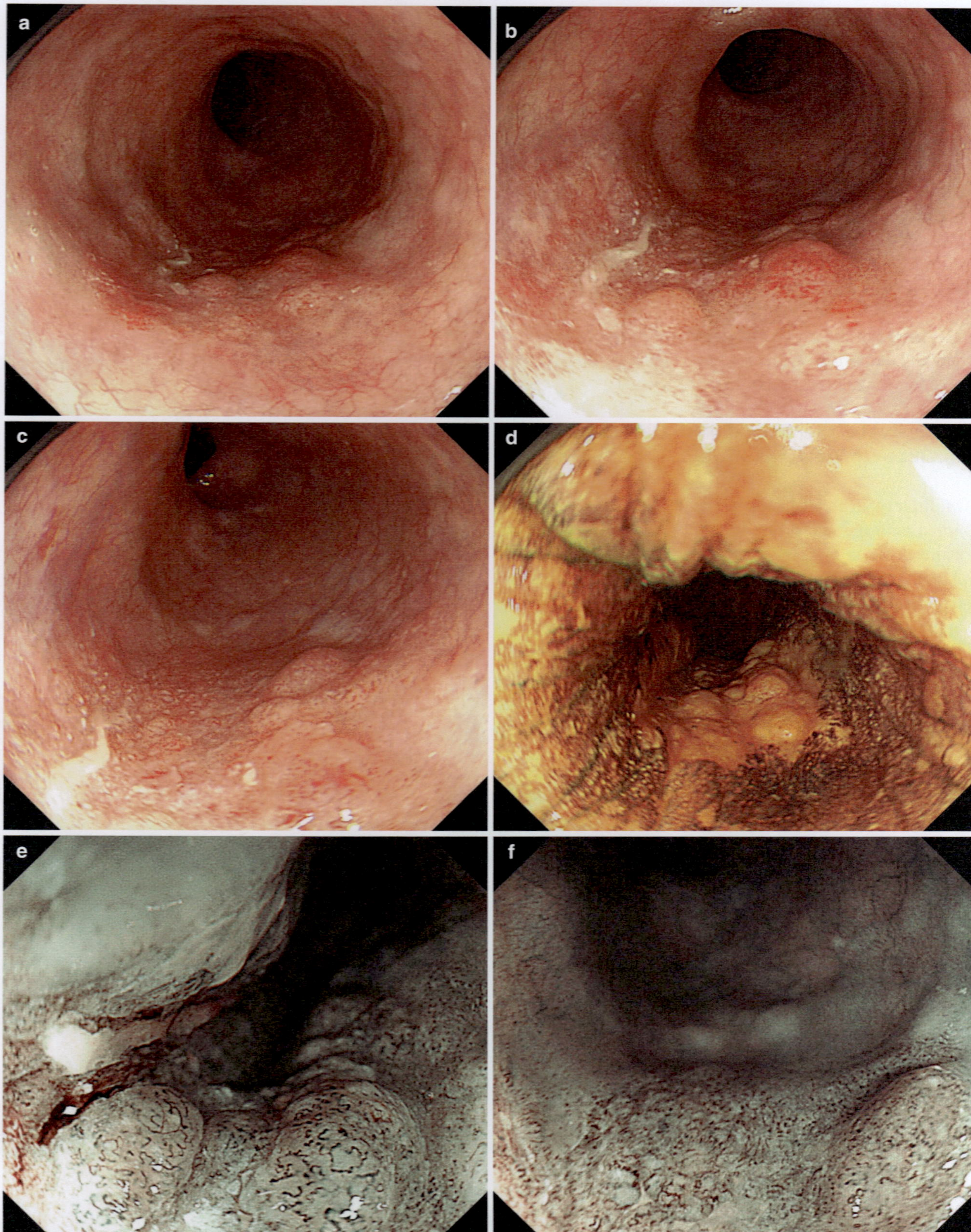

Fig. 16.2 Explanations start from the next page

16.2 Let's Observe the Following Six Images Carefully

Let's Note the Morphology (Fig.16.3a)

- A depressed lesion with partly whitish and partly reddish areas was noted in the upper thoracic esophagus.
- The surface is rough, and the oral margin was clearly demarcated and irregular, as shown by white arrows, and can be diagnosed as cancer.
- With air inflation, there were multiple small elevations within the depressed area, suggestive of submucosal invasions.

What Should Be Done Next (Fig.16.3a)

- The nature of the raised and depressed parts of the lesion should be observed with close-up view, adjusting air volume to evaluate for morphological changes.

Let's Evaluate the Raised and Depressed Parts with Close-Up View (Fig. 16.3b)

- Multiple pale reddish raised areas of varied sizes were noted with the tallest and largest one marked by yellow arrows.
- Although noted with white exudates on the left side of the depressed area, the nature of the depressed surface appeared to be about the same.
- Based on the above observation, the area of the marked raised part was thought to have the deepest invasion.

Let's Confirm Morphological Changes of the Lesion with Air Volume Adjustments (Fig. 16.3c)

- With mild deflation of air, the depressed area including the part with white exudates was noted with vertical creases traversing within, suggesting unlikeliness of submucosal fibrosis, supportive of an intramucosal lesion.
- The central raised part of the lesion did not have a vertical crease traversing through, suggesting a possibility of submucosal invasion.

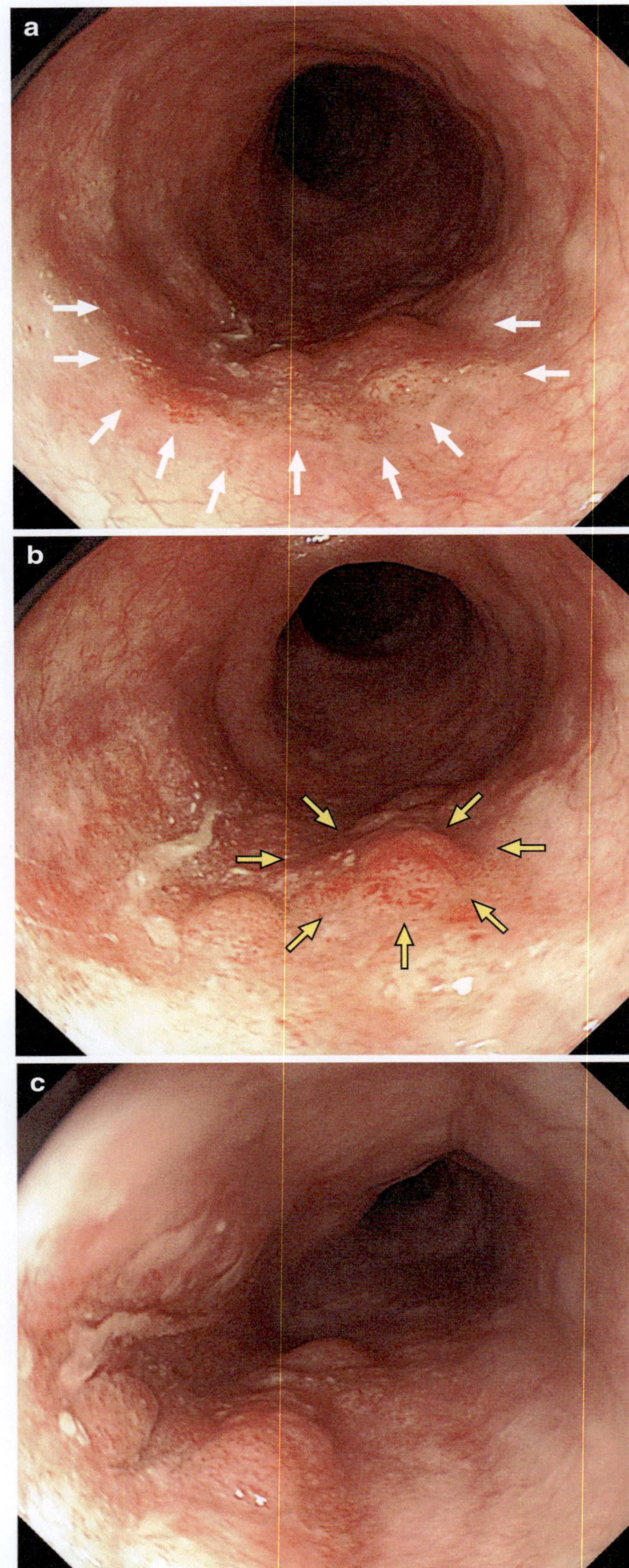

Fig. 16.3 Same images as Fig. 16.2

Let's Note Firmness of Various Parts by Observing Peristalsis After Iodine Dye Staining (Fig. 16.3d)

- After iodine dye staining, esophageal wall peristalsis becomes stimulated, making vertical creases and "tatami-mat folds" easier to be seen.
- With air deflation, four vertical creases were noted to form within the lesion (dotted lines 1–4). The area containing the largest nodular part was noted to have a wider space between the creases (between lines 3 and 4).
- A possibility of a nodular part preventing mucosal crease formation and a possibility of submucosal invasion and fibrosis formation were considered.
- Based on the above observations, it was considered that submucosal invasion at the largest raised area cannot be denied.

Let's Observe the Nodular Parts with Magnifying NBI (Fig. 16.3e)

- Within the largest nodule and the adjacent nodule on the left, non-loop-forming dilated blood vessels were found consistent with Type B2 blood vessels.
- Although submucosal invasion could not be denied at the largest nodule by white light imaging, invasion depth diagnosis of T1a-MM~T1b-SM1 was made by magnifying NBI.

Let's Observe the Anal Side of the Lesion with Magnifying NBI (Fig. 16.3f)

- The raised part on the right wall side showed dot-like blood vessels and small loop-forming dilated irregular blood vessels.
- The depressed area on the left wall side showed loop-forming dilated irregular blood vessels around multiple small AVAs.
- Based on above findings, the anal side of the lesion including a raised part was diagnosed as T1a-EP~LPM.

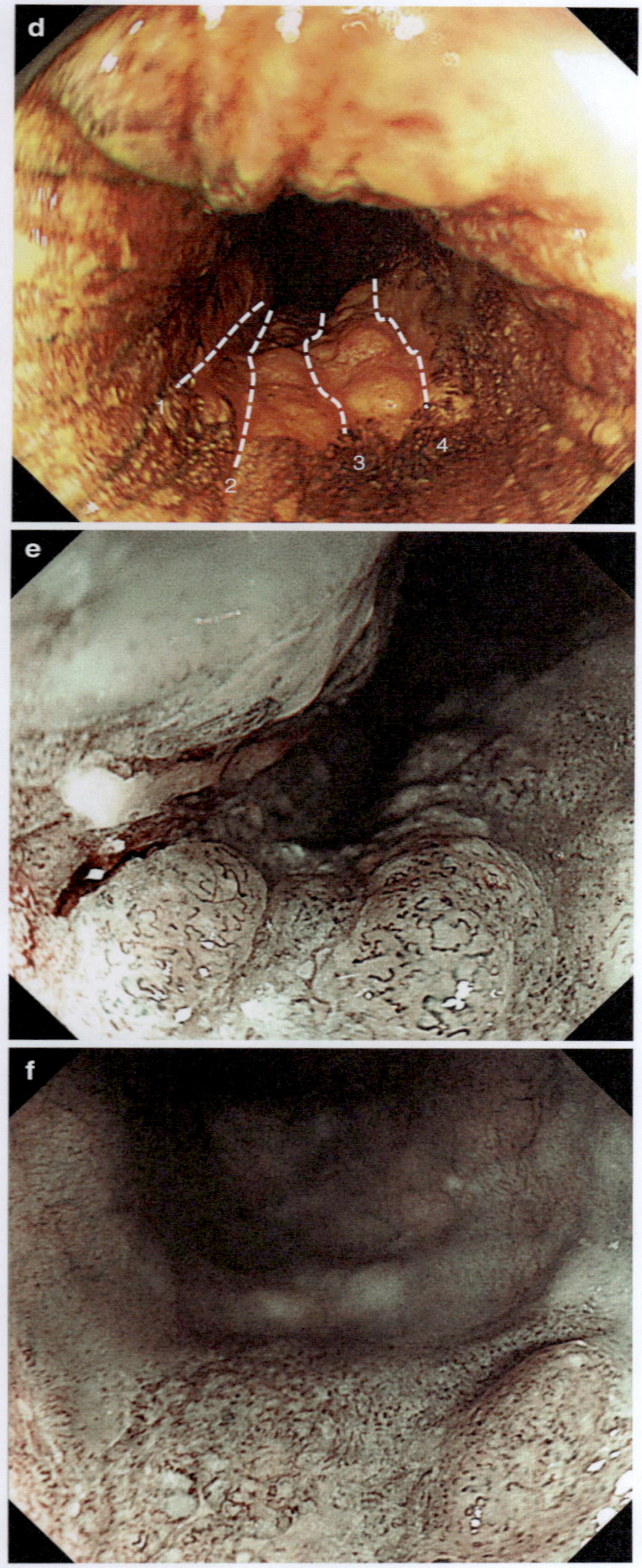

Fig. 16.3 (continued)

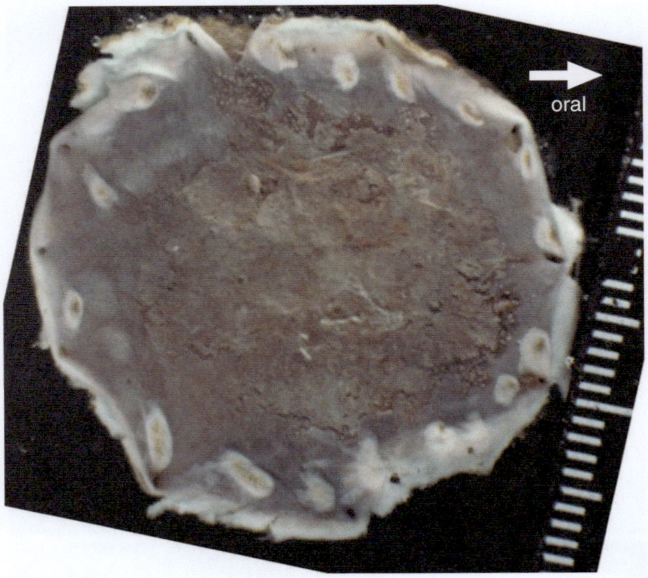

Fig. 16.4 The specimen after fixation with formalin

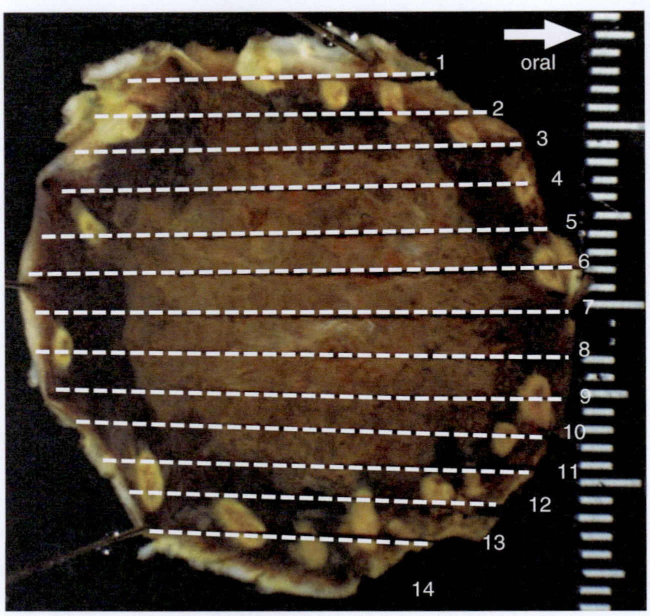

Fig. 16.5 The resected specimen after iodine staining

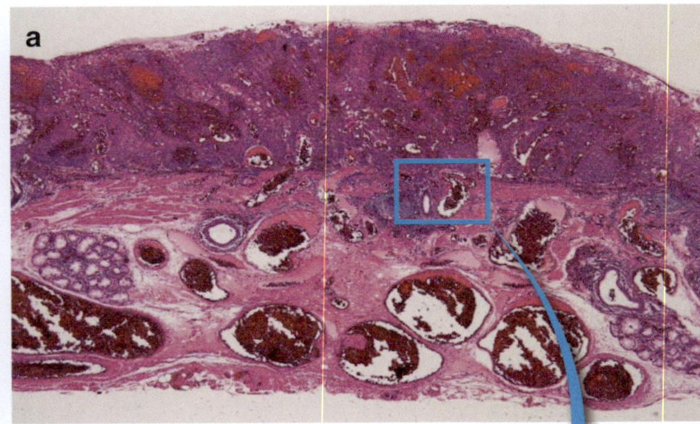

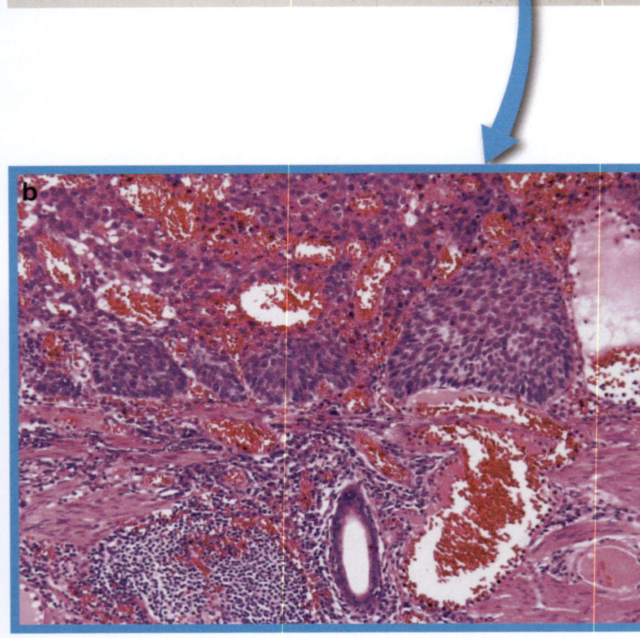

Fig.16.6 (**a**) H&E staining of the most raised part included in the fifth section was viewed under low magnification (×40). (**b**) The area marked by a blue square in the previous image was magnified (×200)

16.3 Let's Compare the Resected Specimen with the Endoscopic Images Towards the Final Diagnosis

Let's Observe the Formalin-Fixed Specimen (Fig. 16.4)

- The lesion had irregularly shaped border, clearly demarcated by color tone and surface structure.
- There are multiple nodular elevations of various sizes within the depressed lesion.

Let's Observe the Iodine Dye-Stained Specimen (Fig. 16.5)

- The lesion was clearly recognized as an irregularly shaped unstained area.
- The markings became clear, allowing easy comparison with endoscopic imaging.

Let's Look at the Histopathological Image (Sect. 5, ×40) (Fig. 16.6a)

- H&E staining of the most raised part included in the fifth section was viewed under low magnification (×40).
- The mucosal layer has thickness due to cancer, but the height of the nodular parts observed with endoscopy was not recognized within the mucosa.
- There were multiple dilated venules observed in the submucosal layer, likely responsible as one of the reasons for the height of the nodular parts.

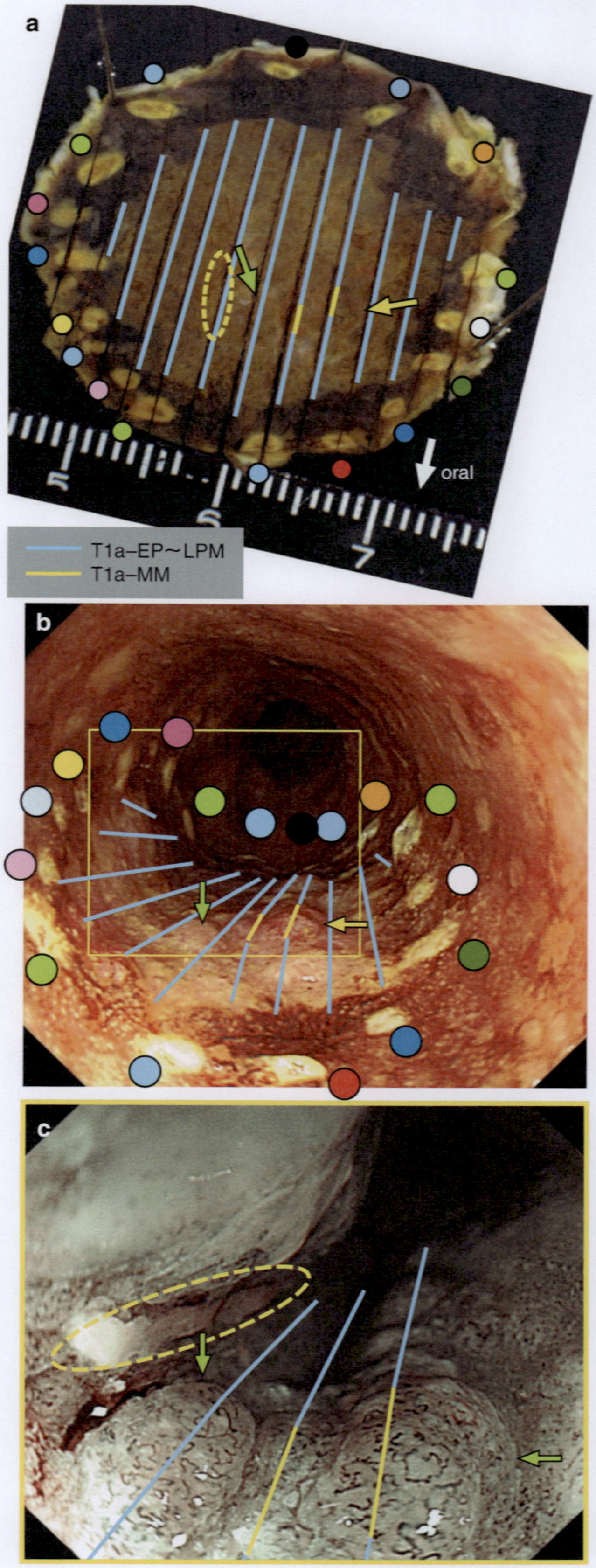

Fig.16.7 (**a, b**) The mapping on the post-slicing iodine dye-stained resected specimen. (**c**) Comparison of the iodine dye staining and magnifying NBI images

Let's Look at the Histopathological Image (Sect. 5, ×200) (Fig. 16.6b)

- The area marked by a blue square in the previous image was magnified (×200).
- The deepest part of the tumor was in contact with the muscularis mucosa, confirming the invasion depth diagnosis of T1a-MM.
- Glandular structures noted beneath the muscularis mucosa are ducts of esophageal gland proper.

Let's Compare with Endoscopic Images and Produce Mappings

- The mapping created on the post-slicing iodine dye-stained resected specimen (Fig. 16.7a) was transposed on the iodine dye-stained endoscopic view shown below in the left image (Fig. 16.7b).
- Comparison of the iodine dye staining and magnifying NBI images showed that invasion depth was deepest at the largest nodular part with invasion depth of T1a-MM (Fig. 16.7c).

Conclusive Diagnosis

Esophageal squamous cell carcinoma, 0-IIc+IIa, T1a-MM, INFα, ly(-), v(-), HM0, VM0, pR0, 26 × 21 mm, Ut, Post.

Summary

Invasion depth diagnosis of esophageal carcinoma must be carefully made by comprehensively evaluating the lesion for its thickness with air inflation, for its firmness with deflation, and for its microvessel pattern typing by magnifying NBI. In this case presentation, the largest nodular part was determined to be the deepest invasion part, but differentiating between T1a-MM~T1b-SM1 and T1b-SM2 was difficult with white light imaging alone, and the correct diagnosis was made after magnifying NBI showing microvessel typing consistent with T1a-MM~T1b-SM1.

16.4 Answer

The correct invasion depth is (2) T1a-MM~T1b-SM1.

17 Question 2: What Is the Invasion Depth?

Tokuma Tanuma

T. Tanuma (✉)
Center for Digestive Diseases, Teine Keijinkai Hospital,
Sapporo, Hokkaido, Japan
e-mail: tokuma@dk9.so-net.ne.jp

T. Oyama (ed.), *Endoscopic Diagnosis of Esophageal Carcinoma for ESD*, https://doi.org/10.1007/978-981-32-9030-3_17

Which Is the Correct Invasion Depth? (Fig. 17.1)

1. T1a-EP~LPM
2. T1a-MM~T1b-SM1
3. T1b-SM2

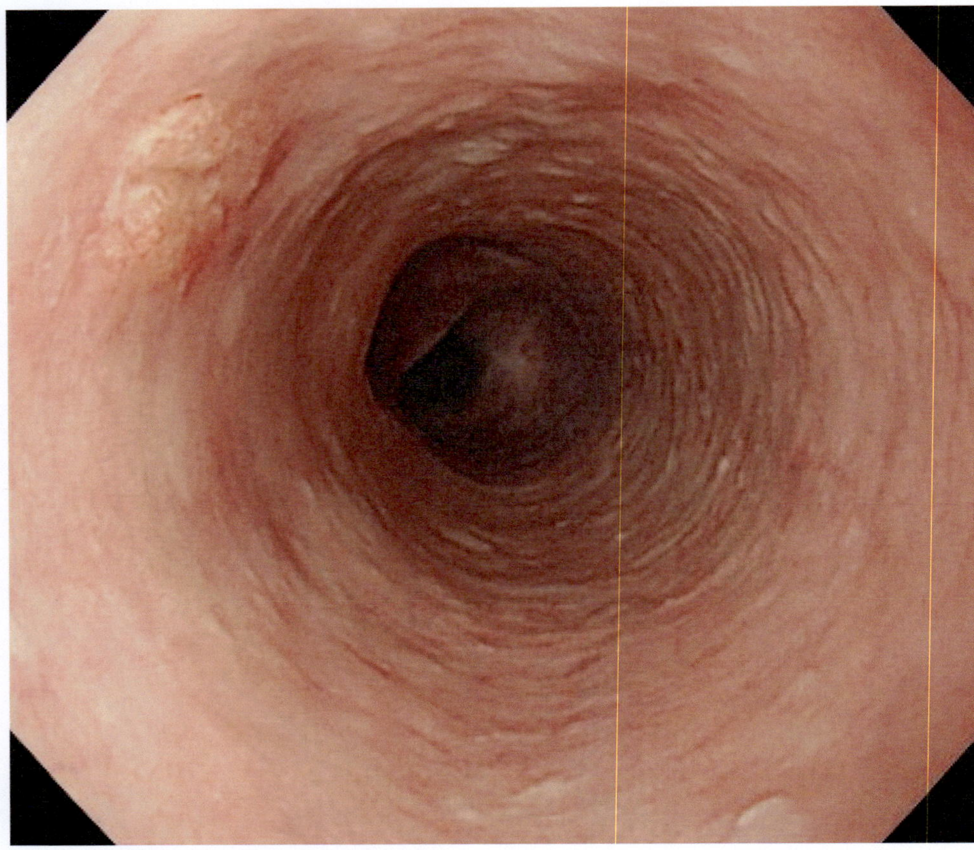

Fig. 17.1 Which is the correct invasion depth?

17.1 Let's Look at These Six Images and Think (Fig. 17.2)

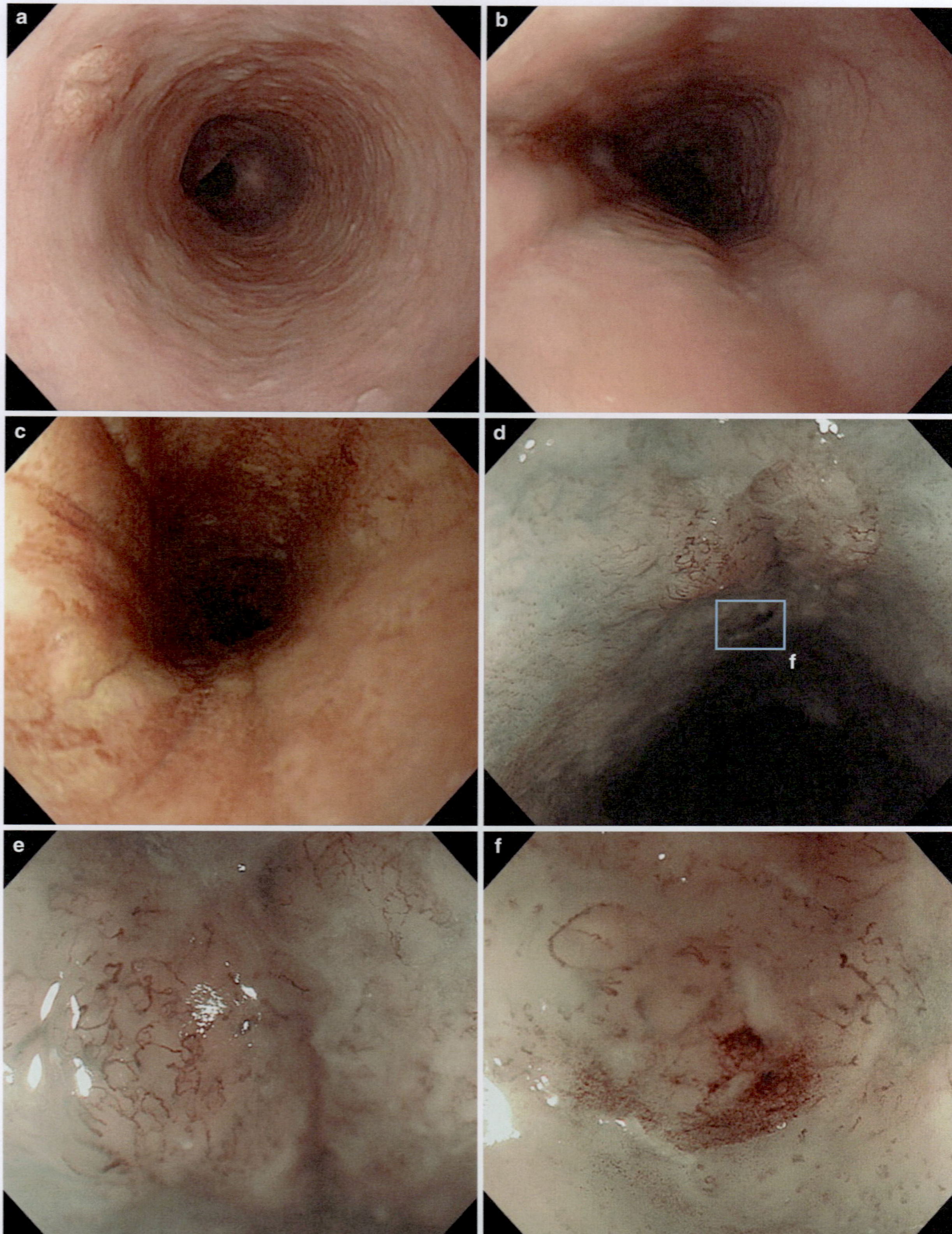

Fig. 17.2 Explanations start from the next page

17.2 Let's Observe the Following Six Images Carefully

Let's Inflate with Air to Extend the Wall (Fig. 17.3a)

- Extensibility of the wall can be evaluated by air inflation by extending the esophageal wall.
- No obvious deformities were noted with this lesion, suggesting the lesion to be T1a-EP~LPM.
- But it should be carefully noted that the lesion seems to have thickness for its size.

Let's Note the Lesion to Change Its Form by Air Deflation (Fig. 17.3b)

- The lesion can be observed to evaluate if its form changes with air deflation.
- The lesions changes its form very easily by air deflation, and its invasion depth was estimated as T1a-EP~LPM.

Let's Observe the Wall with Iodine Dye Staining (Fig. 17.3c)

- The esophageal mucosal folds become easier to be observed with iodine dye staining, and submucosal invasion will be suspected if a disruption of the longitudinal folds is noted.
- The longitudinal folds are traversing the lesion, and invasion depth of T1a-EP~LPM was suspected.

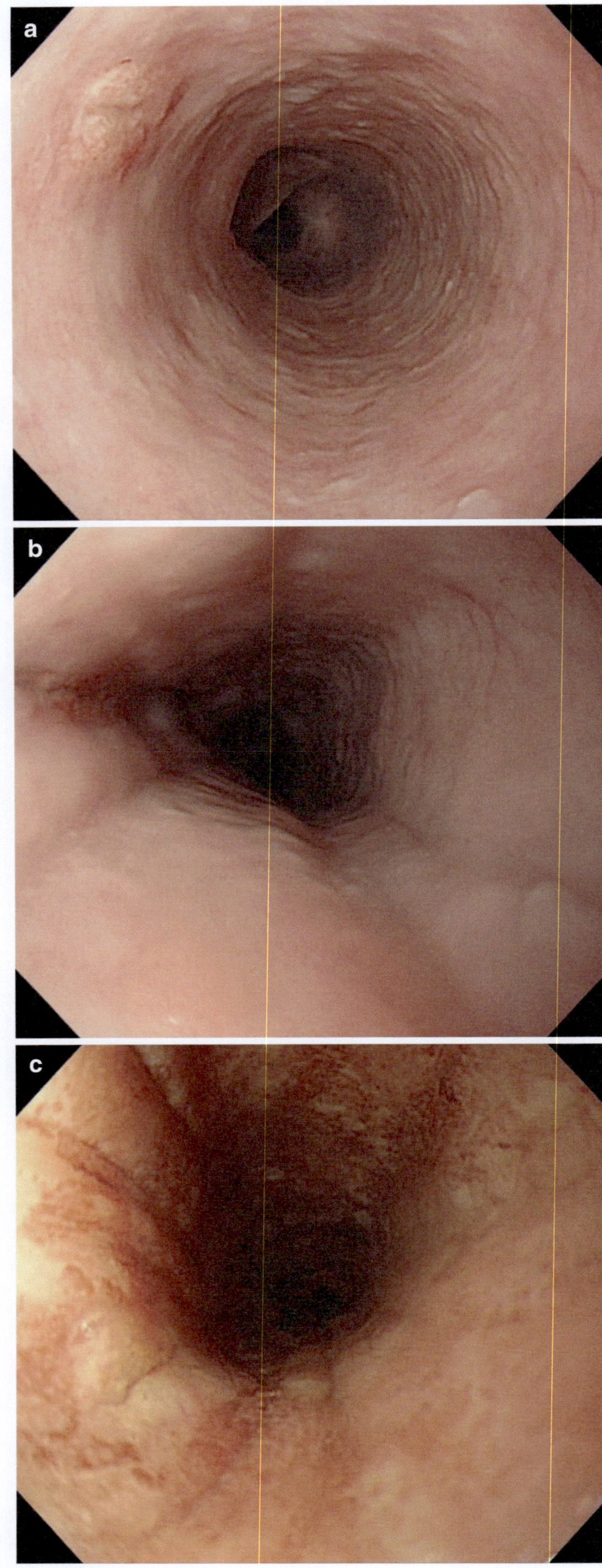

Fig. 17.3 Same images as Fig. 17.2

Let's Switch to NBI (Fig. 17.3d)

- By switching to NBI, the lesion can be identified as a brownish area.
- There are no prominently dilated blood vessels (Type B3) as noticeable by low-magnification NBI.
- A longitudinal fold is marked by a white dotted line to be used as a reference, and a circumferentially traversing fold was marked by a red arrow.

Let's Observe with Magnifying NBI (1) (Fig. 17.3e)

- The oral side of the lesion was observed with magnifying NBI.
- Poorly loop-forming abnormal blood vessels were observed (yellow arrows) and diagnosed as Type B2 blood vessels. Invasion depth of T1a-MM~T1b-SM1 was suggested possible. But no obvious avascular areas (AVA) were recognized.

Let's Observe with Magnifying NBI (2) (Fig. 17.3f)

- The anal side of the lesion was observed with magnifying NBI.
- Loop-forming blood vessels were observed (blue arrows) and diagnosed as Type B1 blood vessels. Invasion depth of T1a-MM~T1b-SM1 was noted consistent with the findings.

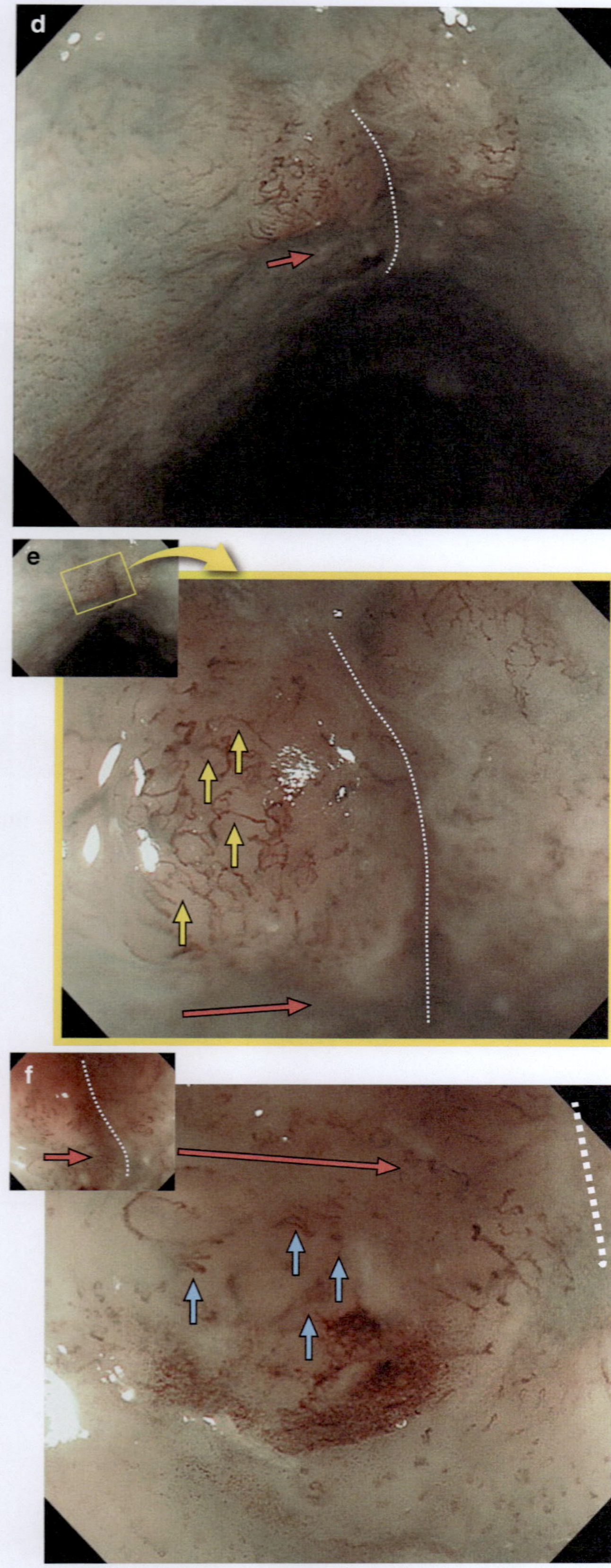

Fig. 17.3 (continued)

17.3 Let's Compare the Resected Specimen with the Endoscopic Images Towards the Final Diagnosis

Magnifying NBI was shown of the area anterior to the dotted white line representing a groove within the lesion (Fig. 17.4a). Histopathological image is shown of the section represented by the yellow line (Fig. 17.4b).

Let's Observe the Histopathological Image (Fig. 17.5)

The oral part of the tumor (Part A) was found to reach the muscularis mucosa by nest forming/pressing fashion, partly invading into the submucosa (50 μm) through a gap between muscularis mucosal plates.

The anal part of the tumor (Part B) remained within the proper mucosal layer (not shown).

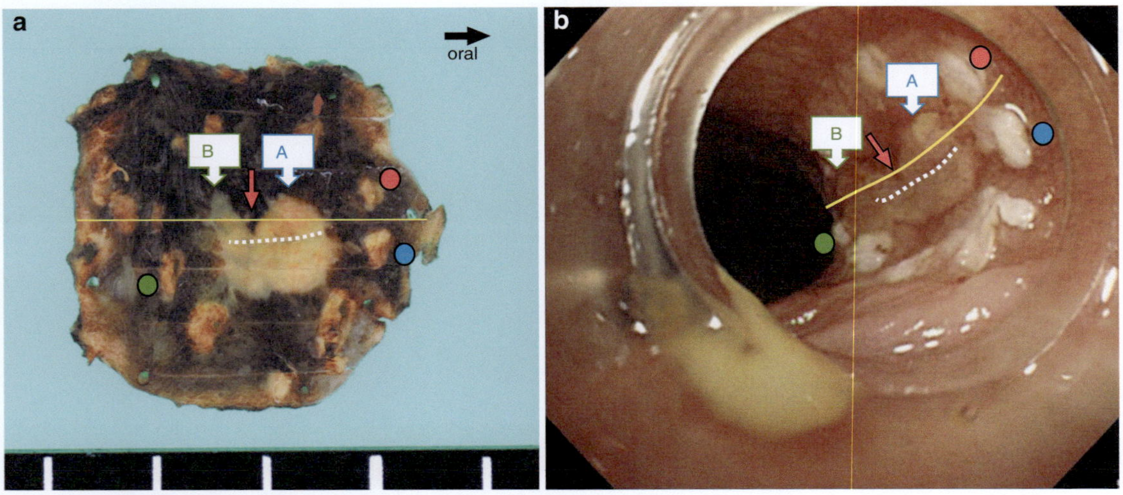

Fig.17.4 (**a**) Image of the sliced iodine dye stained fixed specimen. (**b**) Endoscopic image (180° rotated)

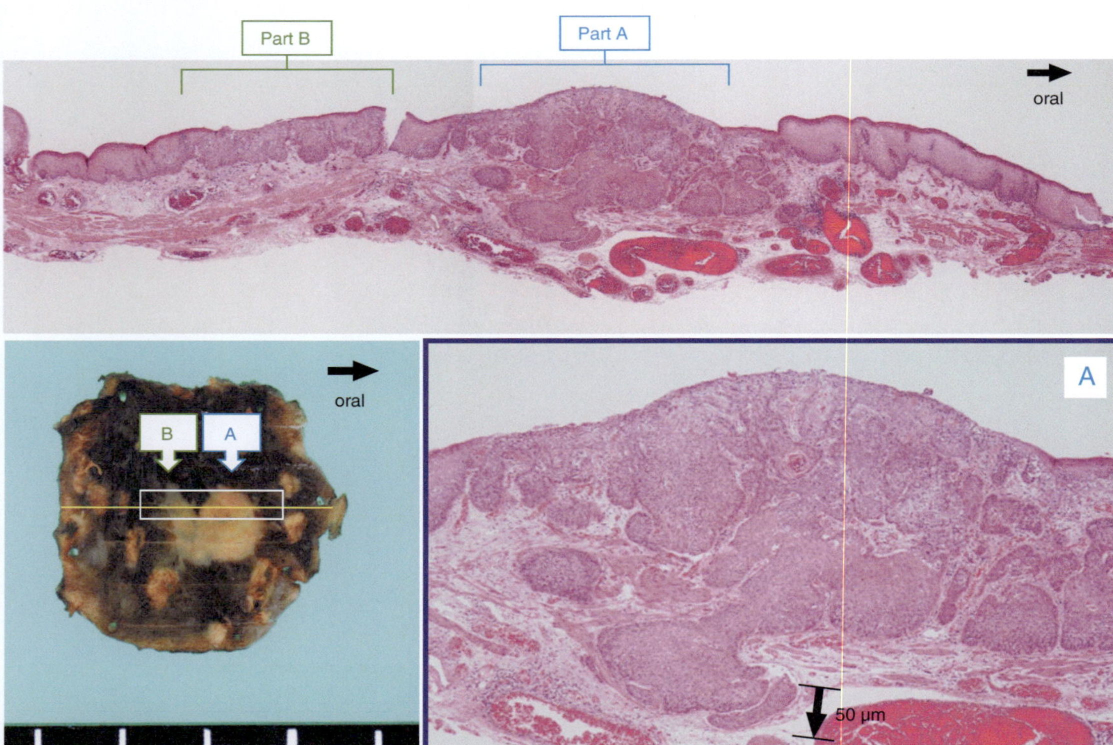

Fig. 17.5 Histopathological image of the resected specimen

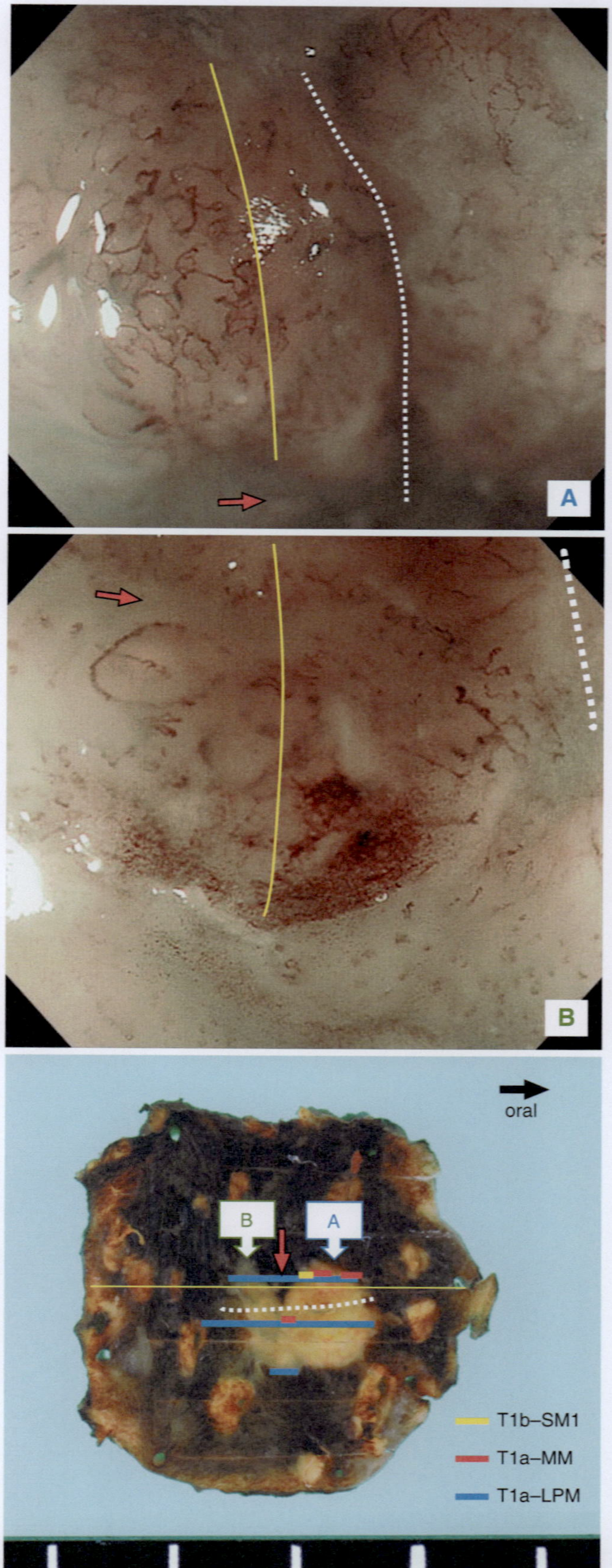

Fig. 17.6 Comparison with the NBI magnified endoscopic images and the resected specimen

Let's Compare with the Endoscopic Images (Fig. 17.6)

From the longitudinal groove and the circumferential groove used as reference points, it was suggested that the yellow line placed would represent the slicing line.

Conclusive Diagnosis
Esophageal squamous cell carcinoma, poorly differentiated, 0-IIa, T1b-SM1(SM:50), INFb, ly(+), (D2-40), v(−), (EvG), HM0, VM0, 7x6mm, pCur C, Ut.

Summary
This lesion was noted to have voluminous appearance for its size by white light imaging, and Type B2 blood vessels were noted in Part A. These findings were clues to invasion depth diagnosis.

17.4 Answer

The invasion depth is (2) T1a-MM~T1b-SM1.

Acknowledgment A special thanks to Dr. Yuko of Omori Department of Pathology at Teine Keijinkai Hospital for helpful discussions and comments on the histopathological findings.

Question 3: What Is the Invasion Depth?

18

Shinichi Furutachi

S. Furutachi (✉)
Department of Gastroenterology, Okayama Medical Center,
National Hospital Organization, Okayama, Japan

T. Oyama (ed.), *Endoscopic Diagnosis of Esophageal Carcinoma for ESD*, https://doi.org/10.1007/978-981-32-9030-3_18

Which Is the Correct Invasion Depth? (Fig. 18.1)

1. T1a-EP~LPM
2. T1a-MM~T1b-SM1
3. T1b-SM2

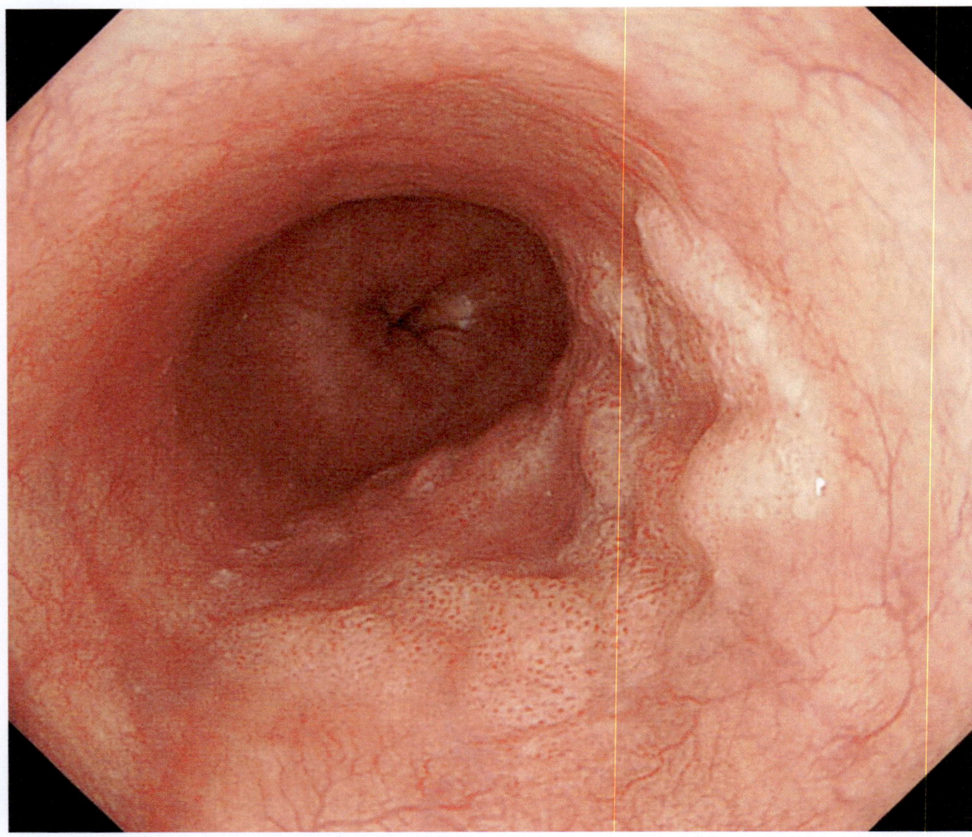

Fig. 18.1 Which is the correct invasion depth?

18.1 Let's Look at These Six Images and Think (Fig. 18.2)

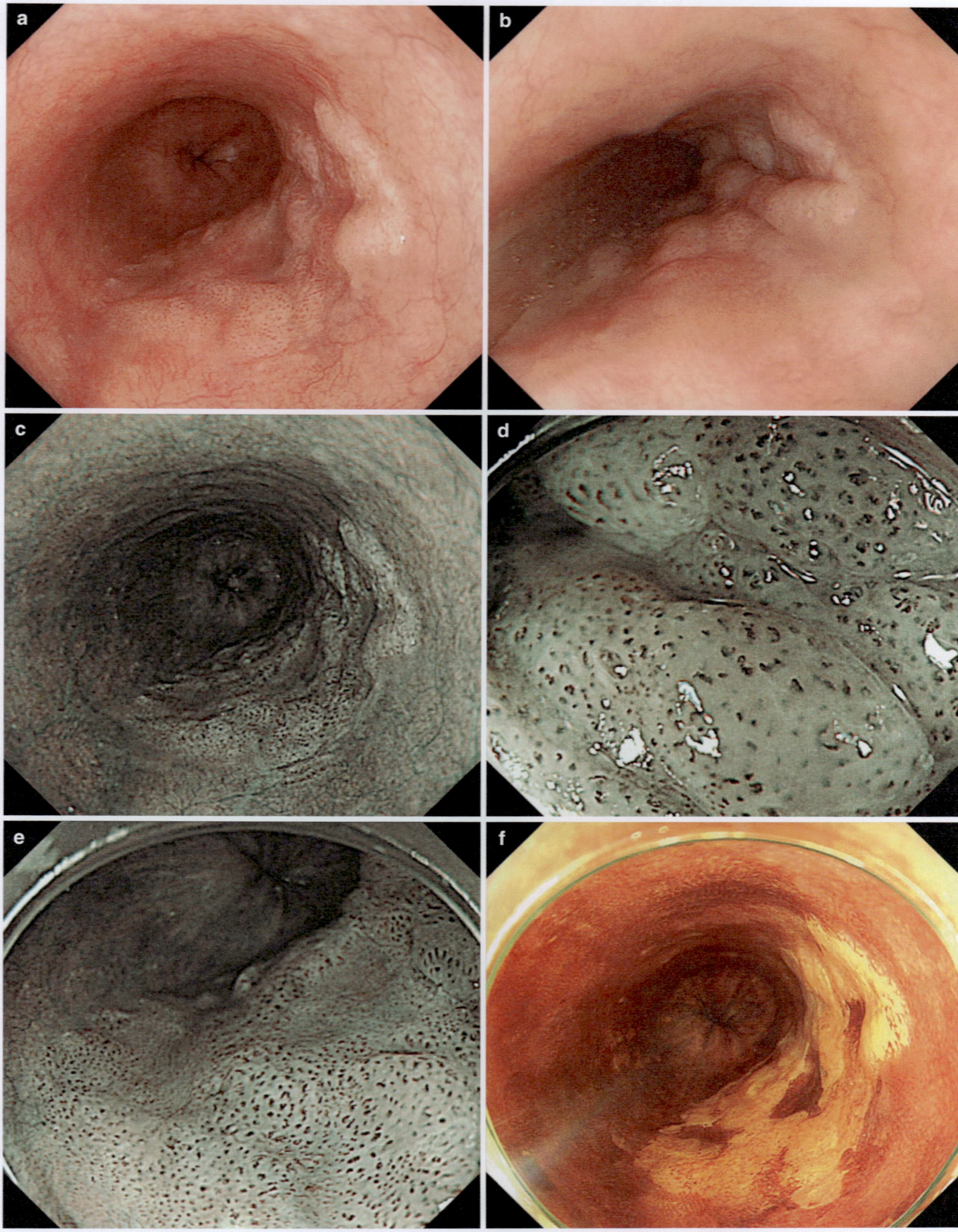

Fig. 18.2 Explanations start from the next page

18.2 Let's Observe the Following Six Images Carefully

Let's Observe with White Light Imaging (Fig. 18.3a)

- There was a slightly reddish raised lesion of the same color tone as the surrounding mucosa, in the lower thoracic esophagus extending from the posterior wall to the right wall. The demarcation of the lesion was clear, and esophageal carcinoma was suspected. Although there were depressed areas within the lesion, the surface appeared to have luster of normal squamous cell epithelium.

Let's Observe with Air Deflation (Fig. 18.3b)

- With air deflation, the raised area became prominent, but a vertical groove was noted to traverse the lesion. (Whether a groove or a fold traverses through the lesion reflects the degree of invasion depth of the lesion.)

Let's Observe with Non-magnifying NBI (Fig. 18.3c)

- Although the background mucosa appeared obscure, dot-like blood vessels were noted in the raised lesion with non-magnifying NBI. When fully insufflated with air, the lesion height became shorter.

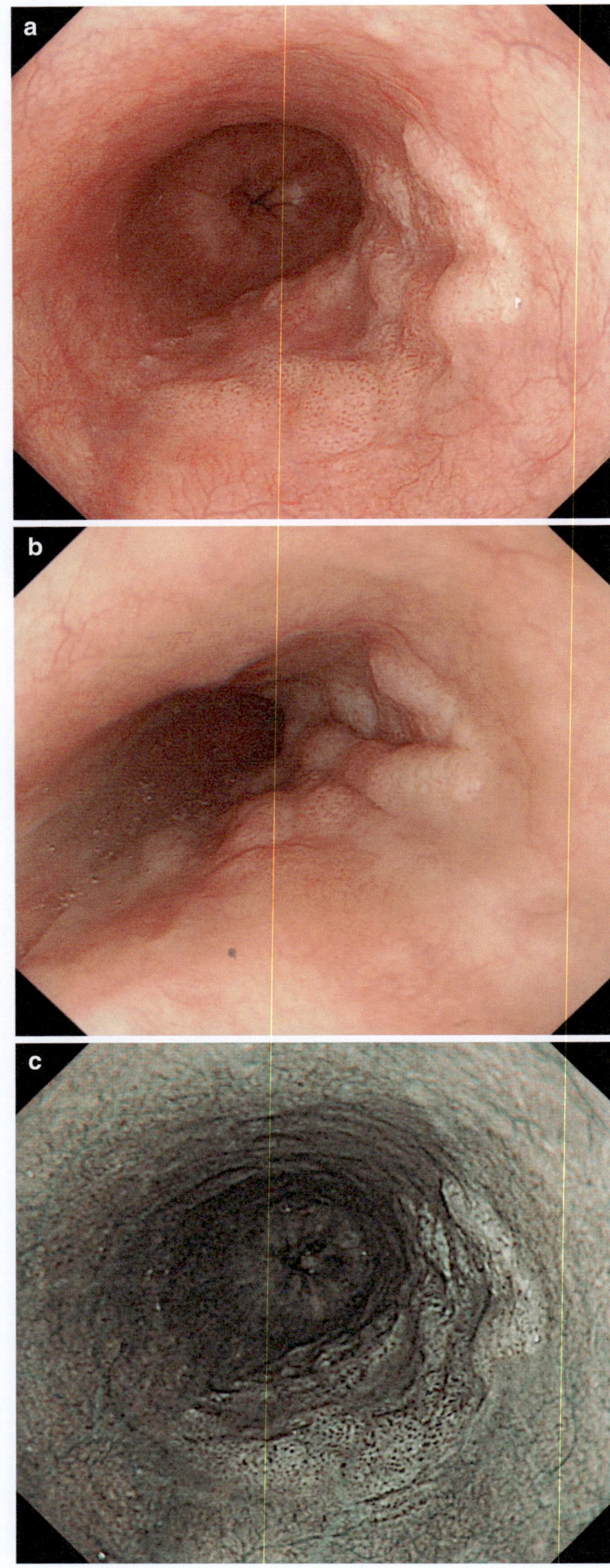

Fig. 18.3 Same images as Fig. 18.2

Let's Observe Within the Lesion with Magnifying NBI (Fig. 18.3d)

- Magnified NBI of the lesion marked by the yellow square was observed. Dilated blood vessels with tortuosity, variable calibers, and shapes were noted confirming diagnosis of squamous cell carcinoma. Loop-forming Type B1 blood vessels were recognized, confirming invasion depth diagnosis of T1a-EP~LPM.

Let's Observe the Posterior Part of the Lesion with Magnifying NBI (Fig. 18.3e)

- The posterior part of the lesion was noted to contain Type B1 blood vessels with low-magnification NBI consistent with invasion depth diagnosis of T1a-EP~LPM.

Let's Perform Iodine Dye Spraying (Fig. 18.3f)

- On iodine dye staining, the raised area became unstained, while normally staining islands of squamous cell epithelium were present, mixed within the lesion.

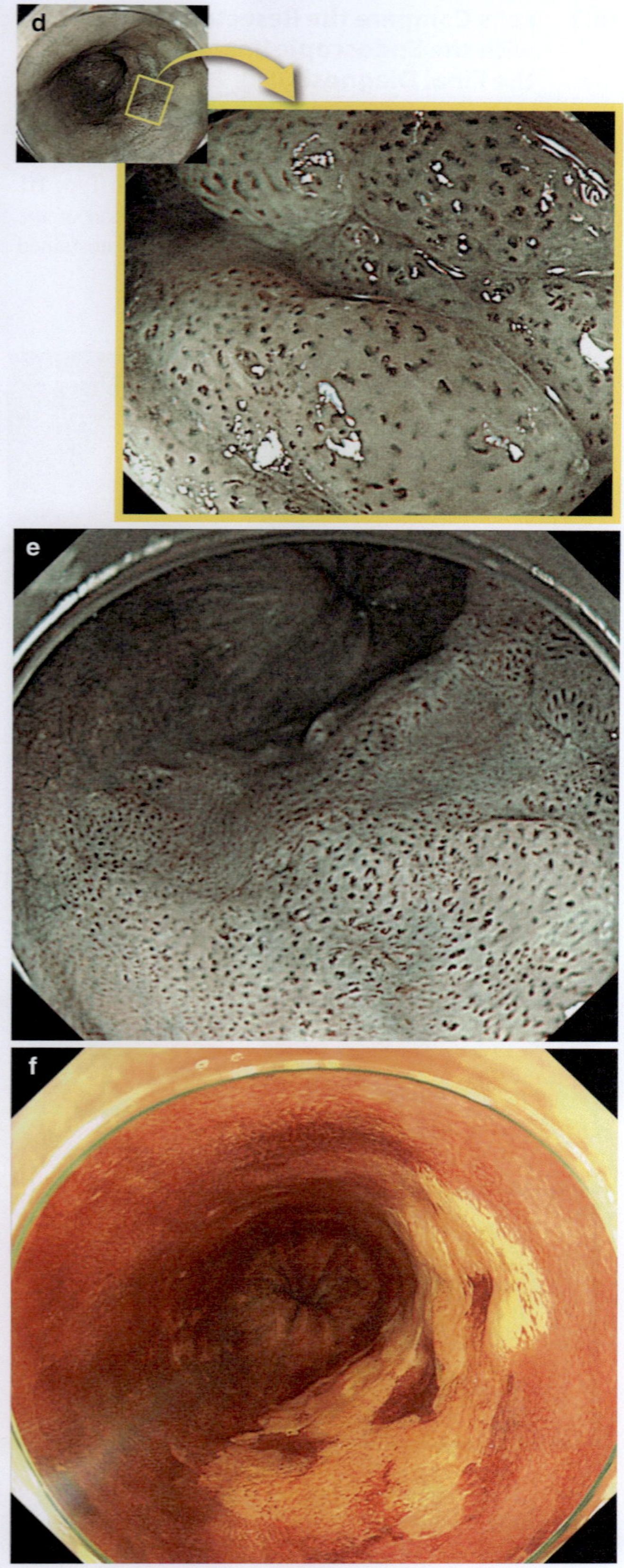

Fig. 18.3 (continued)

18.3 Let's Compare the Resected Specimen with the Endoscopic Images Towards the Final Diagnosis (Fig. 18.4)

The right side is the oral side. A flat raised lesion can be recognized within the freshly resected specimen, with Type B1 blood vessels noted within. Stereoscopic evaluation of the iodine dye stained specimen showed the lesion unstained with stained areas mixed within.

Let's Observe the Histopathological Images (Fig. 18.5)

Histopathological image within the blue square (left image): Enlarged nuclei are filling the full mucosal layer, growing down infiltrating within the mucosal layer, consistent with T1a-LPM. Histopathological image within the red square (right image): This area shows infiltration of the tumor into the submucosa with invasion depth of T1b-SM1 in the area marked by red arrows with the surface covered by an EP cancer.

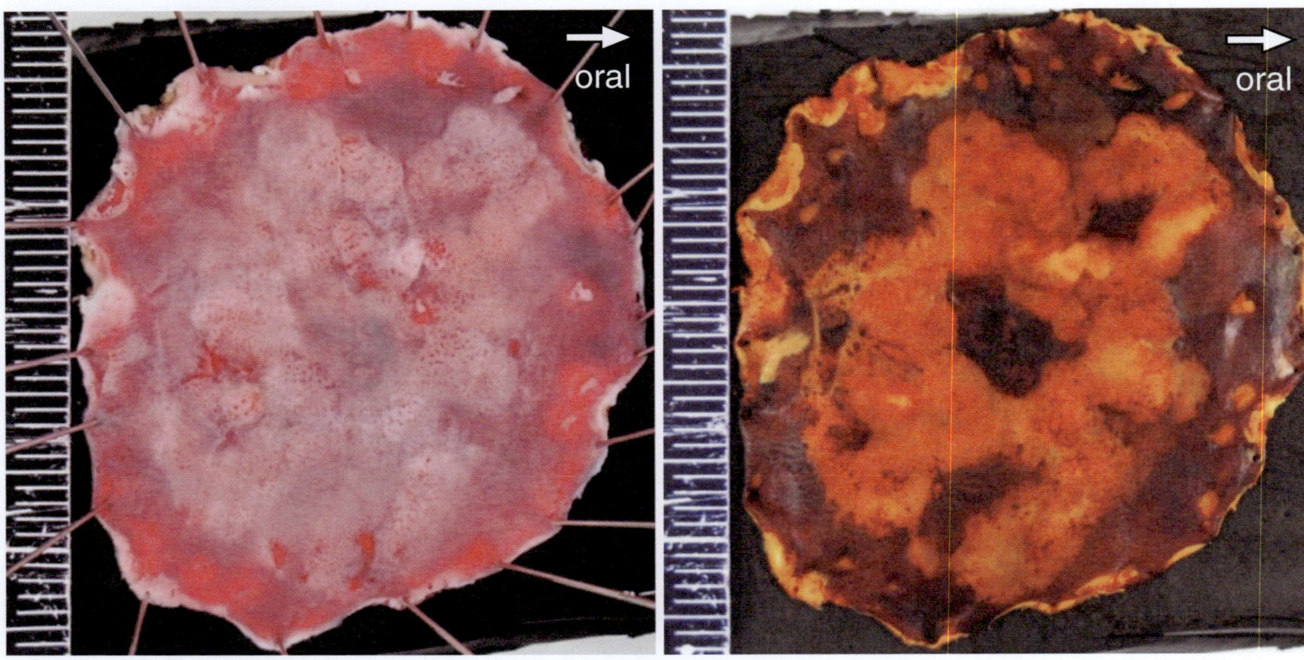

Fig. 18.4 Comparison of fleshly resected specimen and the specimen after staining with iodine

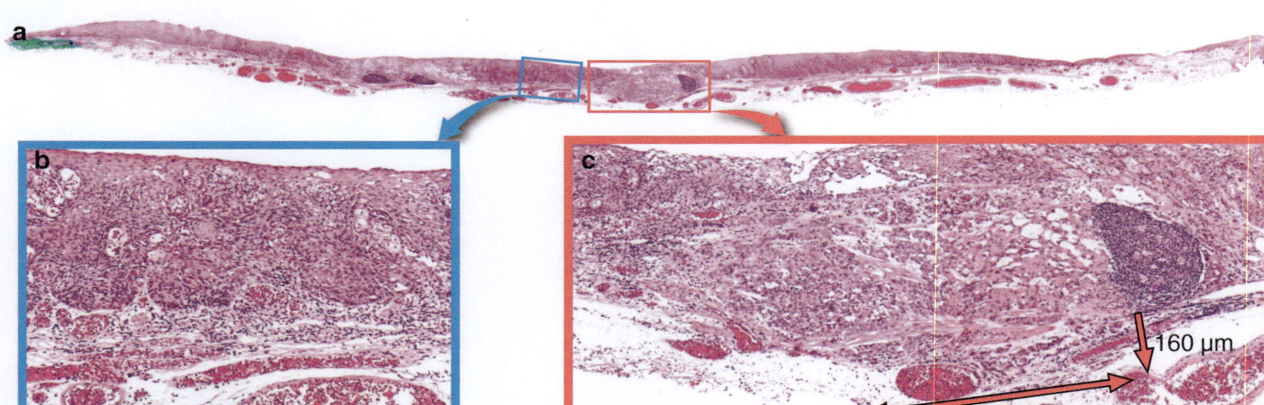

Fig.18.5 (**a**) Histopathological image of the resected specimen. (**b**) Magnified image of the area indicated in blue square. (**c**) Magnified image of the area indicated in red square

Let's Look at the Mapping of the Lesion on the Resected Specimen (Fig. 18.6)

The extent of the tumor matches that of the unstained mucosa, with invasion depth mostly of T1a-EP~LPM, with the exception of one area with T1a-MM~T1b-SM1 measuring 2 mm in width.

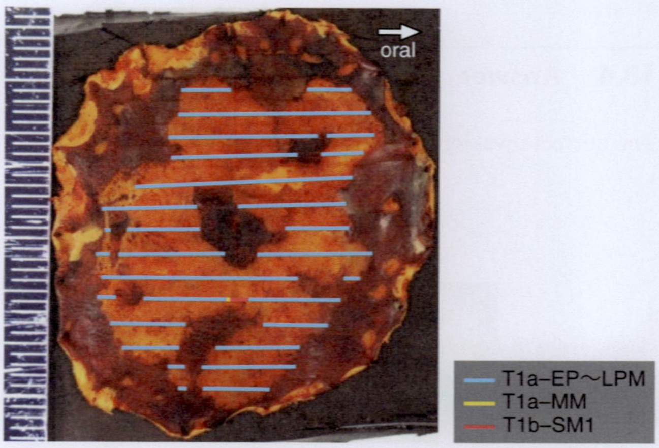

Fig. 18.6 Mapping of the cancer distribution projected on the resected specimen

Conclusive Diagnosis

Esophageal squamous cell carcinoma, 0-IIa, T1b-SM1(160 μm), INFb, ly(−), v(−), HM0, VM0, 31x25mm, pCurA, Lt.

Let's Compare the Mapping with the Endoscopic Images (Fig. 18.7)

In the endoscopic images and the mapping image above, the orally extending part is designated by yellow arrows, and the granular nodule within the lesion is marked by white arrows. Iodine staining areas within the lesion are marked by yellow and white round dots corresponding with each other. The blue line drawn on each of the endoscopic images corresponds with the section with the deepest invasion, and the red line part corresponds to the area with the invasion depth of T1a-MM~T1b-SM1.

Summary

This case was a flat raised lesion without prominently thick areas, containing Type B1 blood vessels within, and its preoperative diagnosis was T1a-EP~LPM. But, a 2 mm area with T1a-MM~T1b-SM1 was noted. This part had its surface covered by EP cancer, and there is a limit to reading invasion depth by blood vessels alone. Invasion depth diagnosis by EUS was thought necessary.

18.4 Answer

The correct invasion depth is (1) T1a-EP~LPM.

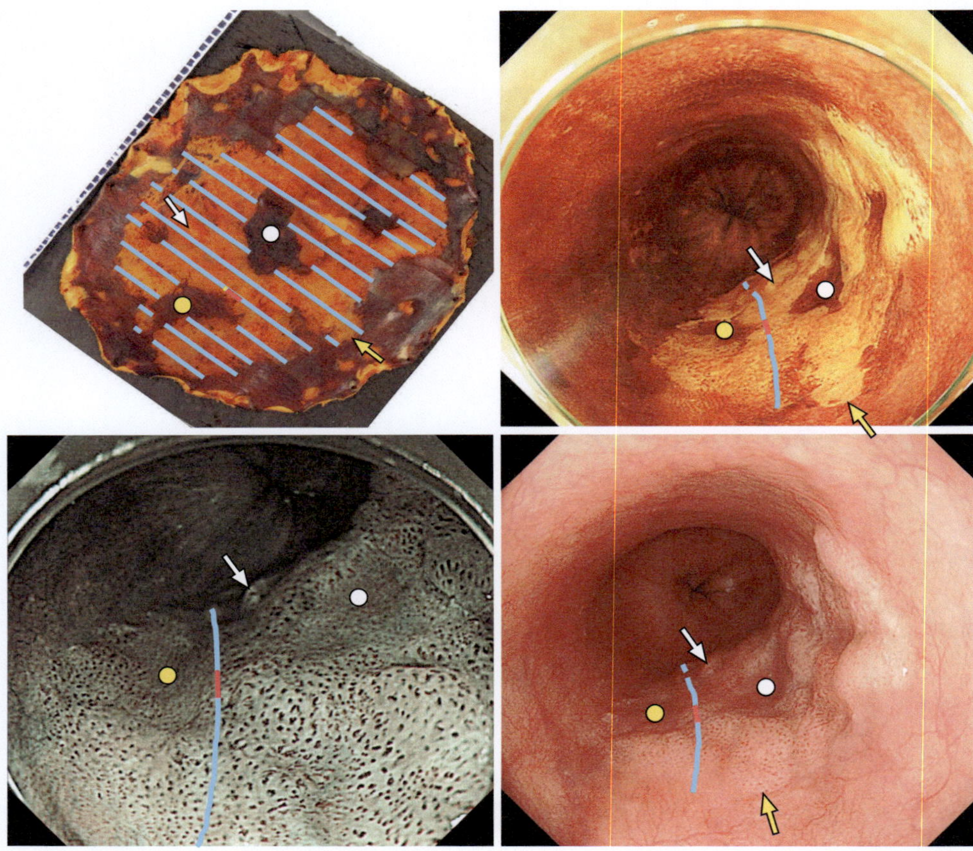

Fig. 18.7 Comparison with the endoscopic images and the resected specimen

19 Question 4: What Is the Invasion Depth?

Keita Funakawa

K. Funakawa (✉)
Department of Gastroenterology, Kagoshima City Hospital,
Kagoshima, Japan
e-mail: kfuna@po.synapse.ne.jp

T. Oyama (ed.), *Endoscopic Diagnosis of Esophageal Carcinoma for ESD*, https://doi.org/10.1007/978-981-32-9030-3_19

Which Is the Correct Invasion Depth? (Fig. 19.1)

1. T1a-EP~LPM
2. T1a-MM~T1b-SM1
3. T1b-SM2

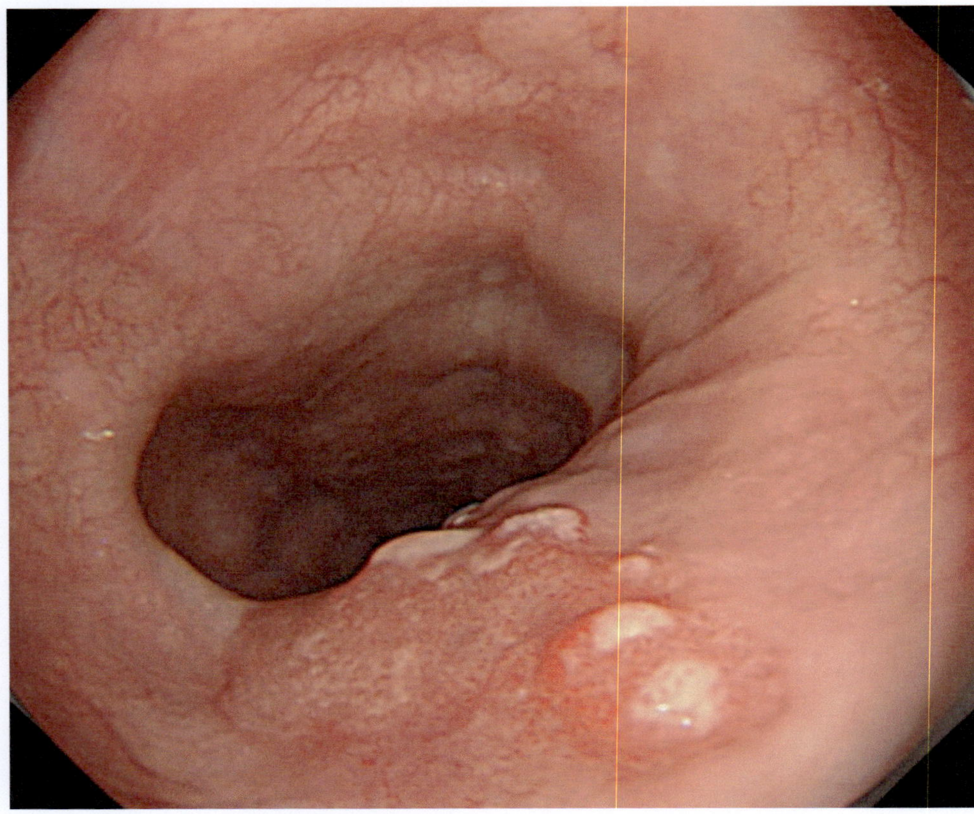

Fig. 19.1 Which is the correct invasion depth?

19.1 Let's Look at These Six Images and Think (Fig. 19.2)

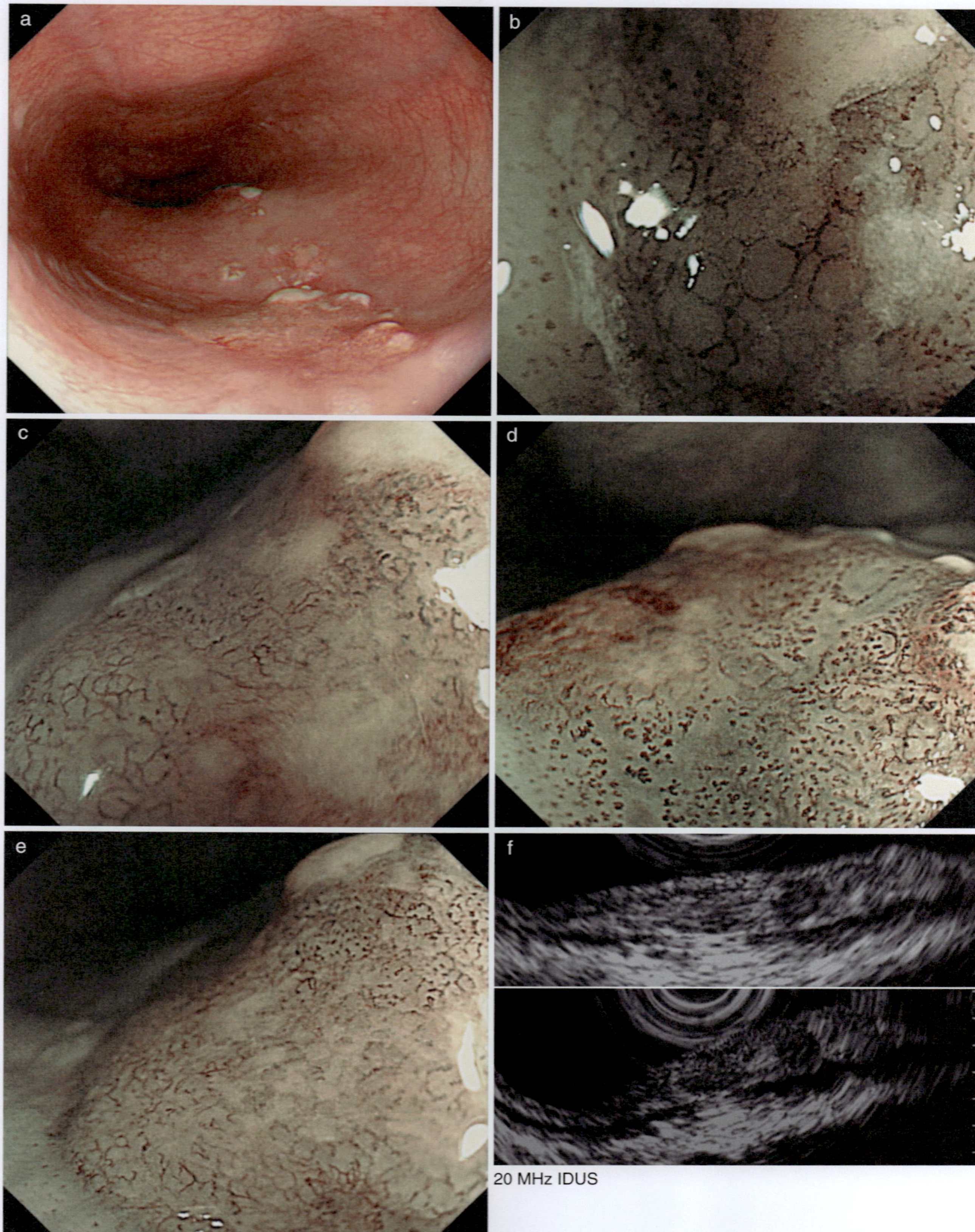

Fig. 19.2 Explanations start from the next page

19.2 Let's Observe the Following Six Images Carefully

Let's Observe the Area with Loss of Vascular Visibility (Fig. 19.3a)

- There was an area with loss of vascular visibility in the thoracic mid-esophagus, coinciding with the area are reddish coarsely granular and slightly raised as a whole. On its surface, focal whitish adhesions and nodular raised areas were noted.
- On the anal side of the lesion, a separate lesion was noted (not considered in this case).
- White exudative adhesions are used as reference points designated by green, yellow, and blue round marks.

Let's Observe with Magnifying NBI of the Area Anal to the Lesion (Fig. 19.3b)

- Although not seen with white adhesions, the blood vessels are noted with non-loop-forming blood vessels. Small AVA was formed with invasion depth of T1a-EP~LMP.

Let's Observe with Magnifying NBI the Left Side of the Lesion (Fig. 19.3c)

- Loop-forming blood vessels are noted in the areas marked by yellow arrows, and non-loop-forming blood vessels are noted traversing in the area marked by a blue arrow. The lesion is gently sloping upwards towards the center of the lesion like an SMT. On the right and lower sides of the image, the surface was covered with white exudates making it difficult to evaluate with NBI.
- Considering SMT like smoothly rising appearance, invasion depth may be deeper, and possibilities of sub-lesional inflammatory changes like lymphoid follicles or submucosal tumor cannot be denied.

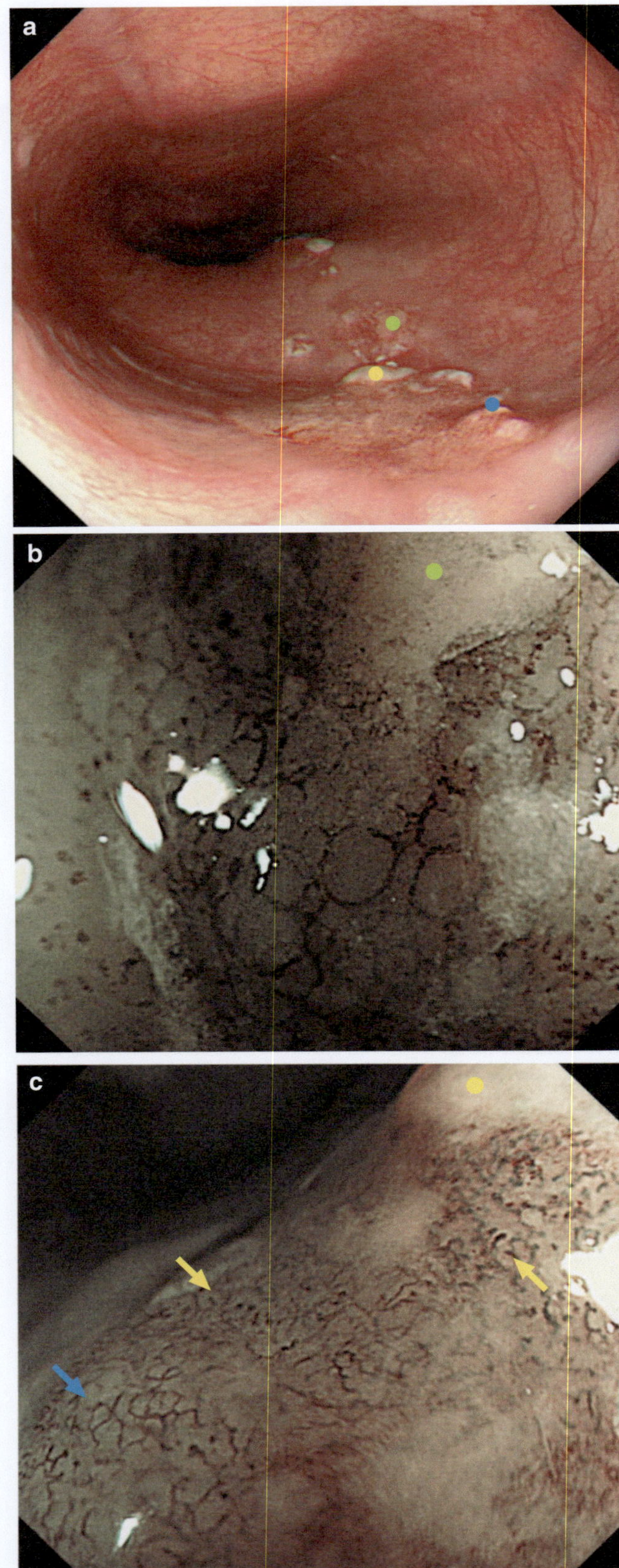

Fig. 19.3 Same images as Fig. 19.2

Let's Observe with Magnifying NBI the Central Part of the Lesion (Fig. 19.3d)

- Most of the observable blood vessels were dot-like to loop-forming types suggestive of invasion depth of T1a-EP~LPM. Adherent whitish exudative materials marked by yellow arrows make it difficult to evaluate blood vessels in the area, but the area as a whole appears to be smoothly rising, and EUS may be a helpful modality in assessment of invasion depth.

Let's Observe with Magnifying NBI the Left Oral Side of the Lesion (Fig. 19.3e)

- Dot-like blood vessels were noted in the area marked by a blue arrow, and traversing non-loop-forming blood vessels were marked by red arrows. Due to coverage by white exudative materials, evaluation of the area marked by yellow arrows was difficult.

Let's Observe with EUS (Fig. 19.3f)

- The muscularis mucosa was seen as three layers out of seven total.
- The third layer (the submucosa) showed low-echoic tumors as marked by yellow arrows or a blue arrow. These may represent inflammatory changes of tumors or lymphoid follicles.

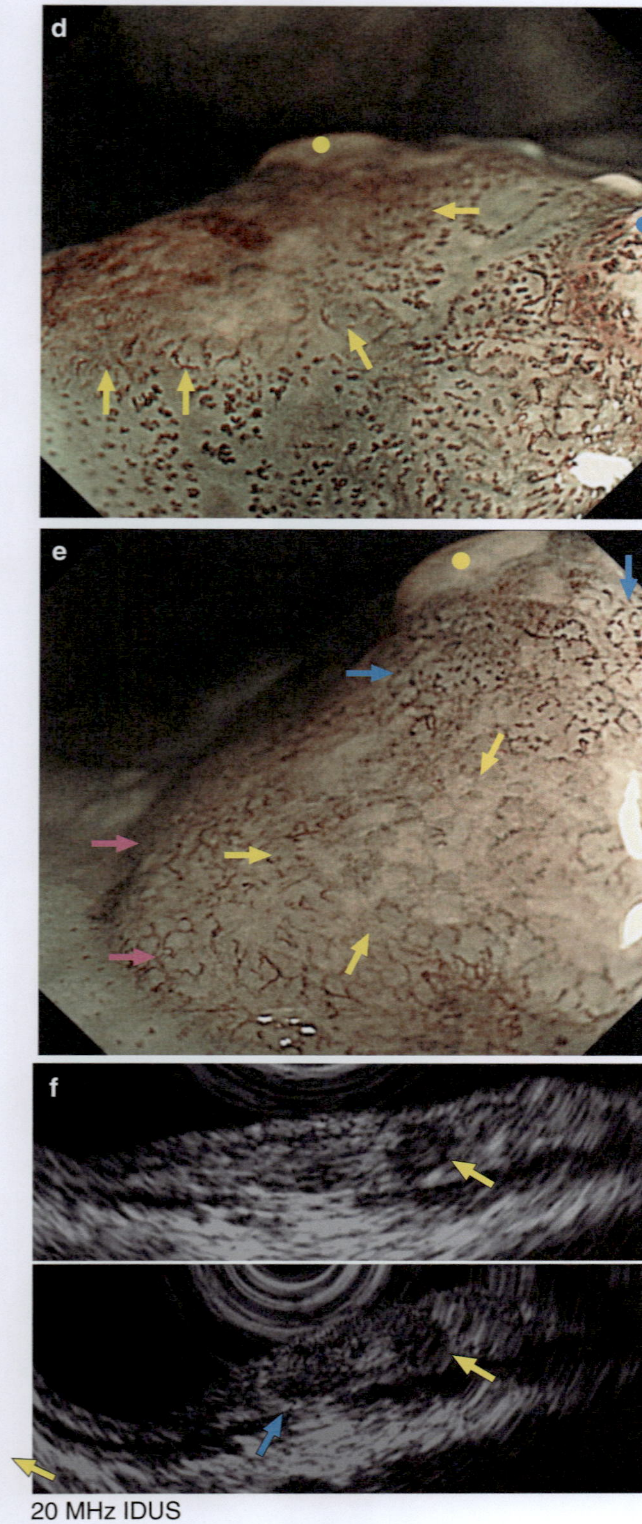

Fig. 19.3 (continued)

19.3 Let's Compare the Resected Specimen with the Endoscopic Images Towards the Final Diagnosis

This is an iodine dye stained freshly resected specimen (Fig. 19.4a). The orientation of the lesion is arranged with the oral side towards the bottom of the image. Two lesions were resected together. The lesion of concern for the current case is the oral lesion towards the bottom of the image. A histopathological image of the anally extending portion is seen in the yellow square below (Fig. 19.4b). The superficial layer shows inflammation consisting mainly of lymphatic cells with cancer nests within the deeper part beneath.

A histopathological image of the oral left wall side is shown where it was difficult to observe surface blood vessels due to adherent white exudative materials. There was an submucosal tumor nest unrelated to the surface carcinoma (Fig. 19.4c).

A histopathological image of the area near the central part of the lesion is shown. The most of the lesion has invasion depth of T1a-LPM. But in two areas, the lesion was found invading submucosa, pressing muscularis mucosa (Fig. 19.4d).

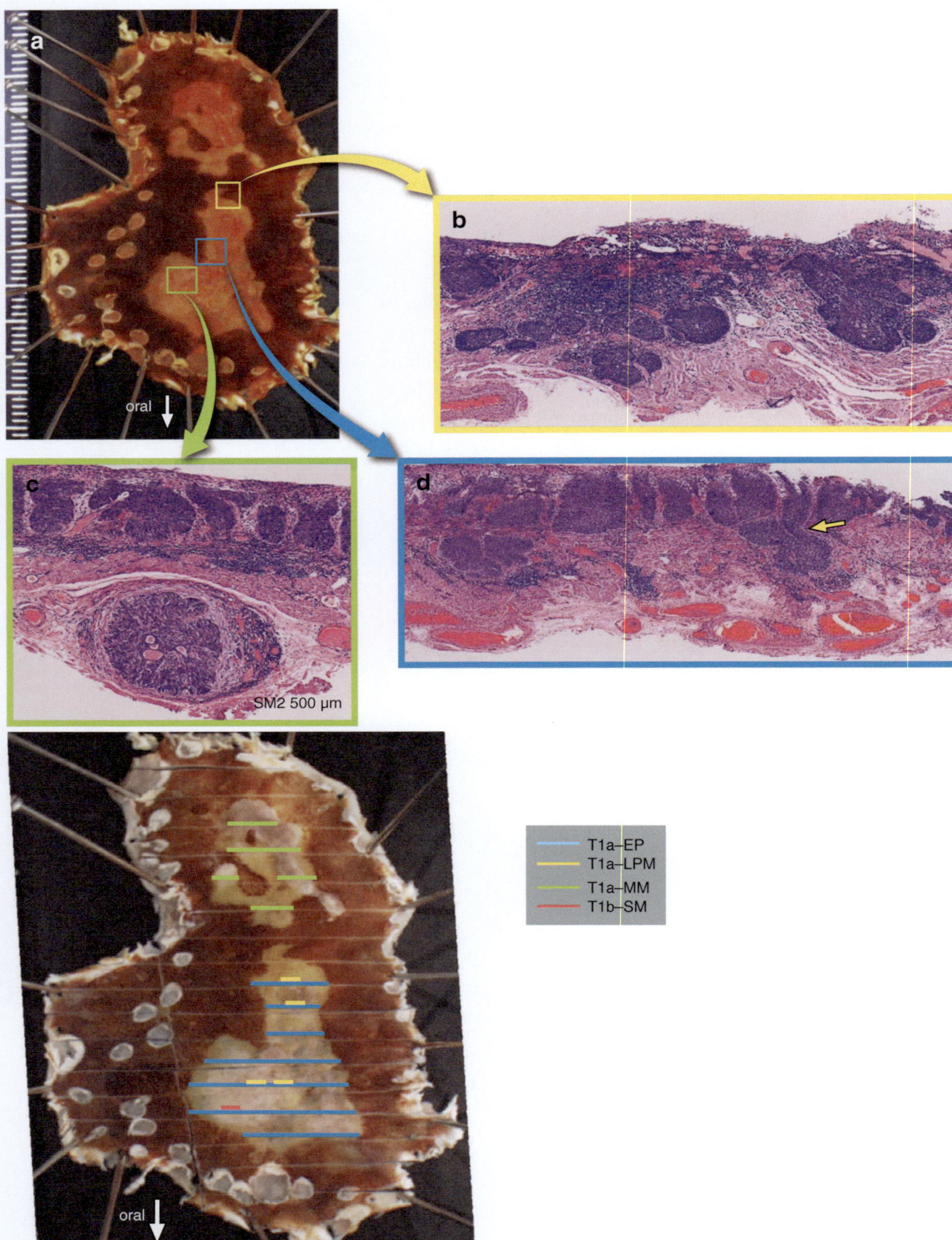

Fig. 19.4 Comparison between the iodine dye-stained resected specimen and histopathological image

Let's Compare the Resected Specimen with Endoscopic Image

The invasion depth of the anally extending part was T1a-MM. By magnifying NBI, this area showed AVA-small and was covered with white exudative materials. The histopathological image had shown cancer nests beneath the superficial inflammatory changes where it was not possible for NBI to detect (Fig. 19.5a).

Both loop-forming blood vessels and non-loop-forming blood vessels are present in this area. Invasion depth diagnosis of the area by NBI was confirmed to be accurate histopathologically (Fig. 19.5b).

This image shows the area one section oral than the previous image. Surface blood vessels appeared the same, but the area covered with adherent exudative materials could not show blood vessels for invasion depth analysis. Histopathological image showed cancer nests in the submucosa separately from the surface cancer, suggesting that the deeper tissue-level information did not manifest on the surface level (Fig. 19.5c).

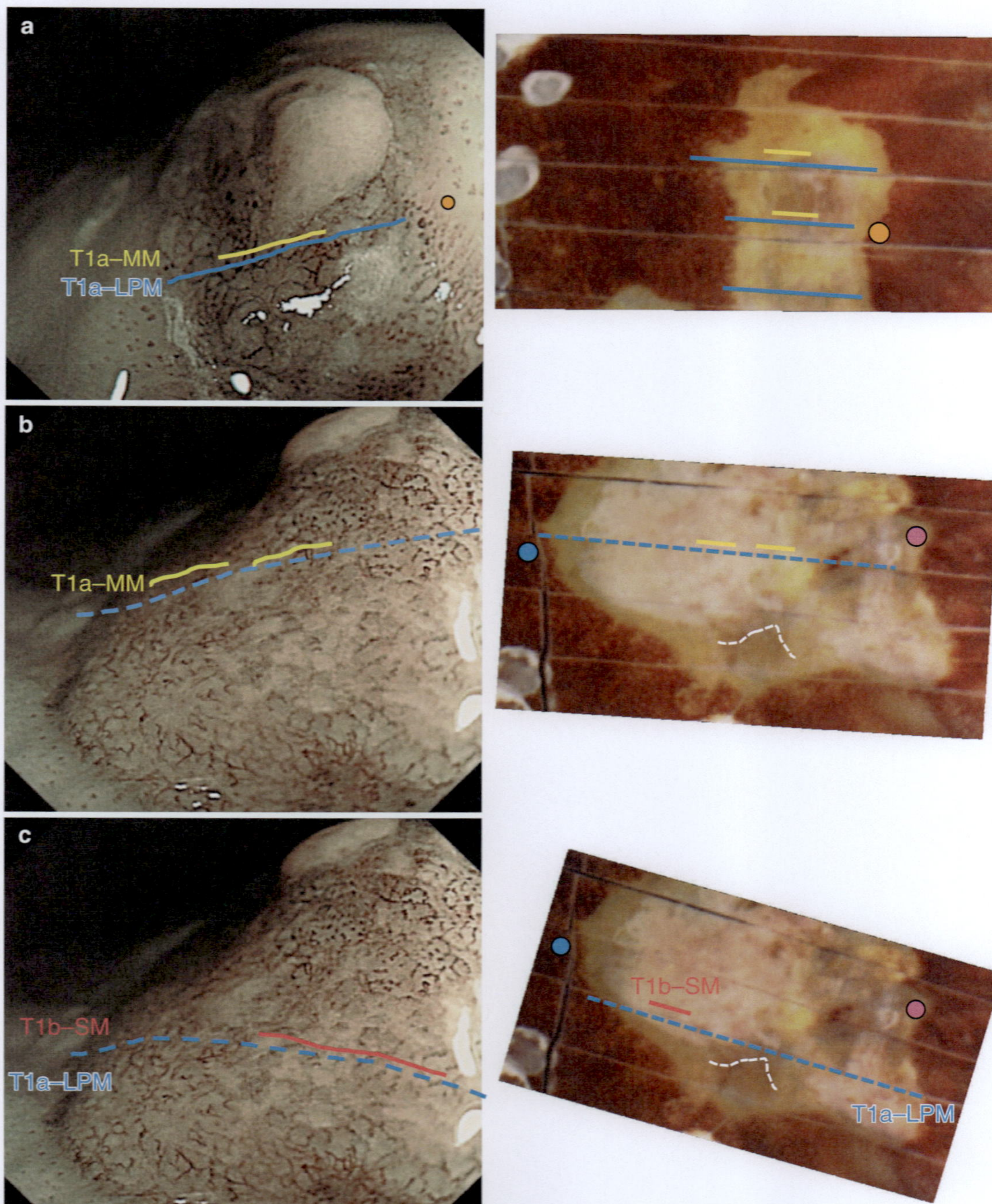

Fig. 19.5 Comparison to the iodine dye-stained resected specimen and NBI magnified endoscopic images

Conclusive Diagnosis

Esophageal squamous cell carcinoma, 0-IIa,T1b-SM2(500 μm), INFb, ly(-), v(-), HM0, VM0, 18x18mm, pCurC, Mt, Post.

Conclusion

Tumor sometimes exists separately in the deeper tissue unrelated to the surface-level tumor. As such information may not manifest as surface-level findings, invasion depth cannot be accurately diagnosed by magnifying NBI. Inflammatory changes at the surface level may also interfere with surface manifestation of deeper level findings. Therefore, it is important to assess whether the lesion has thickness or focally raised parts by white light imaging also, in addition to magnifying NBI. Furthermore, EUS provides helpful findings and should be performed when in question of invasion depth diagnosis.

19.4 Answer

The correct invasion depth diagnosis is (3) T1b-SM2.

20 Question 5: What Is the Invasion Depth?

Keita Funakawa

K. Funakawa (✉)
Department of Gastroenterology, Kagoshima City Hospital,
Kagoshima, Japan
e-mail: kfuna@po.synapse.ne.jp

T. Oyama (ed.), *Endoscopic Diagnosis of Esophageal Carcinoma for ESD*, https://doi.org/10.1007/978-981-32-9030-3_20

Which Is the Correct Invasion Depth? (Fig. 20.1)

1. T1a-EP~LPM
2. T1a-MM~T1b-SM1
3. T1b-SM2

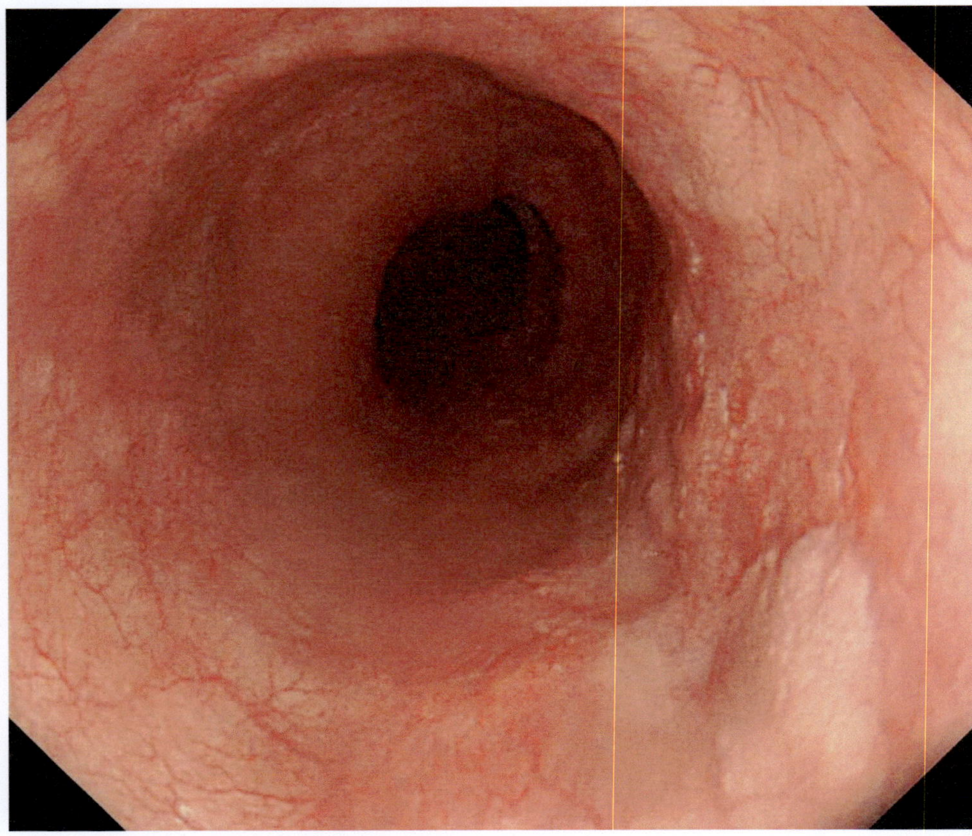

Fig. 20.1 Which is the correct invasion depth?

20.1 Let's Look at These Six Images and Think (Fig. 20.2)

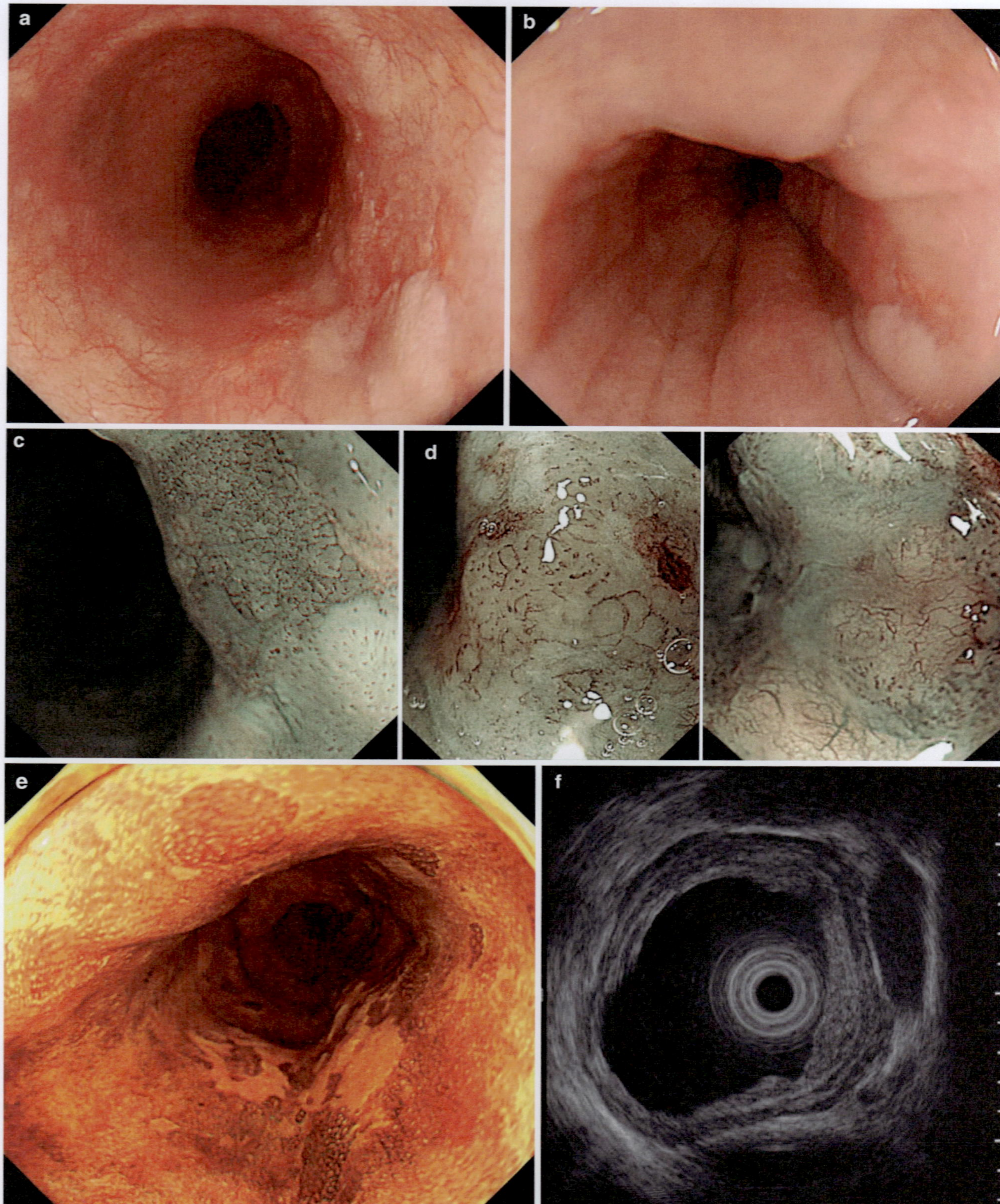

Fig. 20.2 Explanations start from the next page

20.2 Let's Observe the Following Six Images Carefully

Let's Observe Redness and Loss of Vascular Visibility of Mucosa (Fig. 20.3a)

- An irregular depressed lesion was noted in the right wall side of the mid-thoracic esophagus, corresponding with the mucosal area of lost vascular visibility.
- This was obtained with full insufflation, with mild unevenness with relatively smooth depression surface.
- A strongly reddish mucosal area was marked with a yellow round dot, and a light-colored raised part was marked with a blue round dot.

Let's Deflate Air (Fig. 20.3b)

- When deflated, longitudinal folds are traversing through the depressed area, but relatively wider spaces between folds were noted as marked by two sets of yellow arrows, where invasion depth greater than T1a-MM cannot be denied.
- In this case, "tatami-mat"-like patterns of fine horizontal folds were not seen and could not be used for invasion depth diagnosis.

Let's Observe with Magnifying NBI (Fig. 20.3c)

- This image shows mid-magnification NBI of the oral side of the lesion.
- Where observable, dot-like blood vessels or AVA-small were found abundantly. Based on NBI findings, invasion depth up to T1a-LPM was suspected.

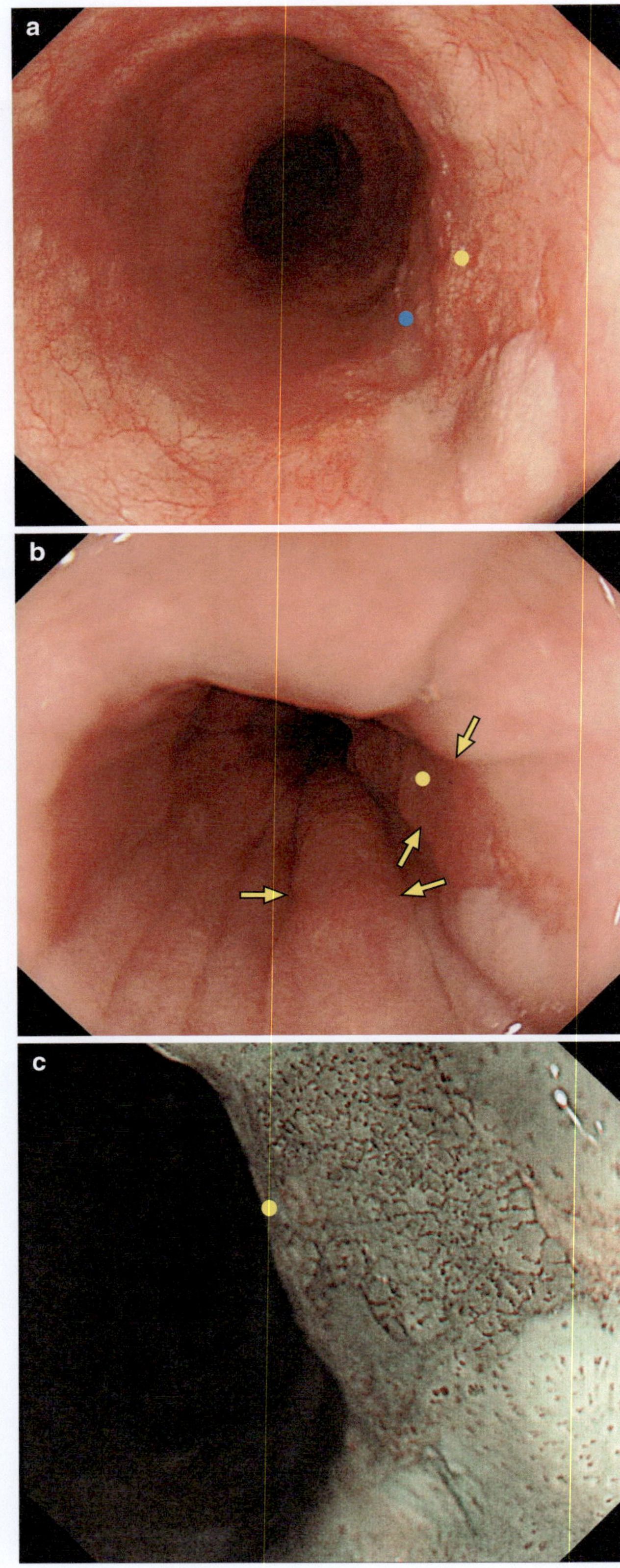

Fig. 20.3 Same images as Fig. 20.2

Let's Observe with Magnifying NBI (Fig. 20.3d)

- Loop-forming blood vessels or AVA-small were noted, and invasion depth was diagnosed as T1a-EP~LPM.
- AVA-middle were noted in the area marked by yellow arrows.
- The right image shows the lesion near its center by magnifying NBI. Fine reticular blood vessels were found in the area marked by yellow arrows. It is suspected possible that poorly differentiated cancer exists immediately beneath the epithelium.
- Although dot-like blood vessels are seen in the area marked by blue arrows, a gently sloping raised area was noted suggestive of a possible lesion beneath the epithelium.

Let's Observe with Iodine Dye Staining (Fig. 20.3e)

- With iodine dye staining, the lesion remains unstained, while the background squamous epithelium and the squamous epithelial islands within became stained.

Let's Observe with EUS (Fig. 20.3f)

- EUS using a mini-probe showed the tumor as a mixture of high-echoic and low-echoic areas in the submucosa as marked by yellow arrows. The muscularis mucosa was found as the third layer, while the tumor existed in the first to the third layers out of seven layers total.

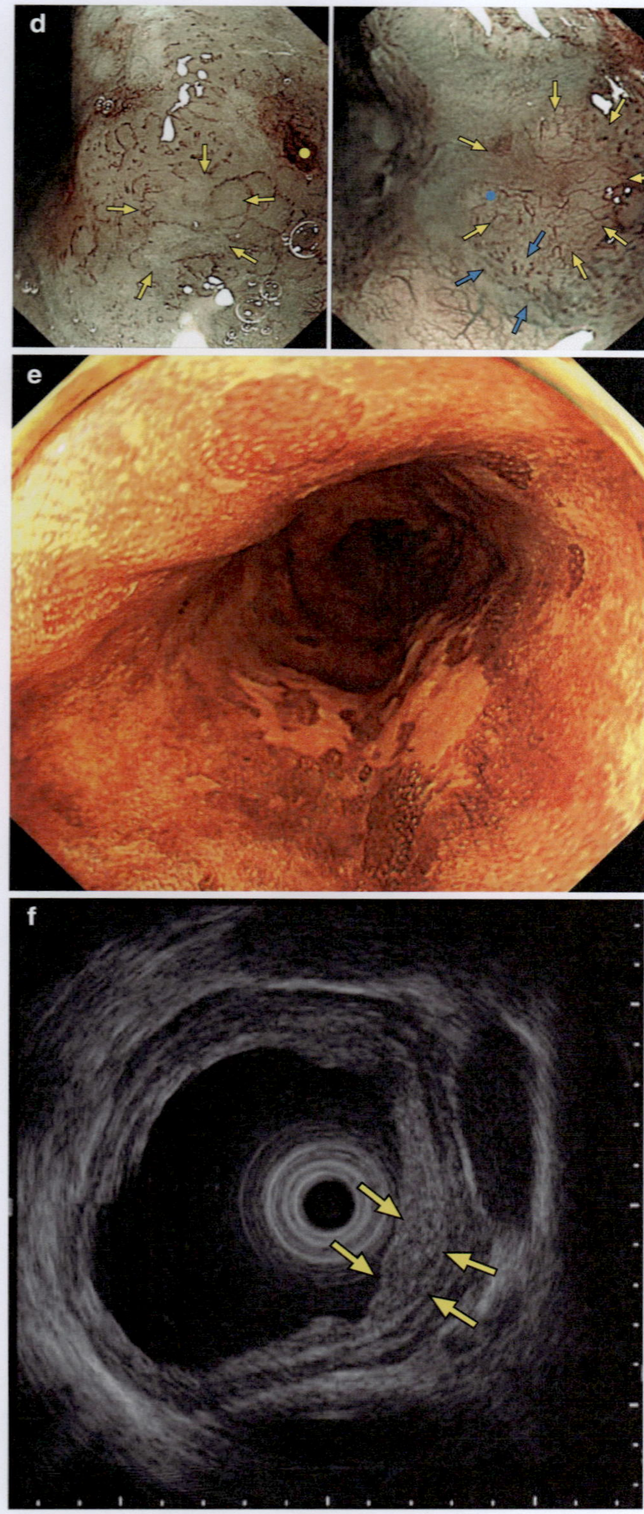

Fig. 20.3 (continued)

20.3 Let's Compare the Resected Specimen with the Endoscopic Images Towards the Final Diagnosis

Figure 20.4a shows the resected iodine stained specimen (sliced into 18 sections). The right side is the oral side.

Figure 20.4b, c is histopathological images for Sect. 10.

There is a large subepithelial tumor and nontumor epithelium and a separate epithelial tumor not connected with subepithelial tumor.

Figure 20.4d, e is histopathological images for Sect. 11.

There is a subepithelial tumor short distance away from the epithelial tumor.

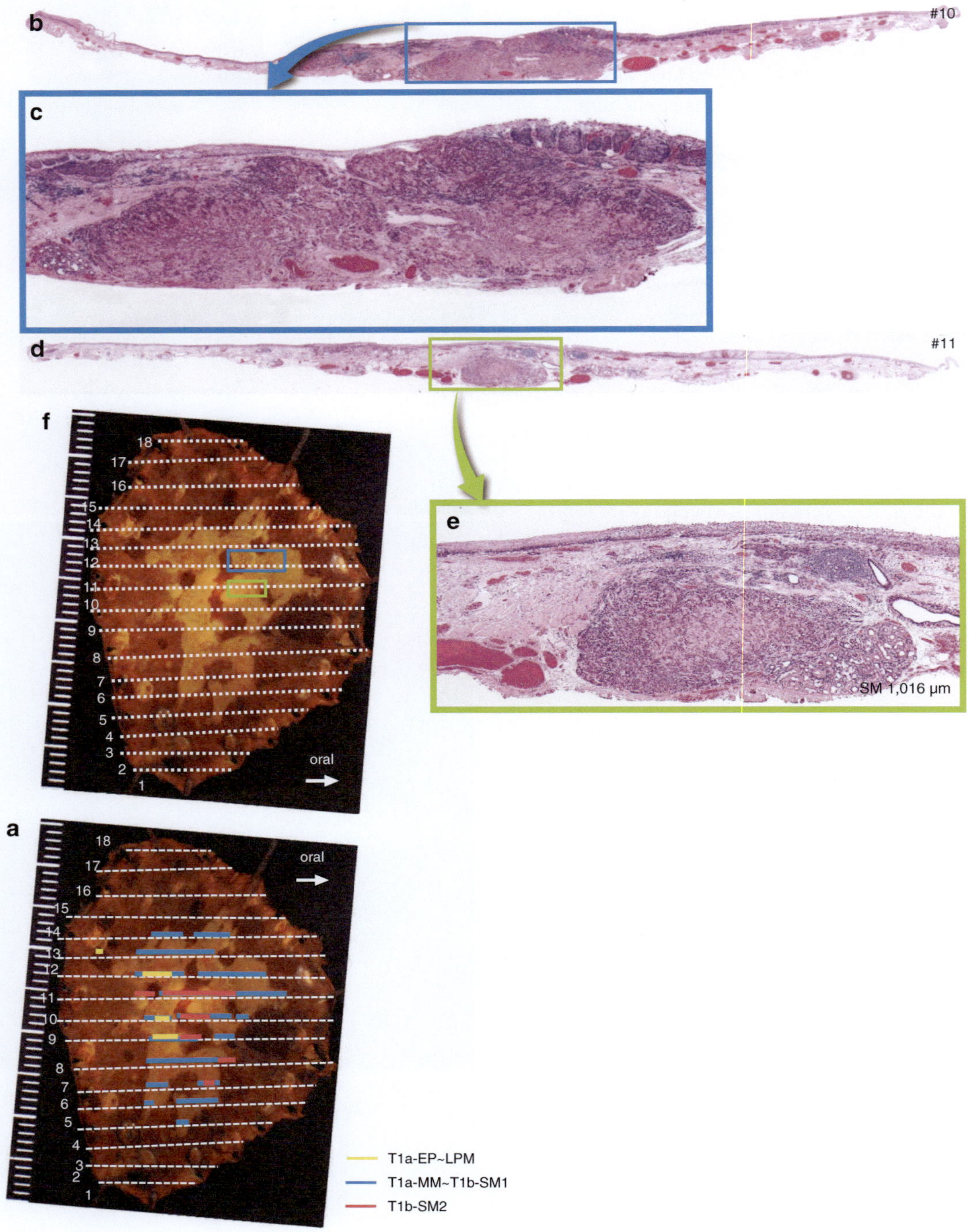

Fig. 20.4 Comparison to the iodine dye-stained resected specimen and the histopathological images

Let's Compare the Histopathological Findings with the Endoscopic Images (Fig. 20.5)

In Part A, immediately beneath the nontumor epithelium, a moderately differentiated squamous cell tumor was noted with the surface structure thought to be showing net-like patterns.

In Part B, block like cancer nests are noted, reflected by AVA-small areas by NBI observation.

In Part C, an epithelial cancer was noted with dot-like blood vessels seen by NBI observation. A deeper tumor was not reflected in surface observation both by the presence of the surface tumor above and by the distance from the surface and the tumor.

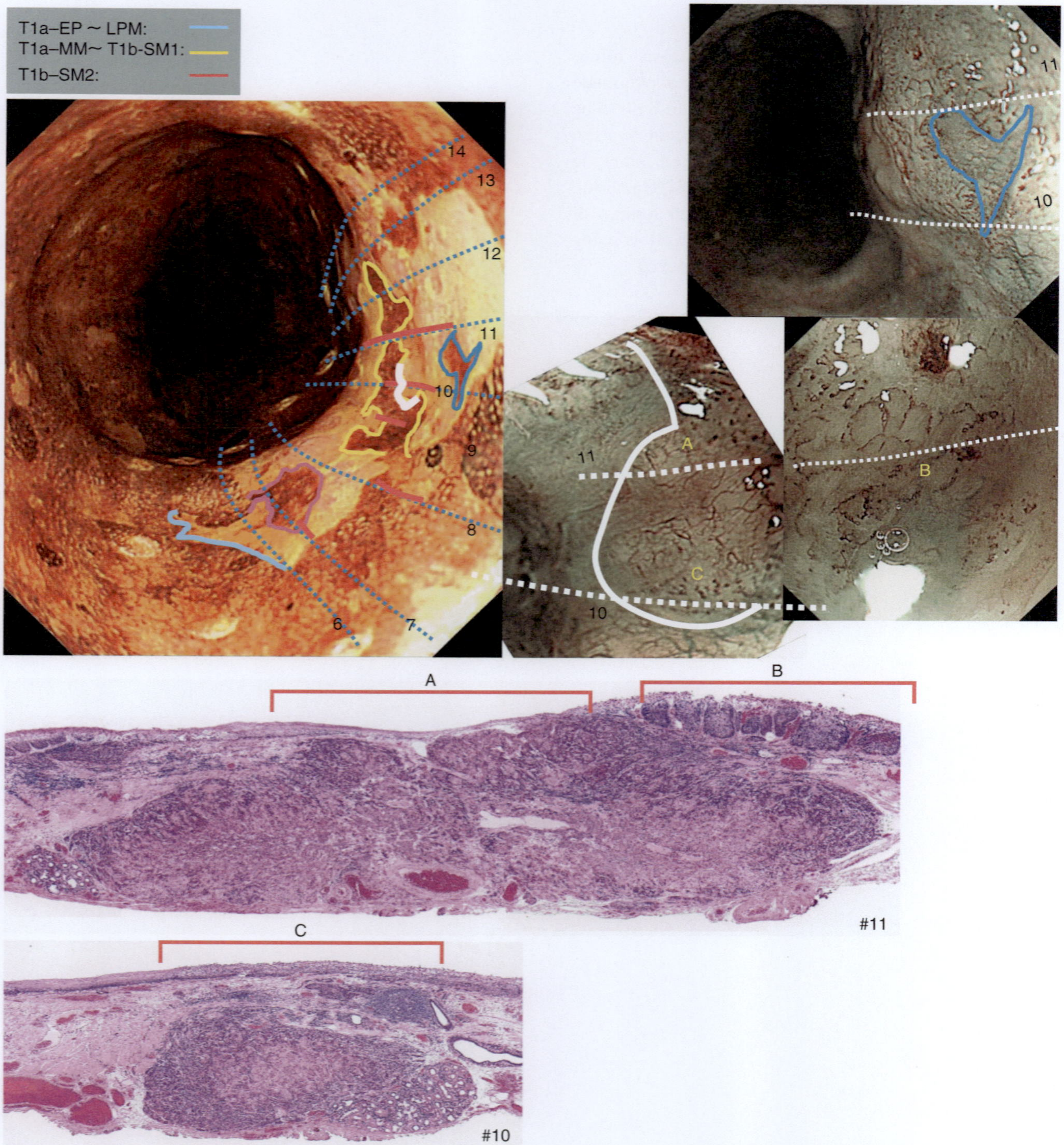

Fig. 20.5 Comparison to the endoscopic images and the histopathological images

Conclusive Diagnosis

Esophageal squamous cell carcinoma, moderately differentiated, 0-IIa+IIb+IIc, T1b-SM2(1,016μm), INFc, ly(+) (D2-40), v(-) (CD31), HM0, VM0, 27x20mm, pCurC, Mt.

Summary

In this case, although a large submucosal tumor existed, another epithelial tumor existing above made the presence of the deeper tumor mostly difficult to be detected. But an area existed where a tumor beneath the nontumor epithelium can be detected, showing blood vessels with network patterns by NBI. Gathering subtle findings suggestive of submucosal tumors of special type of lower differentiation, as well as using EUS, more accurate diagnosis can be achieved.

20.4 Answer

The correct invasion depth diagnosis is (3)T1b-SM2.

Question 6: What Is the Histological Type?

21

Tadashi Miike

T. Miike (✉)
Department of Gastroenterology, Miyazaki University School of Medicine, Miyazaki, Japan
e-mail: tadashi_miike@med.miyazaki-u.ac.jp

T. Oyama (ed.), *Endoscopic Diagnosis of Esophageal Carcinoma for ESD*, https://doi.org/10.1007/978-981-32-9030-3_21

Which Is the Correct Histological Type? (Fig. 21.1)

1. Squamous cell carcinoma
2. Granule cell carcinoma
3. Neuroendocrine cell carcinoma

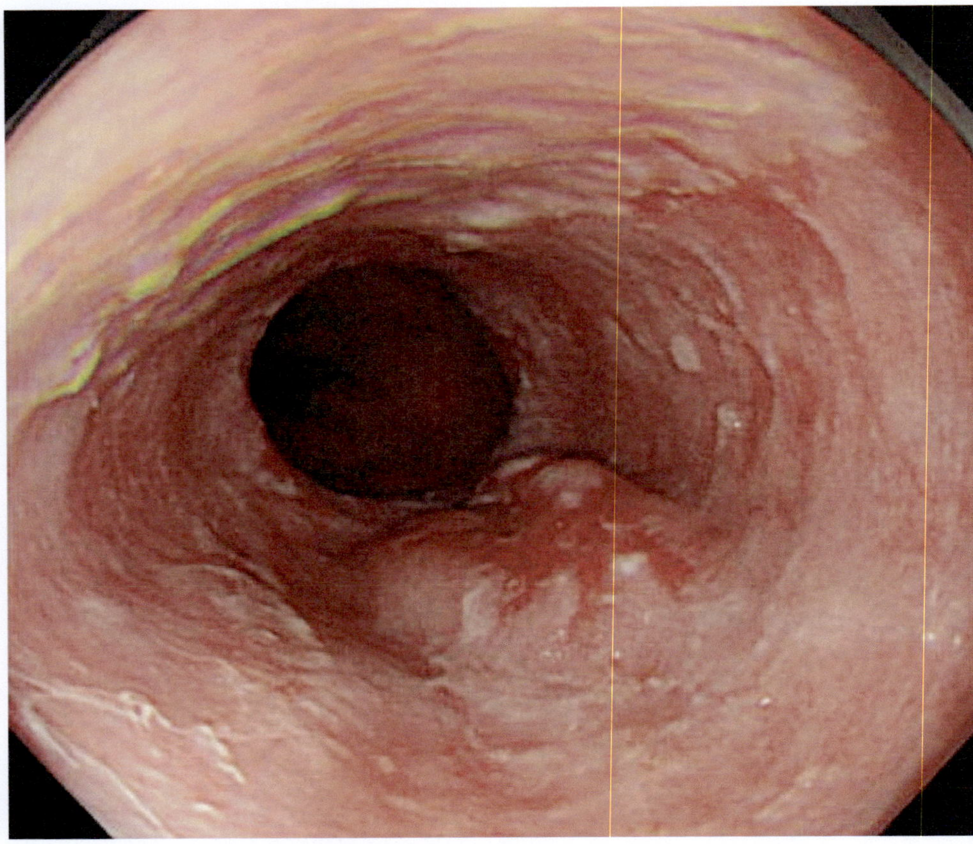

Fig. 21.1 Which is the correct histological type?

21.1 Let's Look at These Six Images and Think (Fig. 21.2)

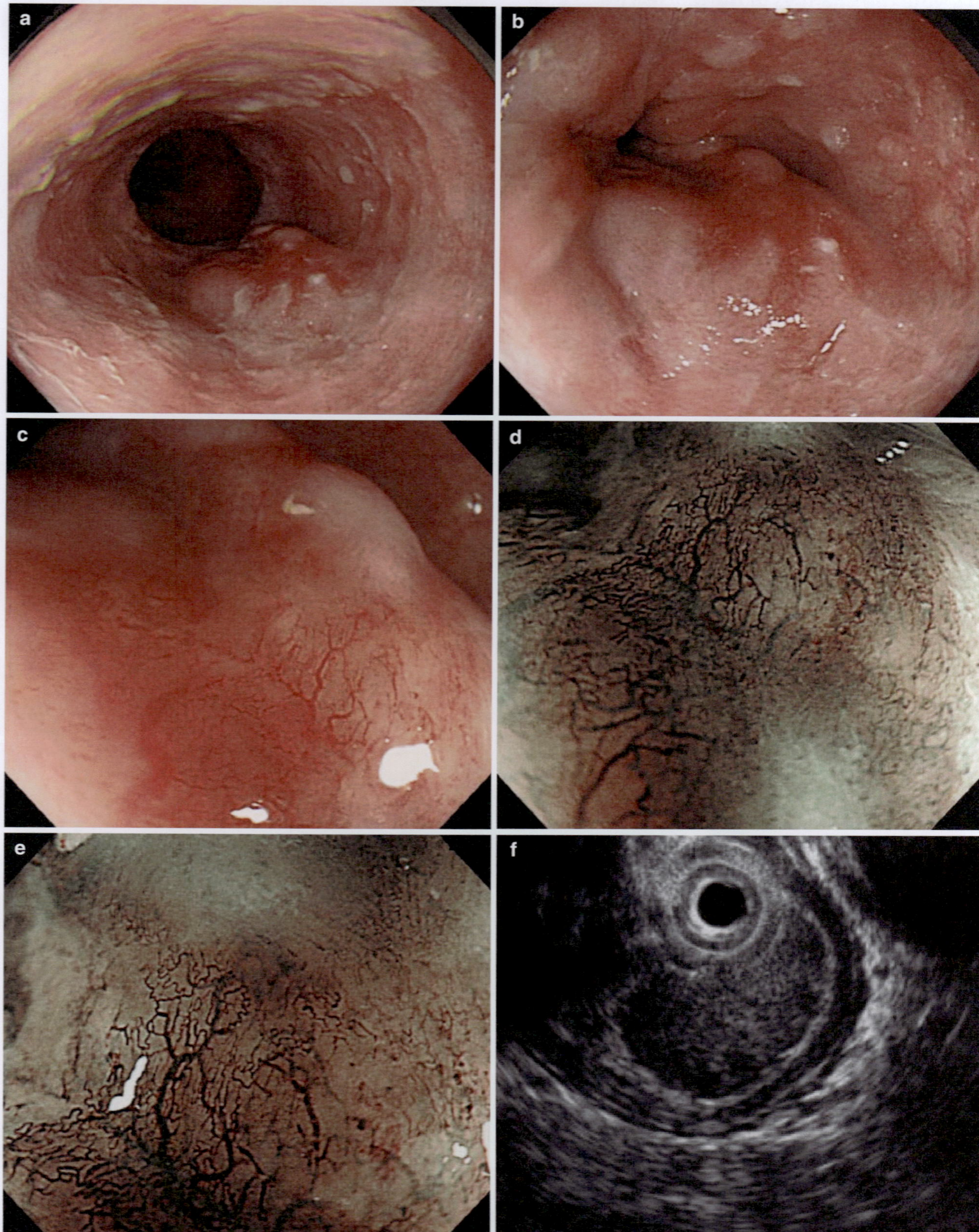

Fig. 21.2 Explanations start from the next page

21.2 Let's Observe the Following Six Images Carefully (Fig. 21.3)

Let's Note the Changes of the Mucosa (Fig. 21.3a)

- The background mucosa showed decreases vascular visibility as well as coarse appearing mucosa. There was a smoothly raised lesion with a shallow depression at the top in the posterior wall of the lower thoracic esophagus.

Let's Observe While Adjusting Air Volume (Fig. 21.3b)

- When air volume is adjusted by deflation, little variation of shape was noted with overall firmness and thick appearance of the lesion as marked by yellow arrows.

How Should the Findings Be Interpreted? (Fig. 21.3b)

- The lesion was a smoothly rising solitary raised tumor of "molar tooth-like" appearance, and granule cell carcinoma was suspected.

Let's Observe Closely with Magnifying White Light Imaging (Fig. 21.3c)

- With a close-up view, dilated blood vessels are noted spreading like nets, traversing horizontally and vertically, with irregular branching.

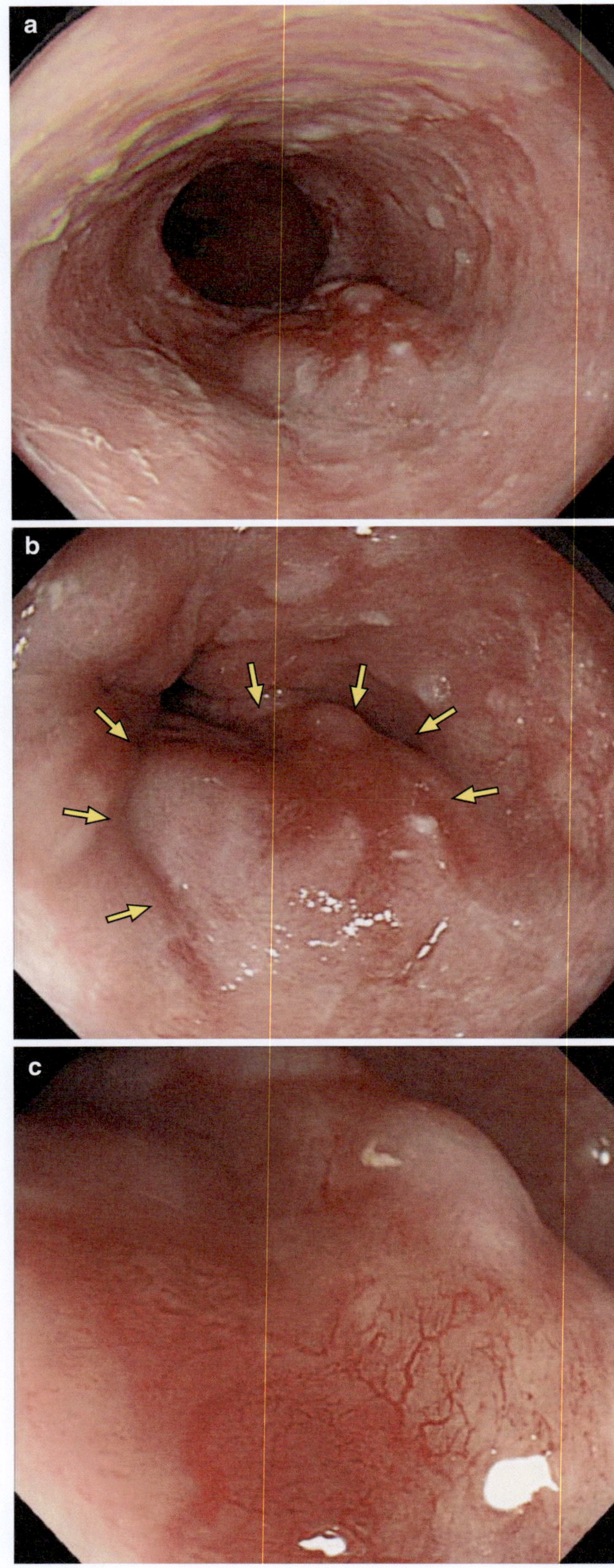

Fig. 21.3 Same images as Fig. 21.2

Let's Observe with NBI (Fig. 21.3d)

- With low-power-magnification NBI, the top level was noted as a faintly brownish area, with dendritic irregularly branching vessels lacking loop formations.

Let's Observe with Magnifying NBI (Fig. 21.3e)

- Irregular dendritic vascular networks lacking loop formations were noted and were diagnosed as Type R blood vessels as marked by yellow arrows.

Let's Observe with EUS (Fig. 21.3f)

- The raised lesion was identified as a low-echoic area with thickness located in the second and the third layers compressing the submucosa as marked by yellow arrows, but without obvious invasions into the muscular layers.
- Based on these findings, the lesion was a submucosal tumor consisting mainly of subepithelial growth, with Type R microvessels irregularly forming net-like patterns, suggesting a special-type esophageal cancer.

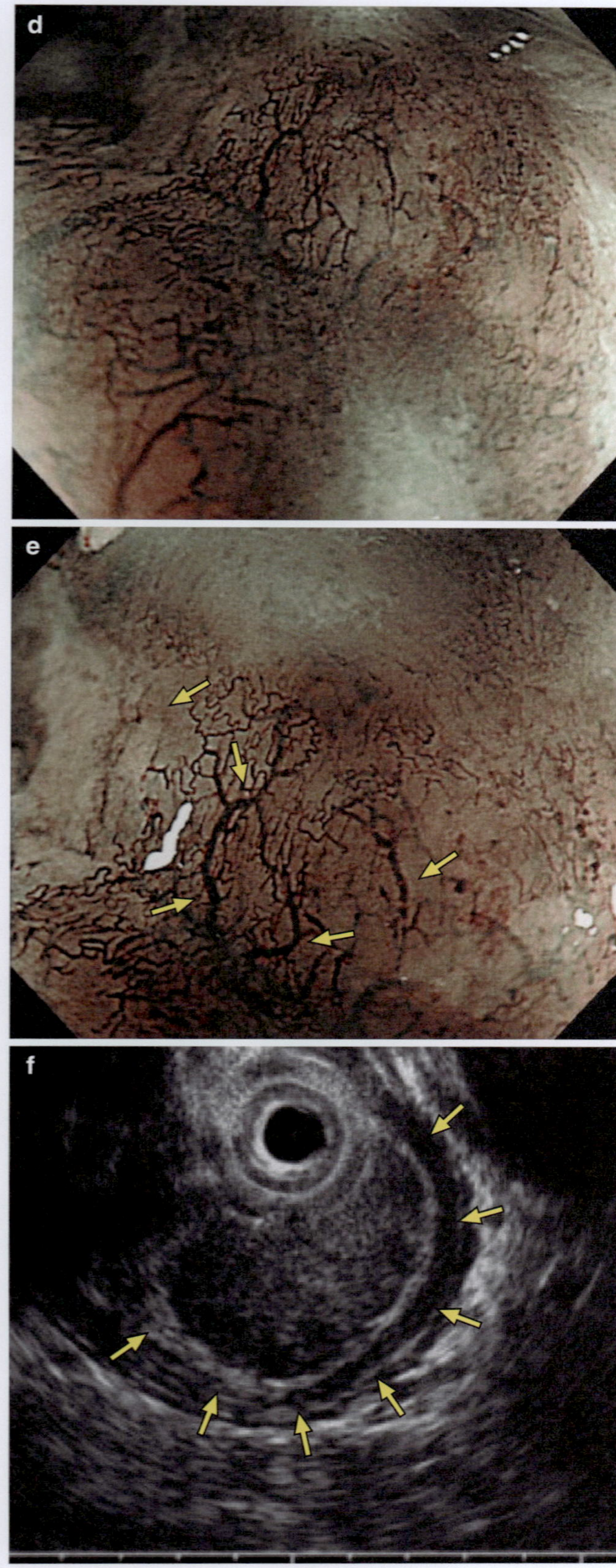

Fig. 21.3 (continued)

21.3 Let's Compare the Resected Specimen with the Endoscopic Images Towards the Final Diagnosis

Let's Observe Histopathology of the Biopsy Specimen (Fig. 21.4)

Top: H&E staining of the stroma showed clusters of cells with high N/C ratio.
Bottom: Immunostaining with chromogranin A and synaptophysin was both positively staining suggesting endocrine-type cancer.

Let's Observe CT to Determine Presence or Absence of Metastases (Fig. 21.5)

The lesion was clearly recognized as an irregularly shaped unstained area.

Let's Confirm the Changes in the Submucosa (Fig. 21.6)

Strong neovascularization and accompanying fibrosis were observed in the submucosa, and a possibility of submucosal

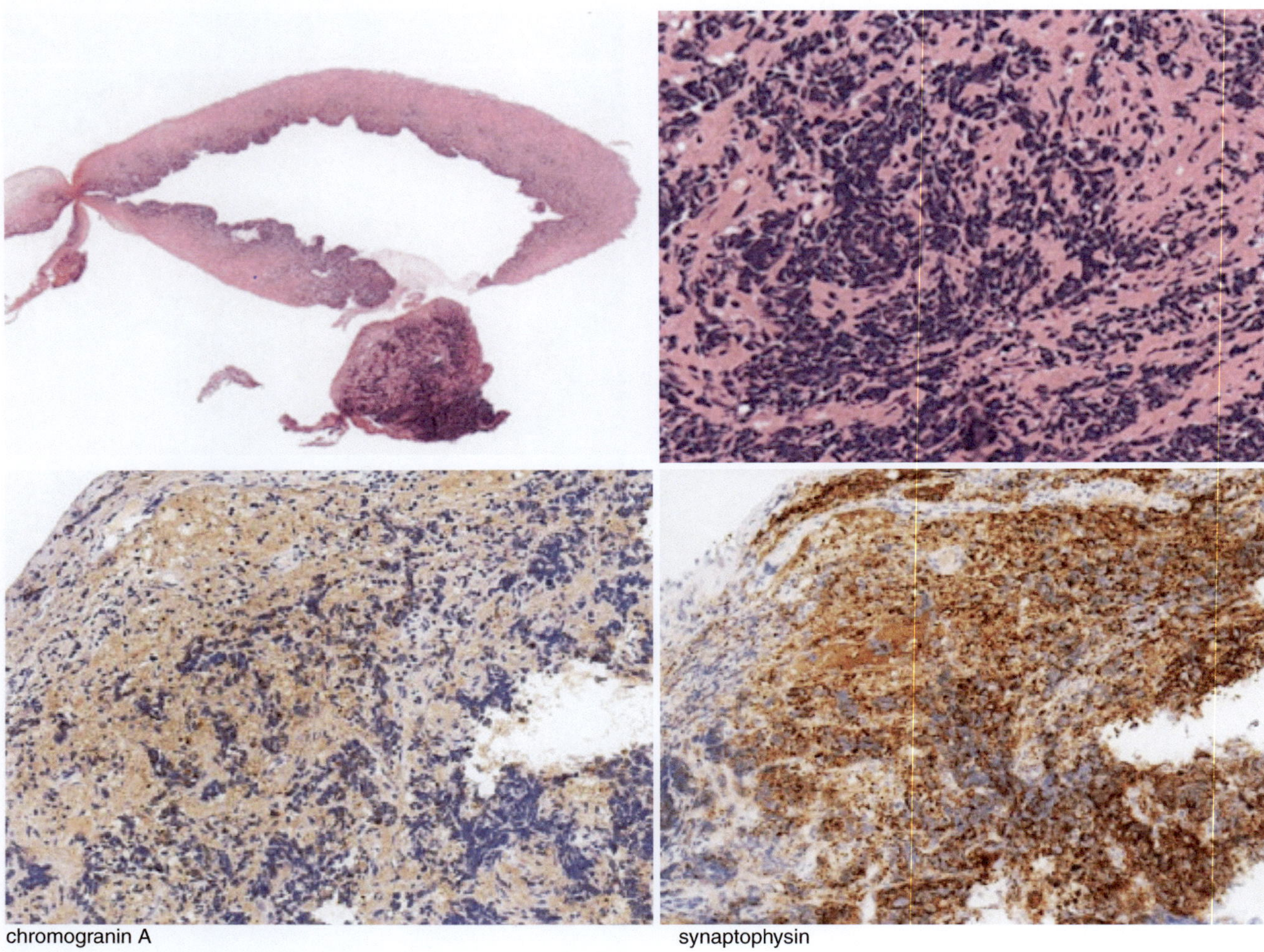

Fig. 21.4 Histopathological images of the biopsy specimens

tumor invasion was suspected. Abundant blood vessels were treated with coagulation hemostasis, exposing the submucosa as transparently as possible, dissecting just above the muscular layer.

Let's Observe the Freshly Resected Specimen

The right side is the oral side. In the center of the smoothly rising elevation, an irregularly shaped reddish depression was noted (Fig. 21.7).

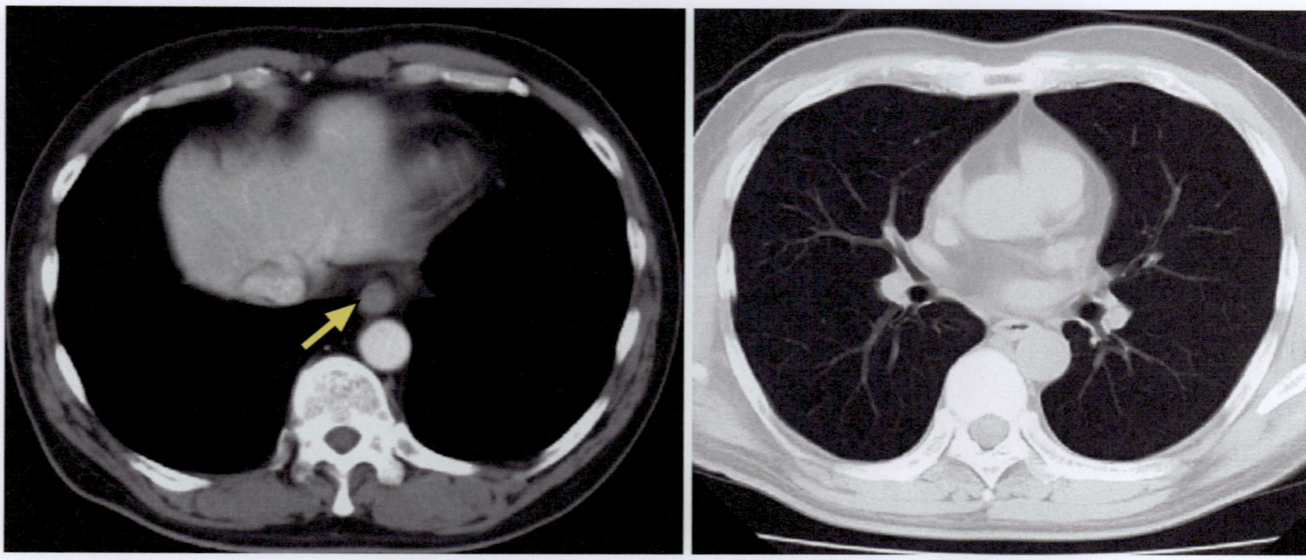

Fig. 21.5 CT images of the chest of the patient

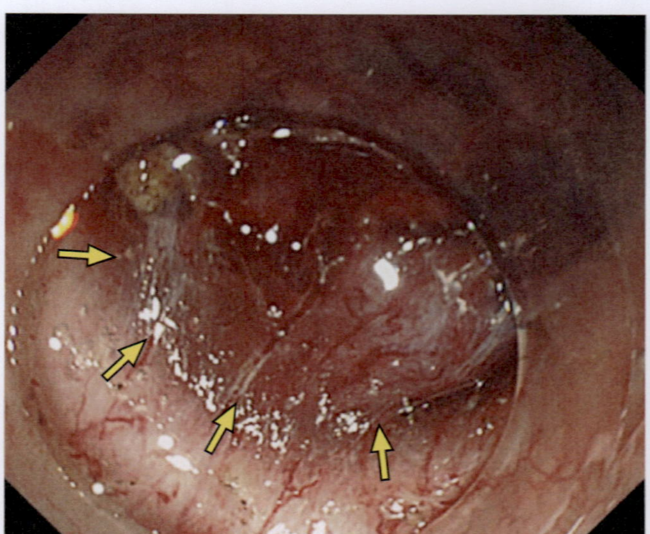

Fig. 21.6 Confirmation of the changes in the submucosa

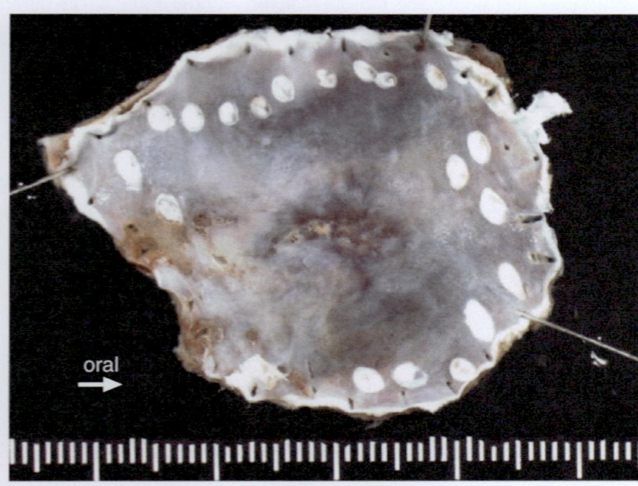

Fig. 21.7 Fleshly resected specimen of the lesion

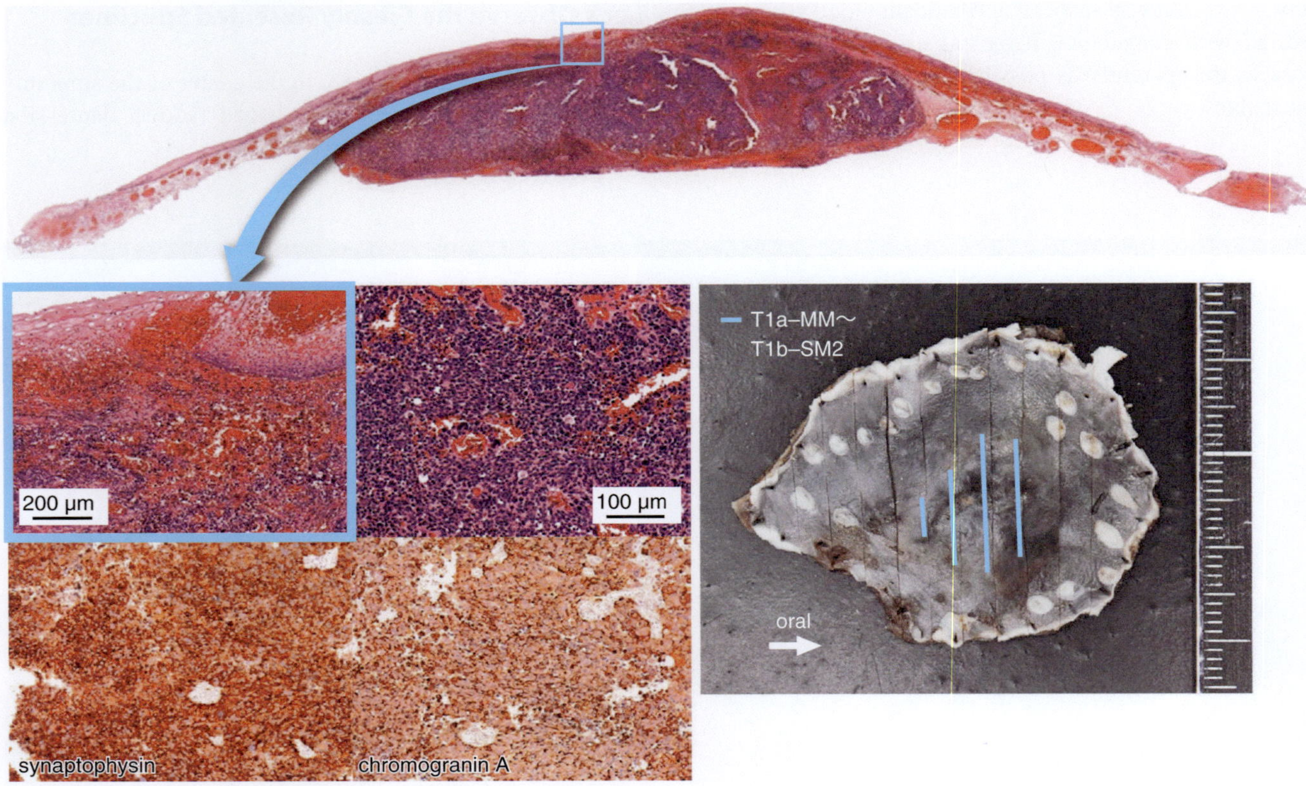

Fig. 21.8 Top/middle left: Observation of H&E staining histopathological images showed tumor cells diffusely existing just beneath the epithelium, forming solid tumor nests mainly in the submucosal layer, infiltrating just above the muscular layer. Middle right: Oval-shaped tumor cells with high N/C ratio proliferated densely. Bottom: Immunostaining for synaptophysin and chromogranin A, both markers for neuroendocrine cells were positive

Let's Compare NBI Findings with Histopathological Image (Fig. 21.9)

Magnifying NBI showed Type R microvessels showing gradually increasing diameters from the surface level to the deeper layer.

Conclusive Diagnosis

Neuroendocrine carcinoma(NEC), 0-Is, T1b-SM2(2,500μm), INFa, Ly(+), v(+), HM0, VM1, 15x11mm, pCurC.

Summary

A smoothly raised lesion with a shallow depression at the top was noted in the lower thoracic esophagus. Observing with white light imaging, granule cell carcinoma was suspected. With magnifying NBI, poorly loop-forming, irregular Type R blood vessels were noted in dendritic fashion. By EUS, the lesion was thick hypoechoic lesion located in the second and the third layers. The lesion was a submucosal tumor with subepithelially growing main body and Type R microvessels in irregular net-like patterns, leading to a diagnosis of special-type esophageal carcinoma, in which magnifying NBI was helpful in providing key diagnostic features. The conclusive diagnosis revealed lymphatic and venous metastases, as well as positive involvement by tumor at vertical margin, but the additional surgical resection with lymph node dissection showed no apparent residual tumor by postoperative histopathological analysis, confirming a completely curative resection.

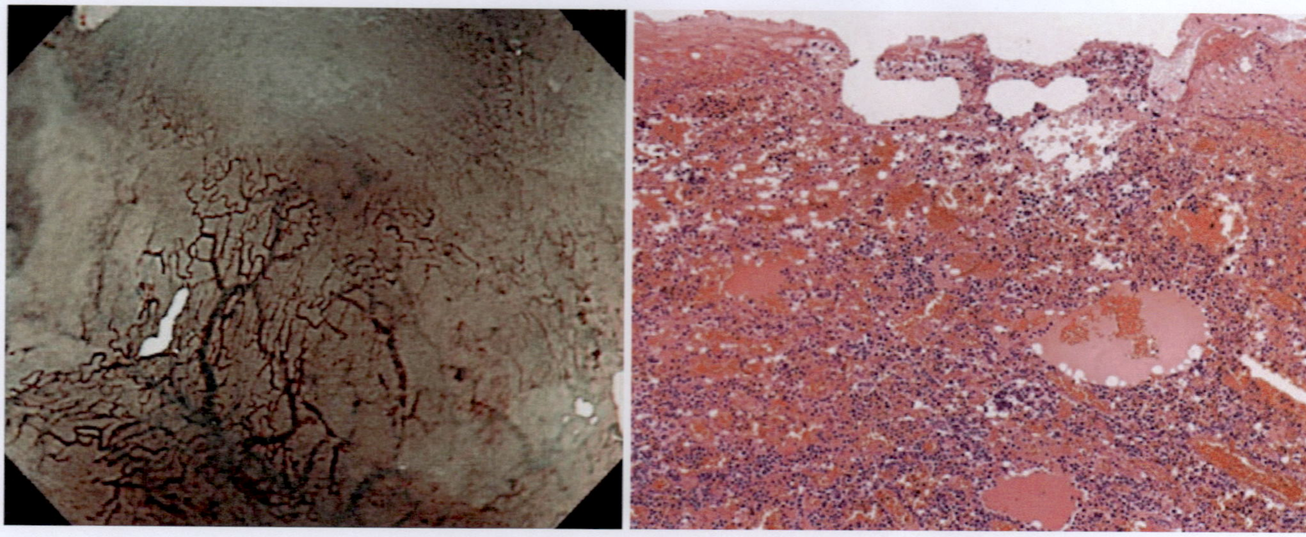

Fig. 21.9 Comparison of NBI findings with histopathological image

21.4 Answer

The correct histological type is (3) neuroendocrine carcinoma.

Acknowledgement A special thanks to Dr Kenji Yorita of Kochi Red Cross Hospital, Department of Pathology, for his guidance in manuscript preparation.

22 Question 7: What Is the Histological Type?

Toshiyuki Kubo

T. Kubo (✉)
Department of Gastroenterology and Hepatology, Sapporo Medical University School of Medicine, Sapporo, Hokkaido, Japan
e-mail: kubo-t@grape.plala.or.jp

T. Oyama (ed.), *Endoscopic Diagnosis of Esophageal Carcinoma for ESD*, https://doi.org/10.1007/978-981-32-9030-3_22

Which Is the Correct Histological Type? (Fig. 22.1)

1. Squamous cell carcinoma
2. Neuroendocrine cell carcinoma
3. Basaloid cell carcinoma

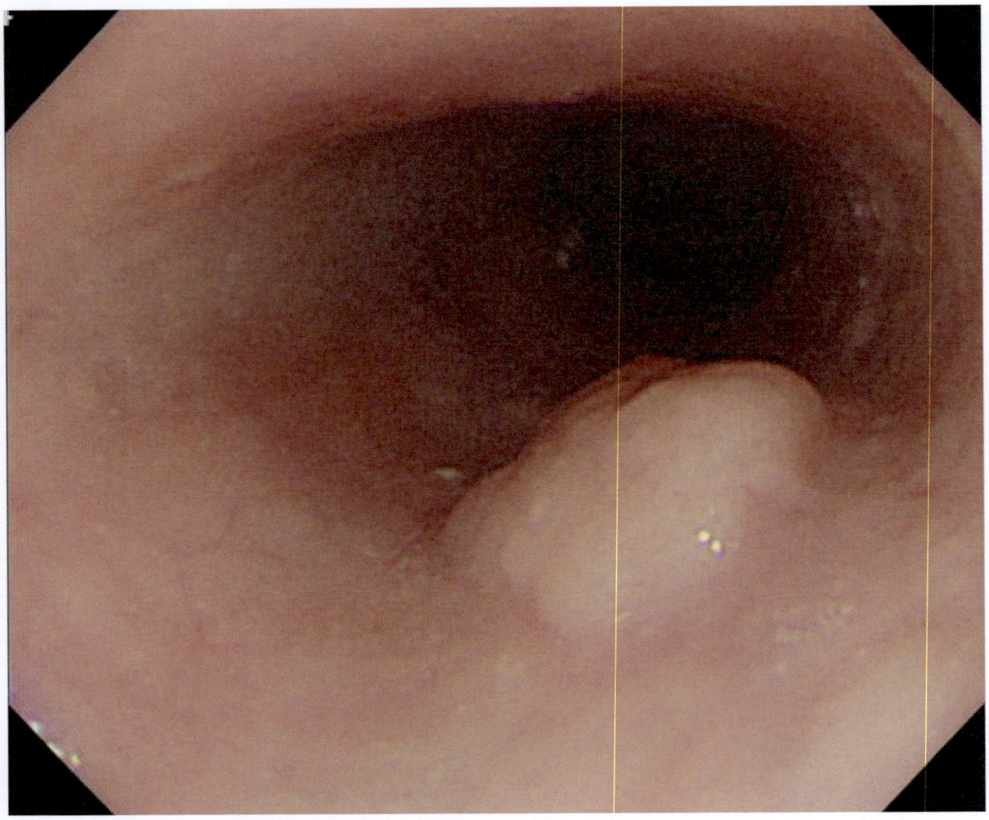

Fig. 22.1 What is the histological type?

22.1 Let's Look at These Six Images and Think (Fig. 22.2)

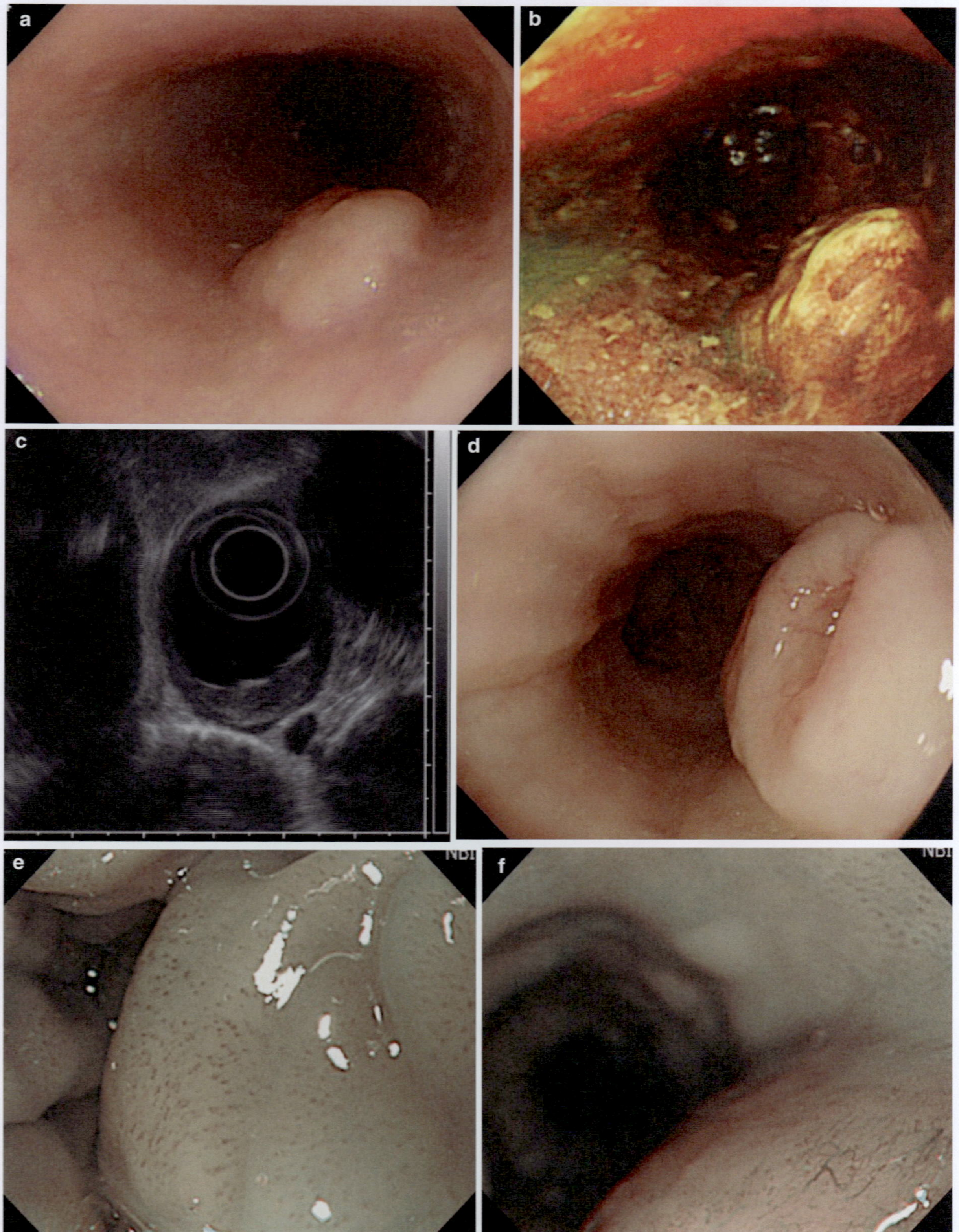

Fig. 22.2 Explanations start from the next page

22.2 Let's Observe the Following Six Images Carefully (Fig. 22.3)

Let's Observe with White Light Imaging (Fig. 22.3a)

- A 20 mm diameter whitish smoothly rising elevated lesion was noted in the posterior wall of the mid-thoracic esophagus. The surface structure was noted with slightly irregular unevenness.

Let's Observe with Iodine Dye Staining (Fig. 22.3b)

- When iodine dye staining was applied, much of the elevated part was stained with iodine, showing much of the lesion surface covered with nontumor squamous cell epithelium.

Let's Observe with EUS (Fig. 22.3c)

- EUS was performed with a dedicated EUS scope. A relatively uniformly low-echoic tumor located in the second and the third layer was identified. The submucosal layer was thinned, but without apparent invasion, the depth of invasion was diagnosed as SM massive.

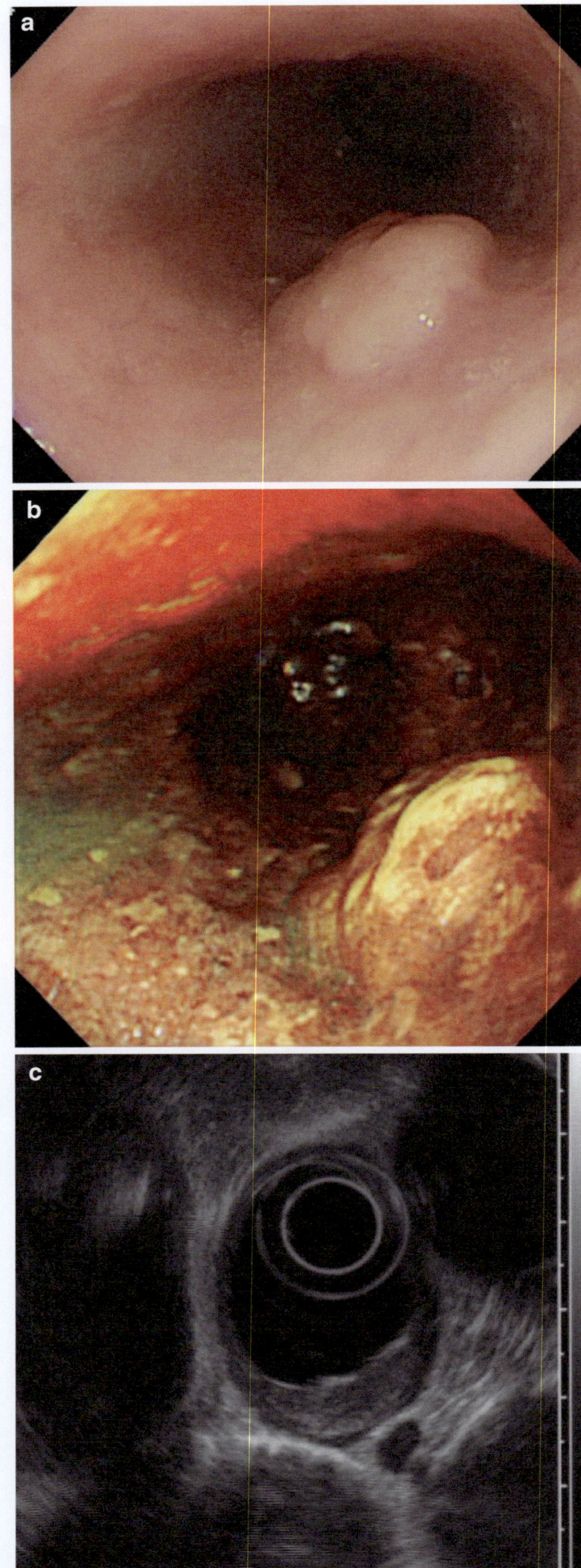

Fig. 22.3 Same images as Fig. 22.2

Histopathological Image of Biopsies Obtained with EUS (Fig. 22.3d)

- Boring biopsies obtained from the iodine dye-unstained area showed proliferating abnormal epithelial cells with an increased N/C ratio (suggestive of basal cell carcinoma or adenoid cystic carcinoma). Chest and abdominal CT showed no apparent distant metastases leading to the diagnosis of T1b, N0, M0, cStage I.

On the Day of EUS (Fig. 22.3d)

- A partially depressed area was noted in the oral side of the lesion as the result of the biopsies.

Let's Observe with Magnifying NBI

- The oral side of the lesion was observed with loop forming blood vessels, without dilation, tortuosity, caliber variation, or uneven shapes (Fig. 22.3e).
- On the anal side, a faintly brownish area was noted. Observation with higher magnification revealed non-loop-forming tortuous blood vessels (Fig. 22.3f).

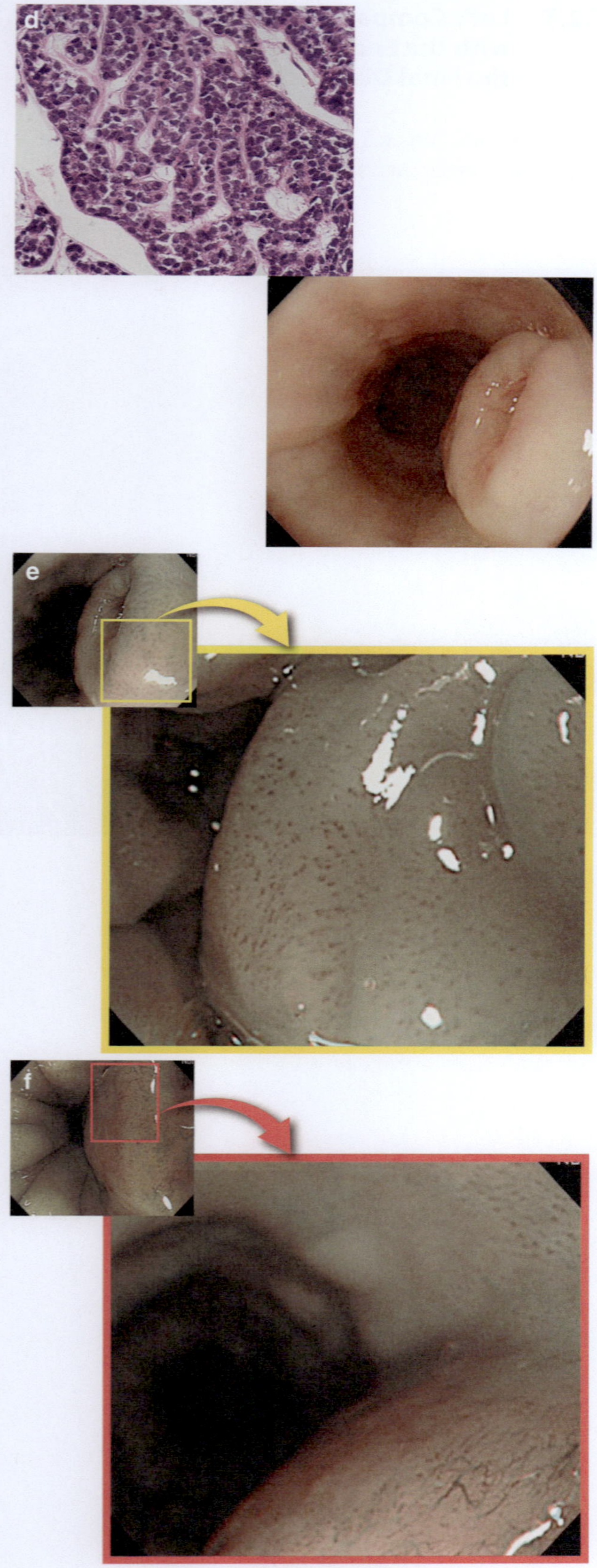

Fig. 22.3 (continued)

22.3 Let's Compare the Resected Specimen with the Endoscopic Images Towards the Final Diagnosis

The lesion was resected en bloc by ESD as shown on the left side and was sectioned as shown on the right side (Fig. 22.4).

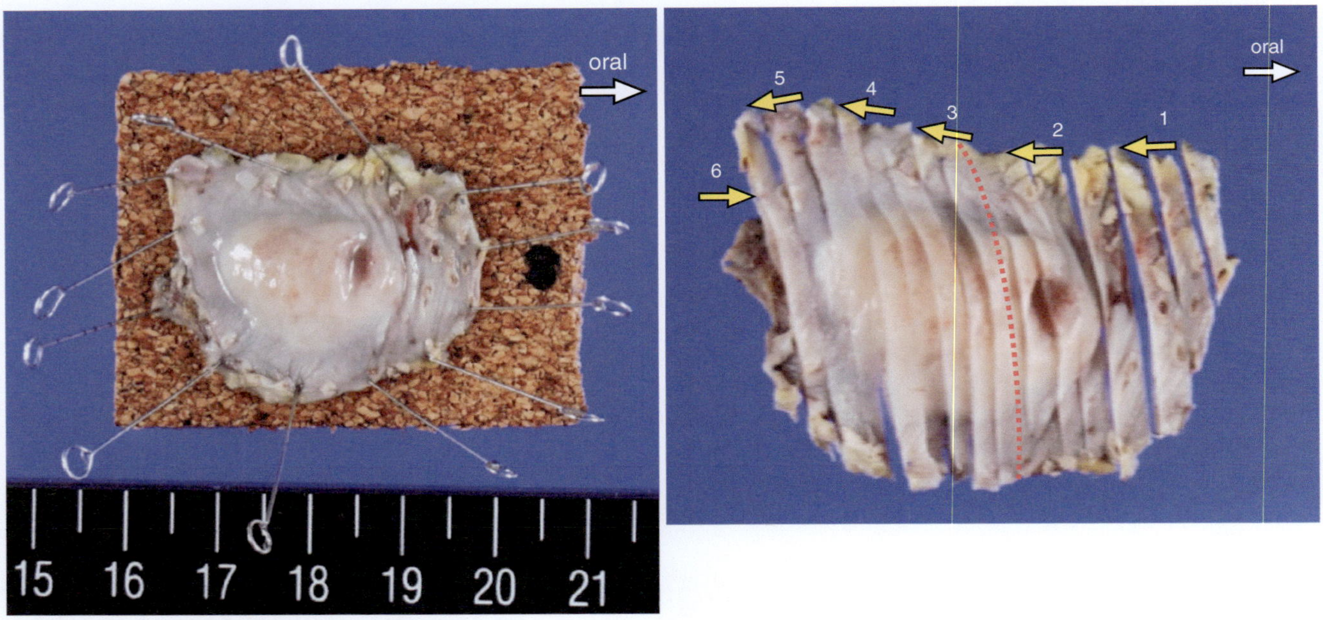

Fig. 22.4 Fleshly resected specimen of the lesion

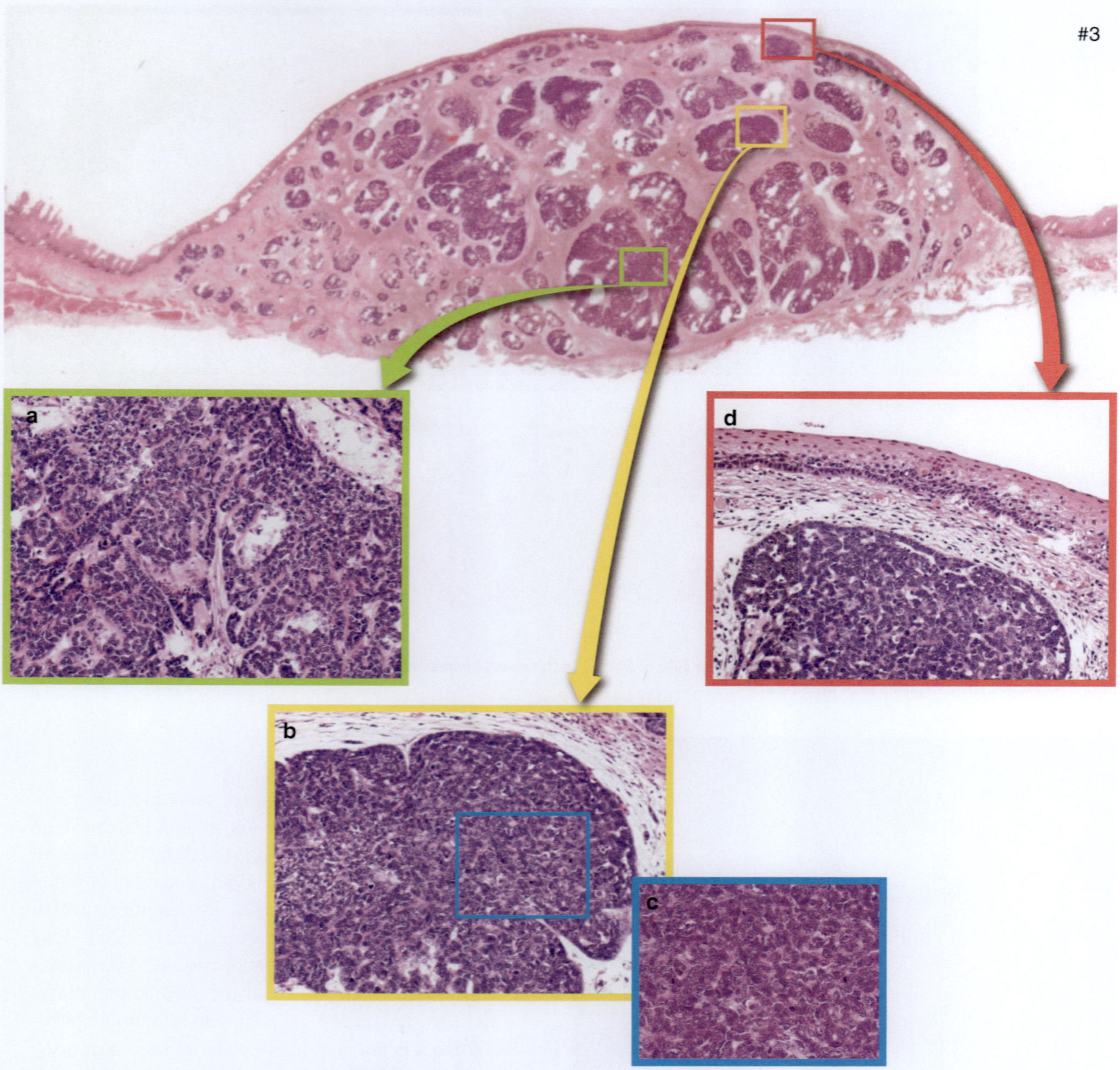

Fig. 22.5 (**a**) Focused image in which surrounded by green square. Multiple locations within tumor nests showed depositions of glass-like (basement membrane-like) materials. Also, immunostaining to differentiate from adenoid cystic carcinoma, S-100 staining, vimentin staining, and a-SMA staining was negative, showing no myoepithelial cells. Based on these findings, the lesion was diagnosed as basaloid squamous cell carcinoma. (**b**) Focused image in which surrounded by yellow square. Tumor cells similar to the cells of the basement membrane with increased N/C ratio were noted to form proliferating solid tumor nests. (**c**) The image in which surrounded by blue square in (**b**). Tumor cells contained increased amount of delicate chromatins with small nucleoli. (**d**) Focused image surrounded by red square. Most of the surface was covered with nontumor squamous cell epithelium

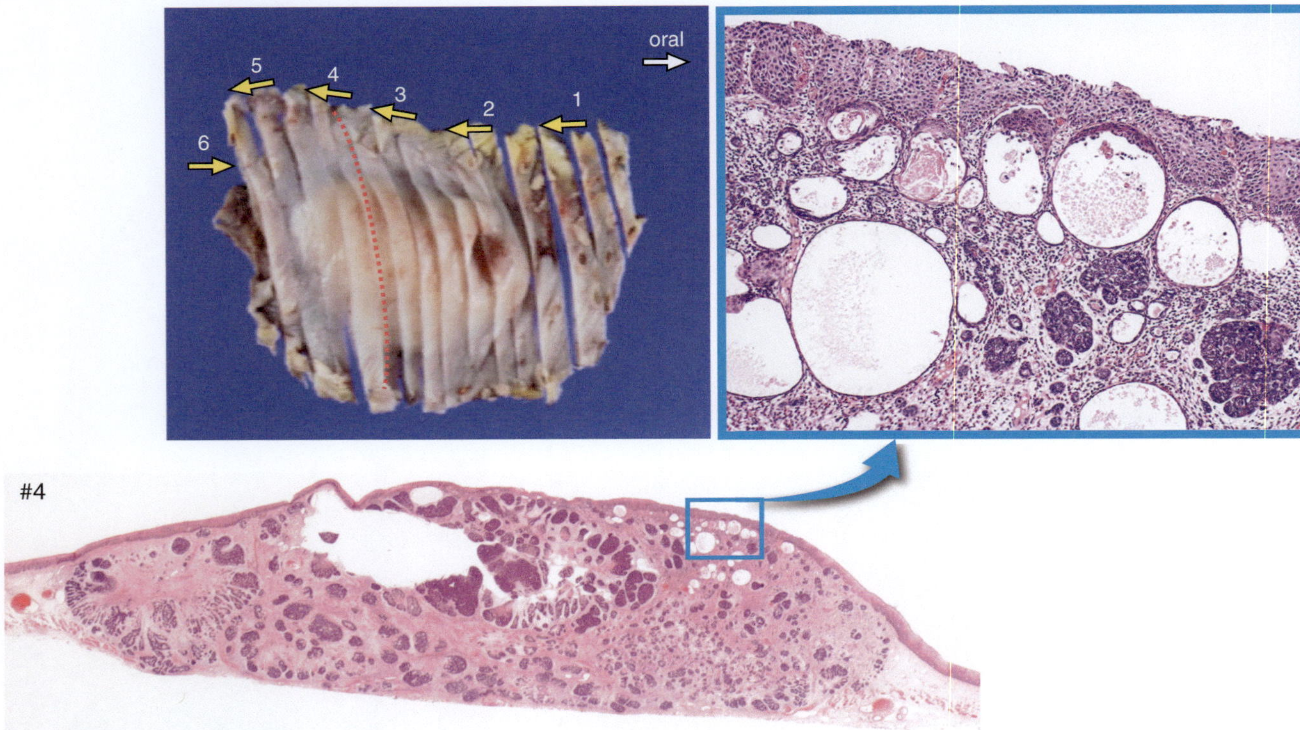

Fig. 22.6 Histopathological images on the right upper side of Sect. 4 in the resected specimen in which surrounded by blue square. A part of the tumor was noted to be exposed near the surface

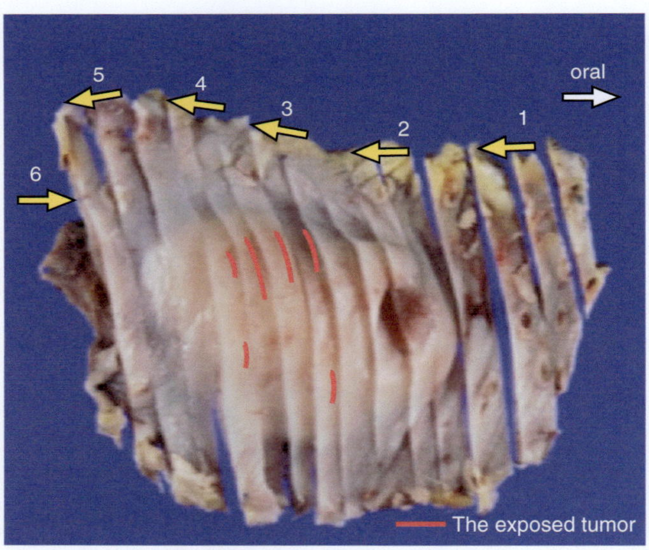

Fig. 22.7 Mapping of the cancer distribution projected on the freshly resected specimen

Conclusive Diagnosis (Fig. 22.7)
Basaloid squamous cell carcinoma (BSCC), 0-Is, T1b-SM2 or deeper, INFb, ly(-), v(-), IM0, HM0, VMX (the tumor was seen to be exposed to the deep resection surface), 20x14mm, Mt, Lt.

Summary
Superficial-type tumors often are smoothly rising submucosal tumors. The surface is smooth covered with nontumor epithelium, accompanied by erosions or depressions at the top. Depending on a case, observation of a tumor exposed area by magnifying NBI makes diagnosis possible. Advanced cancers may present with various forms accompanied by erosions or ulcers on the surface, with the surrounding elevations characteristically covered with nontumor epithelia. When it is not possible to make a diagnose, boring biopsies or EUS-FNA may confirm a diagnosis. It is important to decide on treatment strategies based on comprehensive evaluations utilizing contrast-enhanced studies or EUS.

22.4 Answer

The correct histological type is (3) basaloid cell carcinoma.

The patient is surviving with no recurrence approximately 6 years since ESD.

23 Question 8: What Is the Histological Type?

Takaaki Kishino

T. Kishino (✉)
Department of Gastroenterology, Nara City Hospital Center for Digestive Diseases, Nara, Japan

T. Oyama (ed.), *Endoscopic Diagnosis of Esophageal Carcinoma for ESD*, https://doi.org/10.1007/978-981-32-9030-3_23

Which Is the Correct Histological Type? (Fig. 23.1)

1. Squamous cell carcinoma
2. Neuroendocrine cell carcinoma
3. Basaloid cell carcinoma

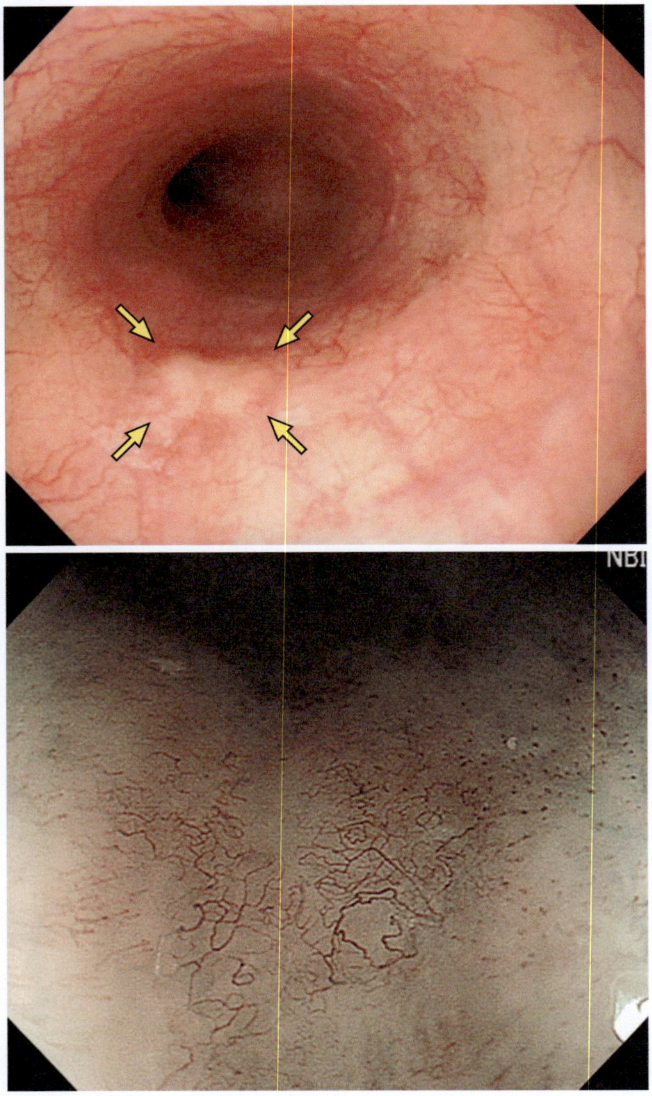

Fig. 23.1 What is the histological type?

23.1 Let's Look at These Six Images and Think (Fig. 23.2)

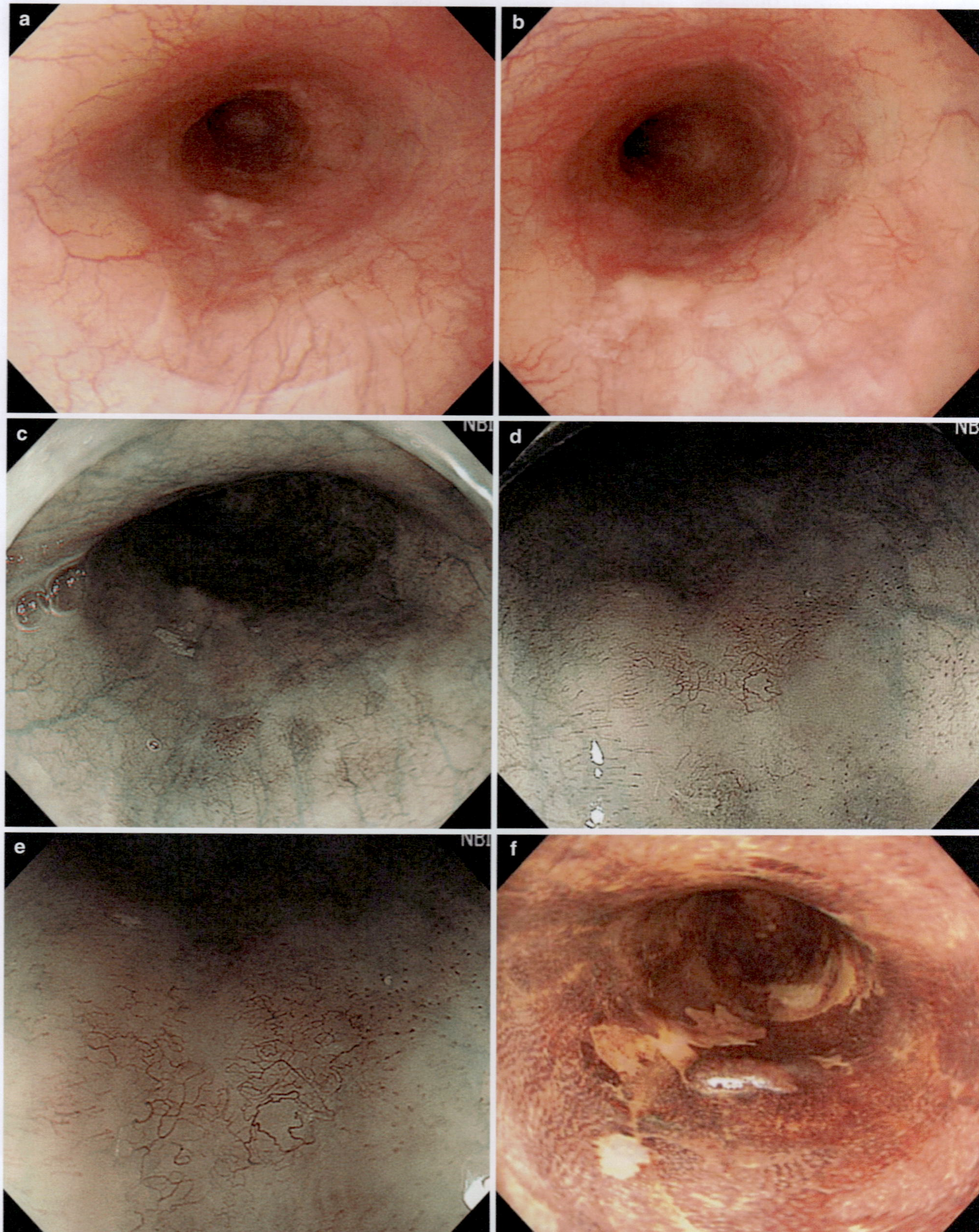

Fig. 23.2 Explanations start from the next page

23.2 Let's Observe the Following Six Images Carefully (Fig. 23.3)

Let's Note Vascular Visibility and Color Tone (Fig. 23.3a)

- There was an area of decreased vascular visibility (indicated in white triangles).
- To the left side, a small reddish area (the yellow arrow) and a faded colored flat raised lesion (the blue arrow) were noted.

Let's Observe the Surface Properties (Fig. 23.3b)

- The flat raised lesion showed a smooth surface with gradual rising.
- The anal side of the flat raised lesion showed a coarse area located in the posterior wall and the right wall.

Let's Observe with Non-magnifying NBI (Fig. 23.3c)

- The area noted with decreased vascular visibility by white light imaging was noted as a brownish area (BA).
- The reddish area noted by white light imaging showed dilated blood vessels (the yellow arrow). The flat raised lesion was noted as a faintly brownish area (the blue arrow).

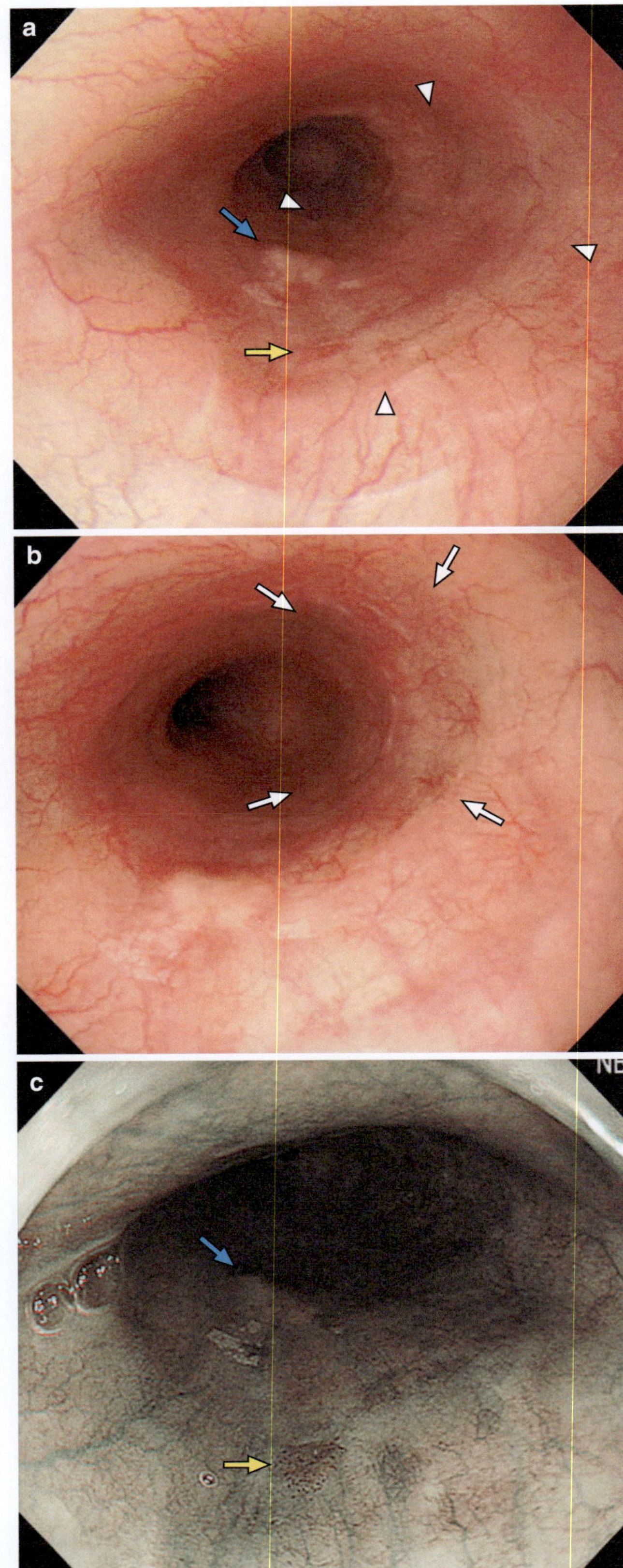

Fig. 23.3 Same images as Fig. 23.2

Let's Observe with Intermediate-Magnification NBI (Fig. 23.3d)

- With intermediate-magnification NBI, the top part of the flat raised lesion showed non-loop-forming blood vessels.
- To the right side of the flat raised lesion, dot-like dilated blood vessels were noted.

Let's Observe with High-Power-Magnification NBI (Fig. 23.3e)

- The top part of the flat raised lesion showed irregularly branching and traversing dilated non-loop-forming abnormal blood vessels consistent with Type R blood vessels.

Let's Observe with Iodine Dye Staining (Fig. 23.3f)

- Note: The raised area marked by the green arrow was a hematoma caused when observing with magnification NBI.
- The small reddish area noted by white light imaging was unstained by iodine as marked by the yellow arrow.
- An unstained area by iodine extended from the top of the flat raised lesion to the right side, but the left wall side stained dark with iodine dye as marked by the blue arrow.
- The anal side of the flat raised lesion showed an area with mixture of iodine dye-unstained and lightly stained areas.

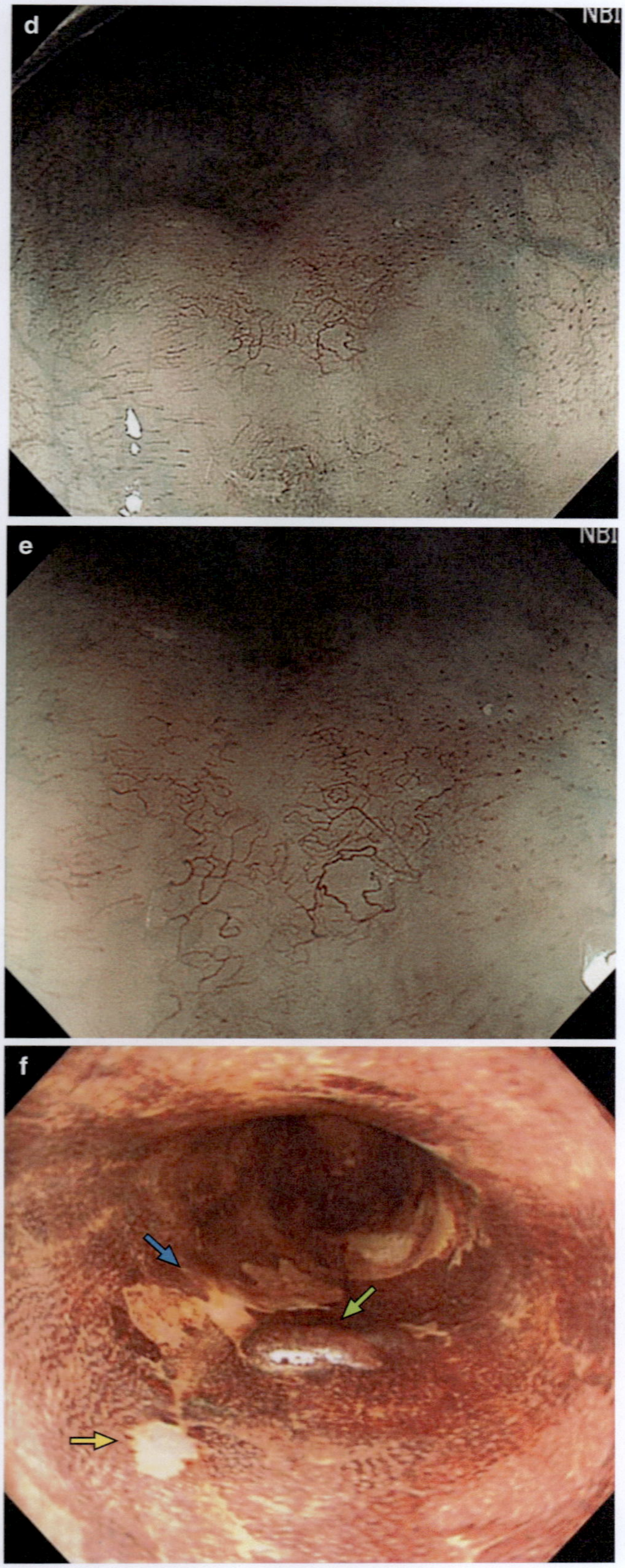

Fig. 23.3 (continued)

23.3 To Confirm the Final Diagnosis, Let's Compare with the Resected Specimen (Fig. 23.4)

The small red area, the flat raised lesion, and the hematoma corresponded with the yellow, the blue, and the green arrows, respectively (Fig. 23.4a–f).

The freshly resected specimen (Fig. 23.4d): The small red area was faintly reddish, and the flat raised part was noted as a whitish elevation.

The fixed resected specimen (Fig. 23.4e): The areas marked by the yellow and the blue arrows showed more distinct demarcations than the freshly resected specimen.

The iodine dye-stained specimen (Fig. 23.4f): The lesion showed geographic unstained to lightly stained parts, and the flat raised part was noted unstained.

Let's Observe the Resected Specimen (Fig. 23.5)

- As shown in the left image, the specimen was rotated and sliced into pathohistological sections.
- The flat raised part was included in the section marked by the yellow dotted line.

Let's Observe the Histopathological Image (Fig. 23.6)

- The histopathological image of the section marked by the yellow dotted line is shown below.
- The flat raised part shows a smoothly rising elevation.

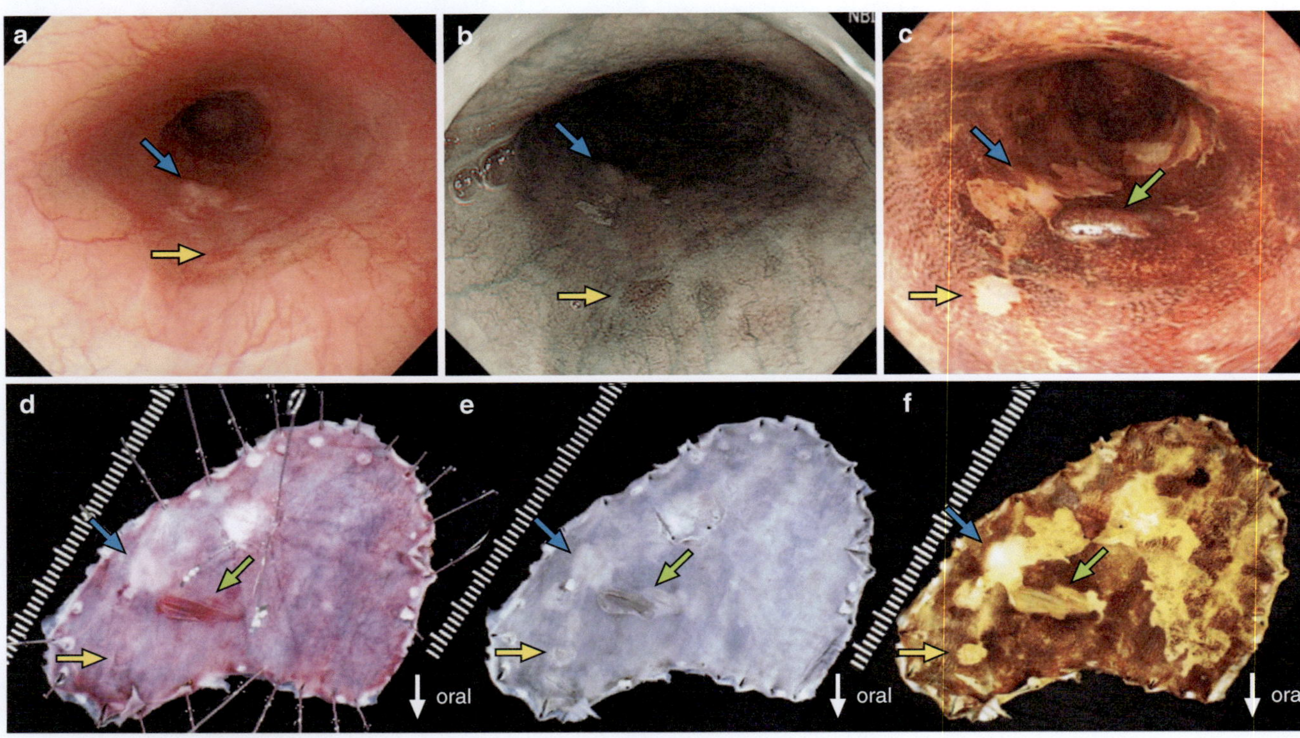

Fig. 23.4 (**a**) White light endoscopic image of the lesion. (**b**) NBI endoscopic image of the lesion. (**c**) Iodine chromoendoscopic image of the lesion. (**d**) Freshly resected specimen of the lesion. (**e**) Fixed resected specimen of the lesion. (**f**) Iodine dye stained specimen of the lesion

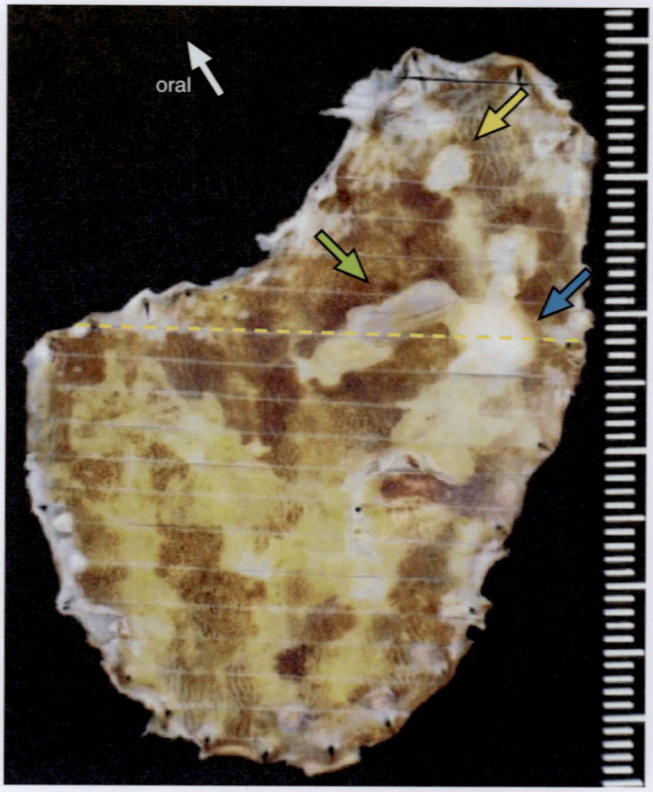

Fig. 23.5 Rotated image of the resected specimen of the lesion

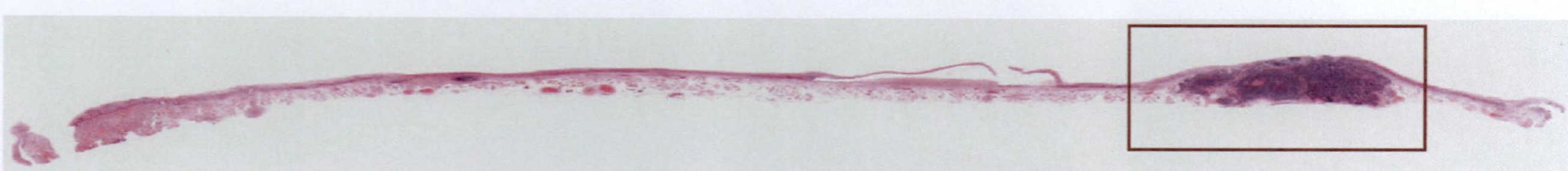

Fig. 23.6 Histopathological image of the resected area indicated with the yellow dotted line on the specimen

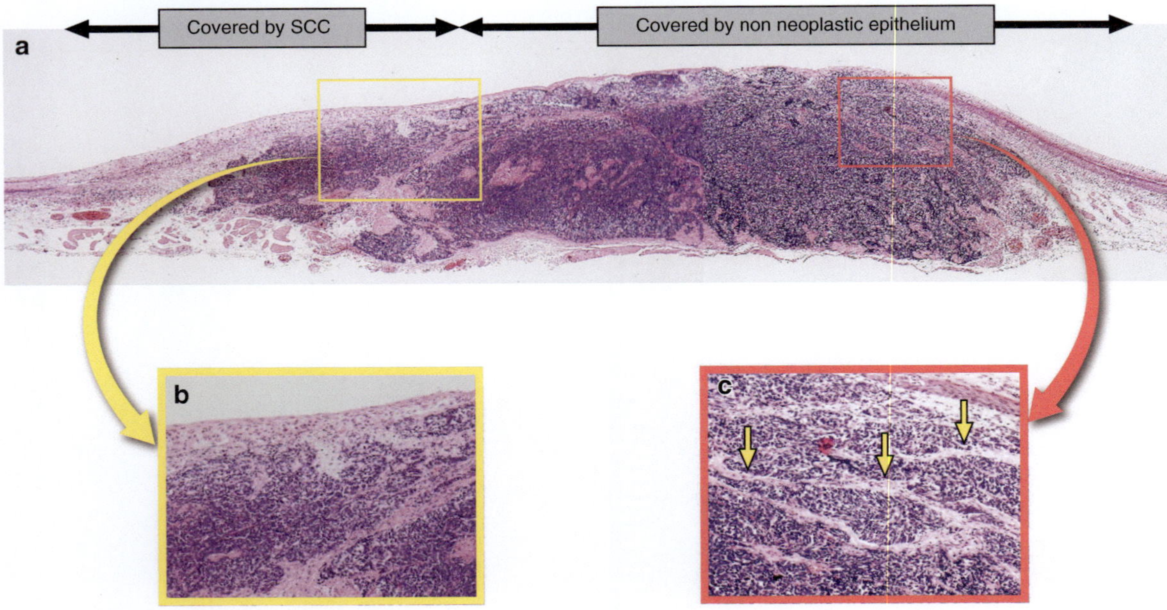

Fig. 23.7 (**a**) The lesion was located mainly within the muscularis mucosa and partly infiltrated the submucosa. The surface was mostly covered by nonneoplastic epithelium, but was partly covered by squamous cell carcinoma with invasion depth of T1a-EP. (**b**) The right wall side of the flat raised area showed squamous cell carcinoma with invasion depth of T1a-EP on the surface. (**c**) With high power magnification, small spindle-shaped tumor cells with high N/C ratio were noted to form solid tumor nests in palisading arrangements. Also, capillary vessels were surrounding the tumor nests in complicated manner as marked by yellow arrows

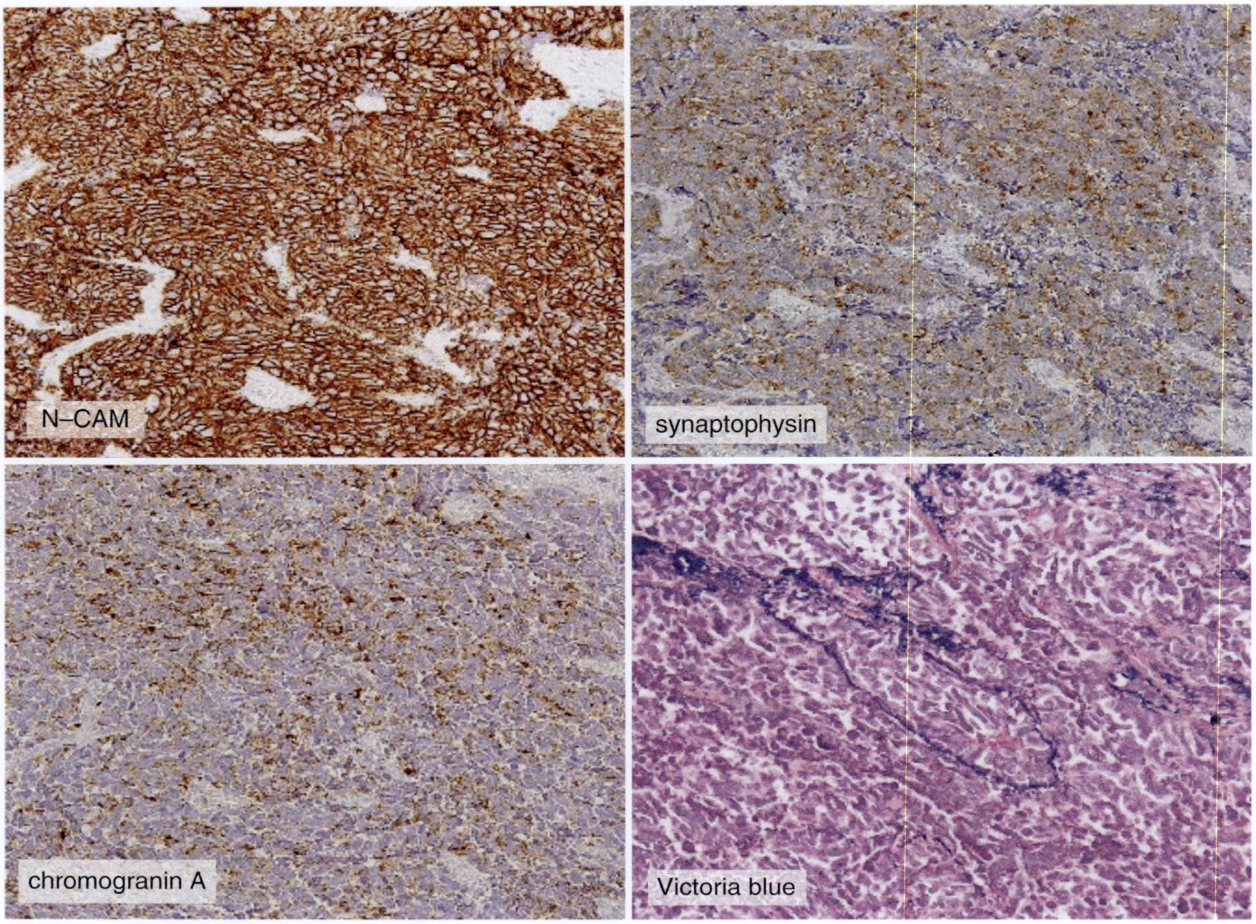

Fig. 23.8 N-CAM-positive, synaptophysin-positive, and chromogranin A-positive tumor cells are diagnosed as endocrine cell carcinoma. Lymphovascular invasions were evaluated by D2-40 and VB immunostains and were found to be ly(–) and v(+)

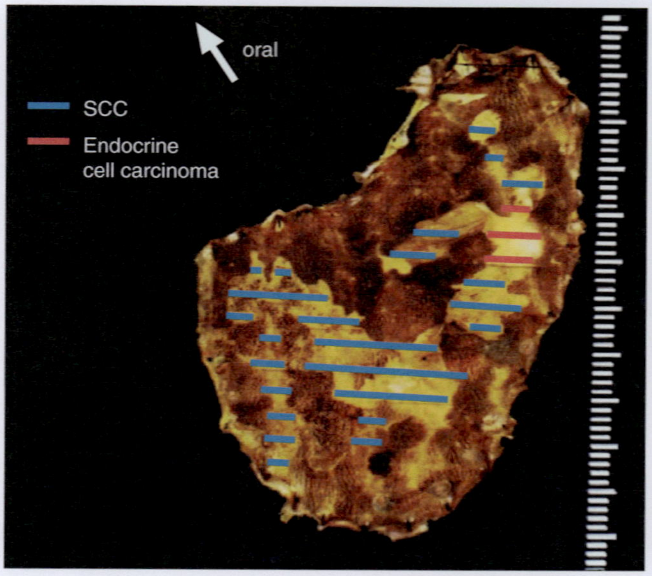

Fig. 23.9 Mapping of the cancer distribution projected on the resected specimen

Conclusive Diagnosis
Endocrine cell carcinoma associated with squamous cell carcinoma, 0-IIa+IIb, T1b-SM2 (250μm), INFb, ly(-), v(+), HM0, VM0, 59x35mm, pCurC, Mt, Post (Fig. 23.9).

Summary
Magnifying NBI of the top of the flat raised part showed Type R blood vessels, thought to reflect the subepithelial capillary networks surrounding the tumor nests. Histologically, Type R vessels are often noted in association with poorly differentiated squamous cell carcinoma or lesions with INFc infiltrative patterns. As endocrine cell carcinoma resembles histologically poorly differentiated squamous cell carcinoma, vascular patterns likely have resembled as well.

23.4 Answer

The correct histological type is (2) neuroendocrine carcinoma.

24 Question 9: What Is the Histological Type?

Kotaro Shibagaki

K. Shibagaki (✉)
Department of Endoscopic Diagnosis and Therapeutics, Shimane University School of Medicine Hospital, Matsue, Shimane, Japan
e-mail: shibagaki@zb.wakwak.com

T. Oyama (ed.), *Endoscopic Diagnosis of Esophageal Carcinoma for ESD*, https://doi.org/10.1007/978-981-32-9030-3_24

Which Is the Correct Histological Type? (Fig. 24.1)

1. Squamous cell carcinoma
2. Special-type esophageal carcinoma
3. Adenocarcinoma

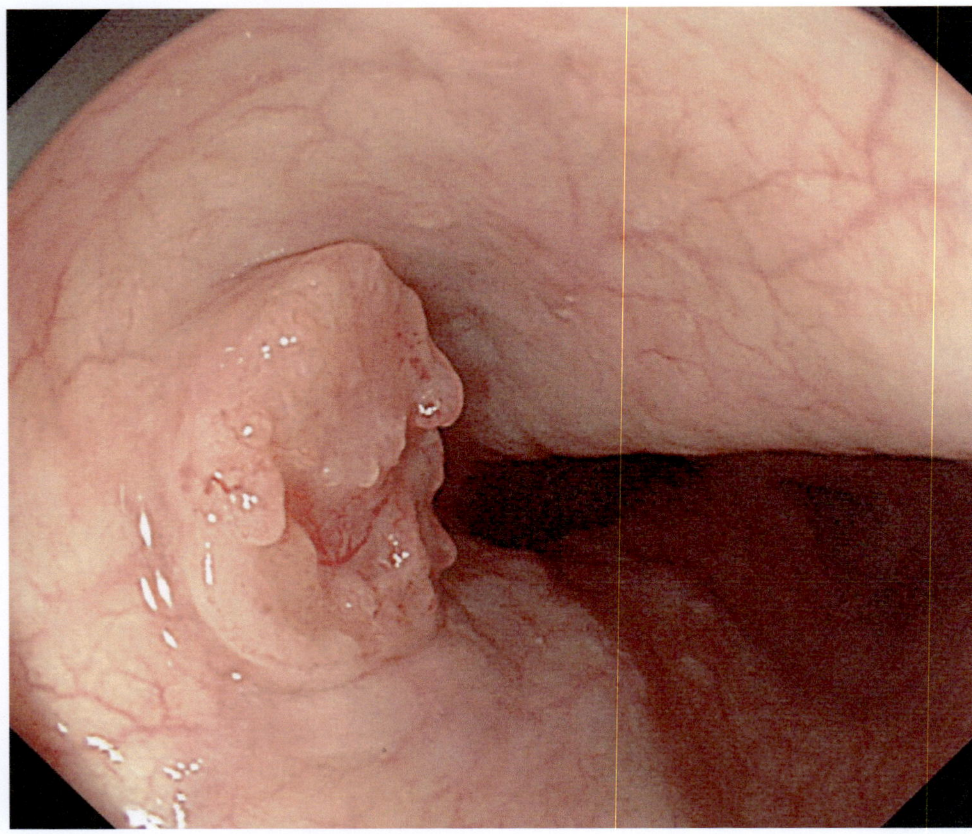

Fig. 24.1 What is the histological type?

24.1 Let's Look at These Six Images and Think (Fig. 24.2)

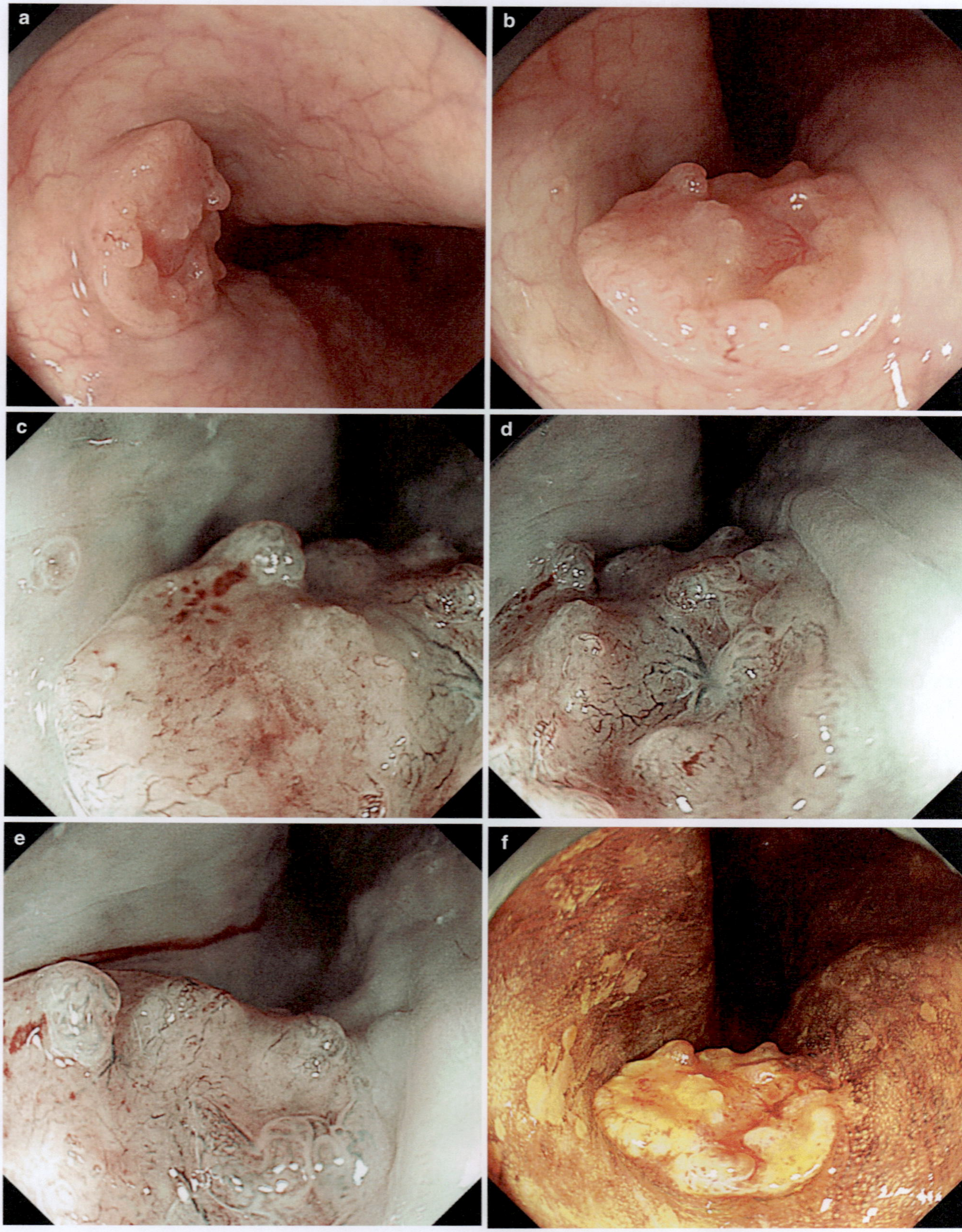

Fig. 24.2 Explanations start from the next page

24.2 Let's Observe the Following Six Images Careful (Fig. 24.3)

Let's Observe the Lesion Shape (Fig. 24.3a)

- There was a pinkish thick raised lesion on the left wall of the second physiological esophageal narrowing in the mid-thoracic esophagus.
- The lesion did not bend by the esophageal narrowing showing itself as a lesion with firmness.
- The raised lesion was irregularly shaped with a distinct rise and irregularly uneven surface supporting the diagnosis of cancer.

Let's Observe the Lesion Closely for Its Surface Properties and Its Rise (Fig. 24.3b)

- On close-up observation, the surface of the raised lesion show multiple small nodules and dilated blood vessels in the right wall side.
- The rising part of the lesion was covered with non-tumor epithelium as marked by the yellow arrows and had an SMT-like appearance.
- Based on these, the lesion was diagnosed as having submucosally infiltrating cancer.

What Should Be Done Next?

- The tumor should be evaluated for its depth of invasion and histological type with magnifying NBI.

Let's Observe with Magnifying NBI the Left Wall Side of the Lesion? (Fig. 24.3c)

- The tumor had brownish color tone with very sparse vascular density only showing dendritic blood vessels extending from the tumor base beneath the non-tumor epithelium.

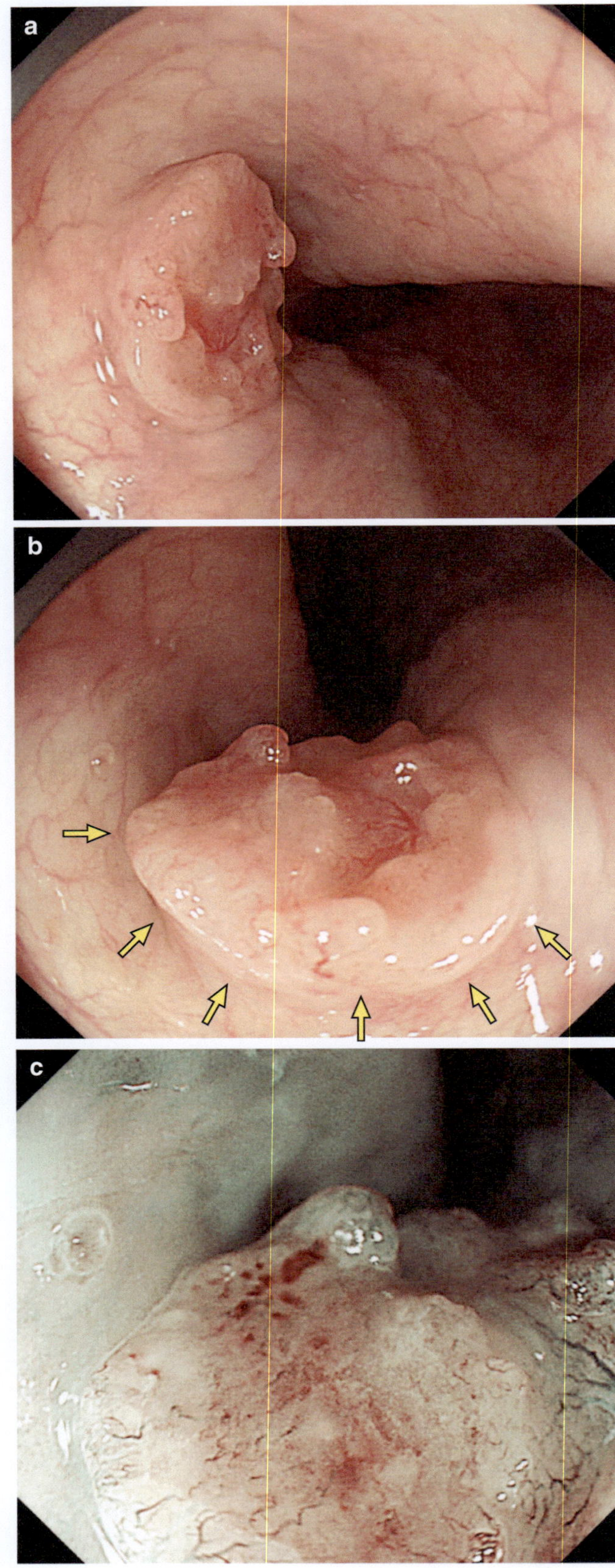

Fig. 24.3 Same images as Fig. 24.2

Let's Observe with Magnifying NBI the Right Wall Side of the Lesion (Fig. 24.3d)

- A prominently dilated dendritic blood vessel was noted, marked by the white dotted circle. The base of the blood vessel had cyan color tone, and the branch ends brown color tone. It was evident that the blood vessel extended from the deeper base to the surface.

Let's Observe with Magnifying NBI the Anal Side of the Lesion (Fig. 24.3e)

- The depressed area surrounded by the yellow arrows did not clearly show SMT-like rising at its base and appeared thinner suggesting a possibility of mucosal cancer.
- The surface structure was unclear; blood vessels were sparsely seen, with only occasional dendritic blood vessels.
- Based on magnifying NBI findings, well-differentiated squamous cell carcinoma and adenocarcinoma were thought unlikely, and the lesion, noted with a SMT-like rise and no apparent intraepithelial extension, was suspected to be a special-type esophageal carcinoma, or poorly differentiated squamous cell carcinoma.

Let's Observe with Iodine Dye Staining to Determine Intraepithelial Extension (Fig. 24.3f)

- The tumor became an unstained area with pink color positivity, and its base was covered with non-tumor epithelium.
- Small iodine dye unstained areas were noted surrounding the tumor, but without continuity with the main lesion and without recognizable intraepithelial extensions.
- Based on above, special-type esophageal carcinoma with the invasion depth of SM or deeper was diagnosed.
- PET-CT showed no apparent metastases, and EUS showed remaining submucosal layer beneath the tumor. Because of significantly high risk of surgery, ESD was performed.

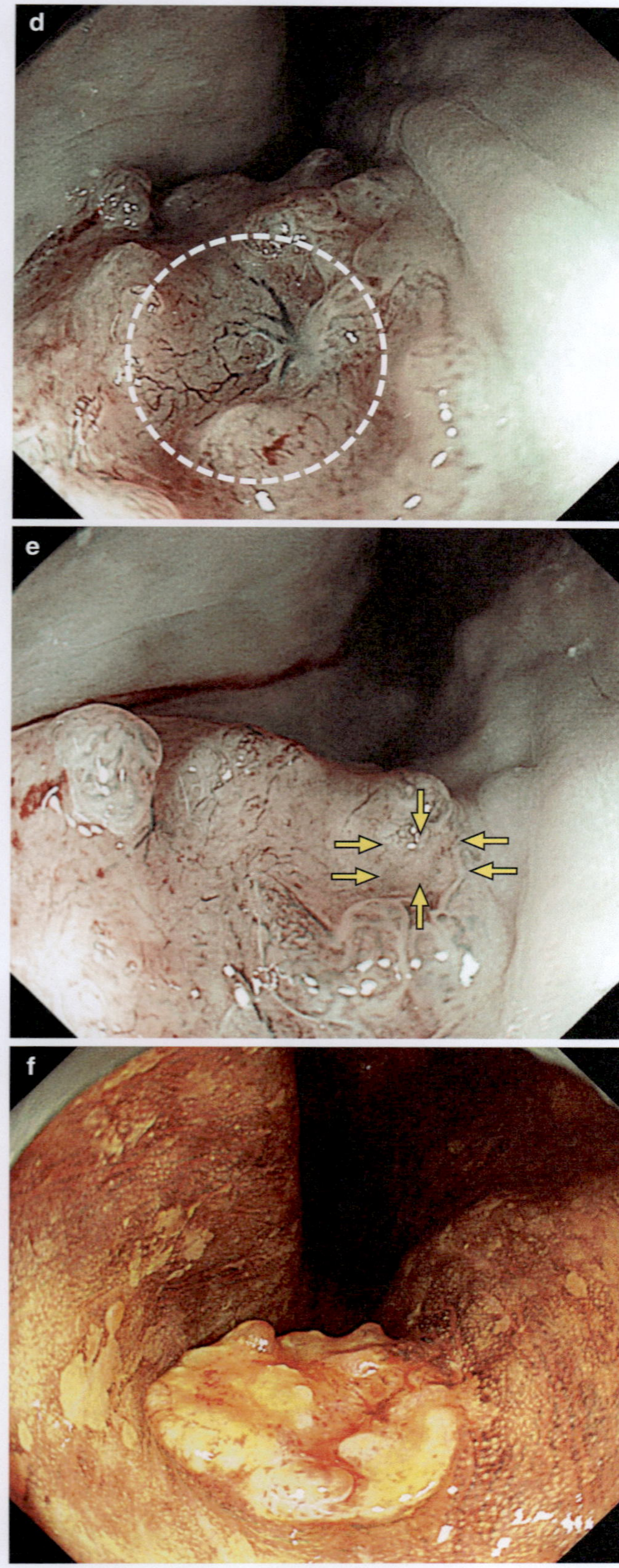

Fig. 24.3 (continued)

24.3 Let's Compare the Resected Specimen with the Endoscopic Images Towards the Final Diagnosis

Let's Observe the Fixed Resected Specimen (Fig. 24.4)

- An irregularly shaped base-like lesion with a clearly rising rim and coarse surface with small nodules were noted.

Let's Observe the Iodine Dye-Stained Specimen (Fig. 24.5)

- The lesion was noted as a clearly demarcated and irregularly shaped unstained area, and no surrounding unstained areas to suggest intraepithelial extensions were noted.

Let's Observe the Histopathological Image

- The tumor showed submucosally expanding growth, but the lesion was resected free of vertical margin involvement. (Fig. 24.6a)
- (Sect. 5, ×100) Sheet-like proliferations of tumor cells were noted without apparent keratinization, and the lesion was diagnosed as poorly differentiated squamous cell carcinoma (Fig. 24.6b).
- (Sect. 8, left front part, ×100) The anal side of the tumor showed intramucosal tumor component (MM) of poorly differentiated squamous cell carcinoma (Fig. 24.6c).

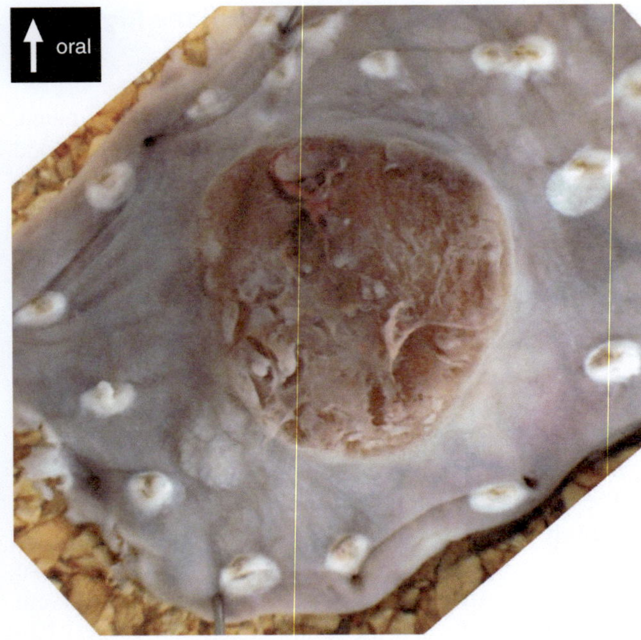

Fig. 24.4 Resected fixed specimen of the lesion

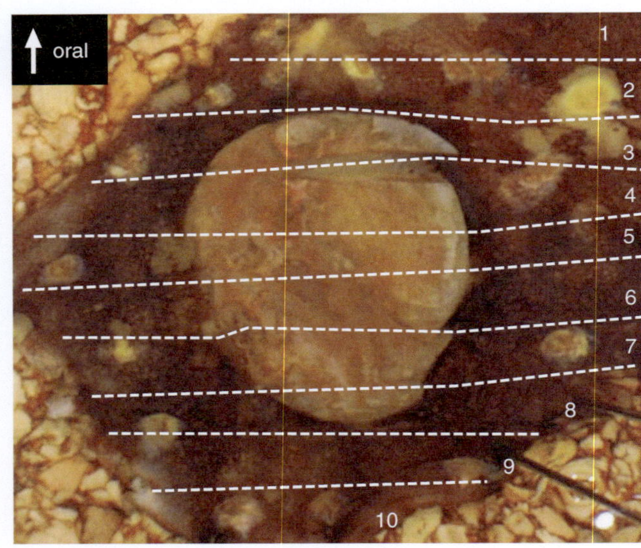

Fig. 24.5 The specimen after staining with iodine

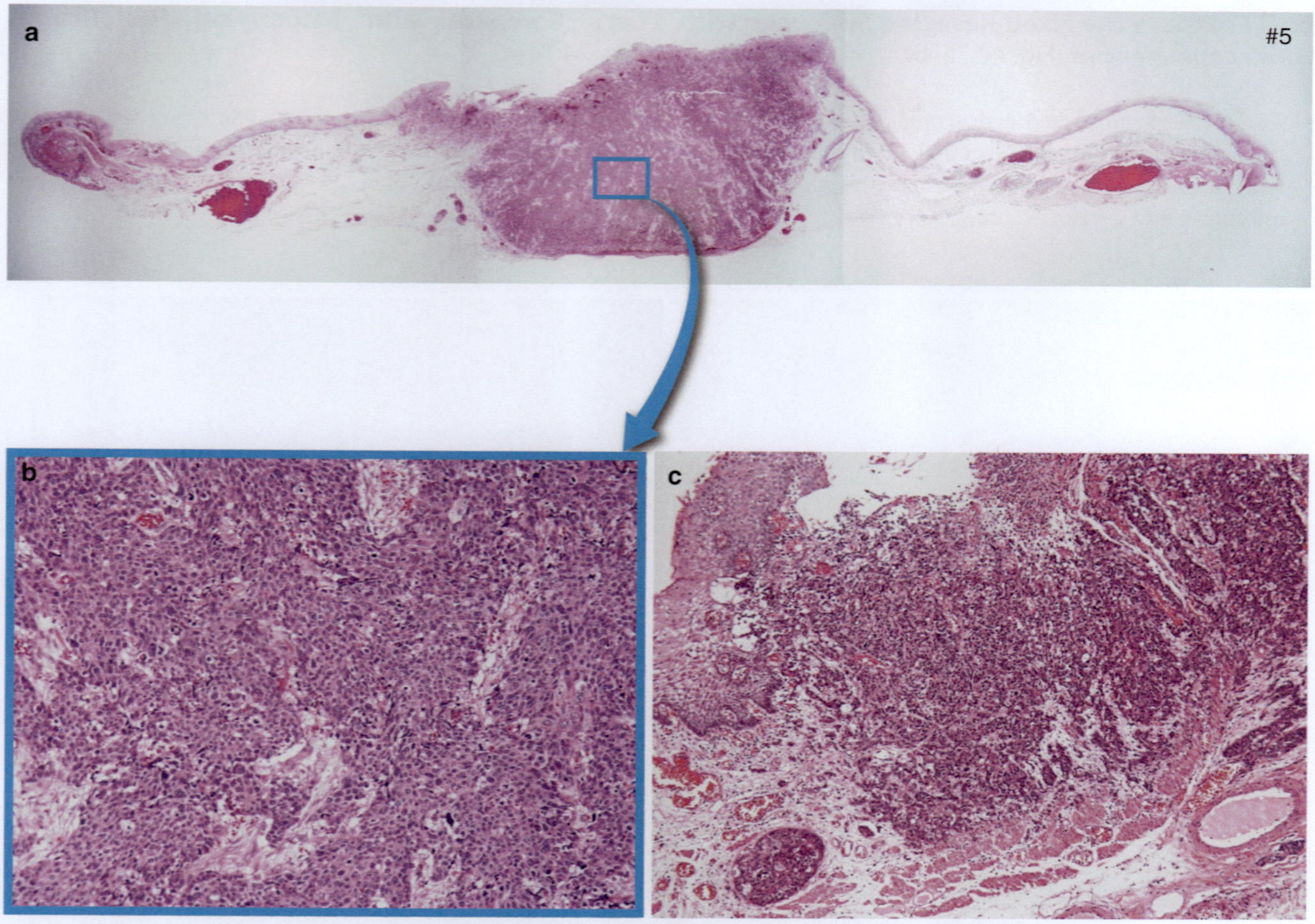

Fig. 24.6 (**a**) Histopathological image of Sect. 5 in the resected specimen in Fig. 24.5. (**b**) Magnified image of the area indicated in blue square. (c) Magnified histopathological image of Sect. 8, left front part in Fig.24.5

Let's Compare the Fixed Resected Specimen with Endoscopic Images (Fig. 24.7a, b)

- The fixed specimen and endoscopic white light imaging were compared with each other and were compared further with magnifying NBI images of the areas marked with a red square and a green square.

Let's Compare with Magnifying NBI Images (Fig. 24.7c, d)

- The thick areas with sparsely visible blood vessels were all poorly differentiated squamous cell carcinoma with submucosal invasion.

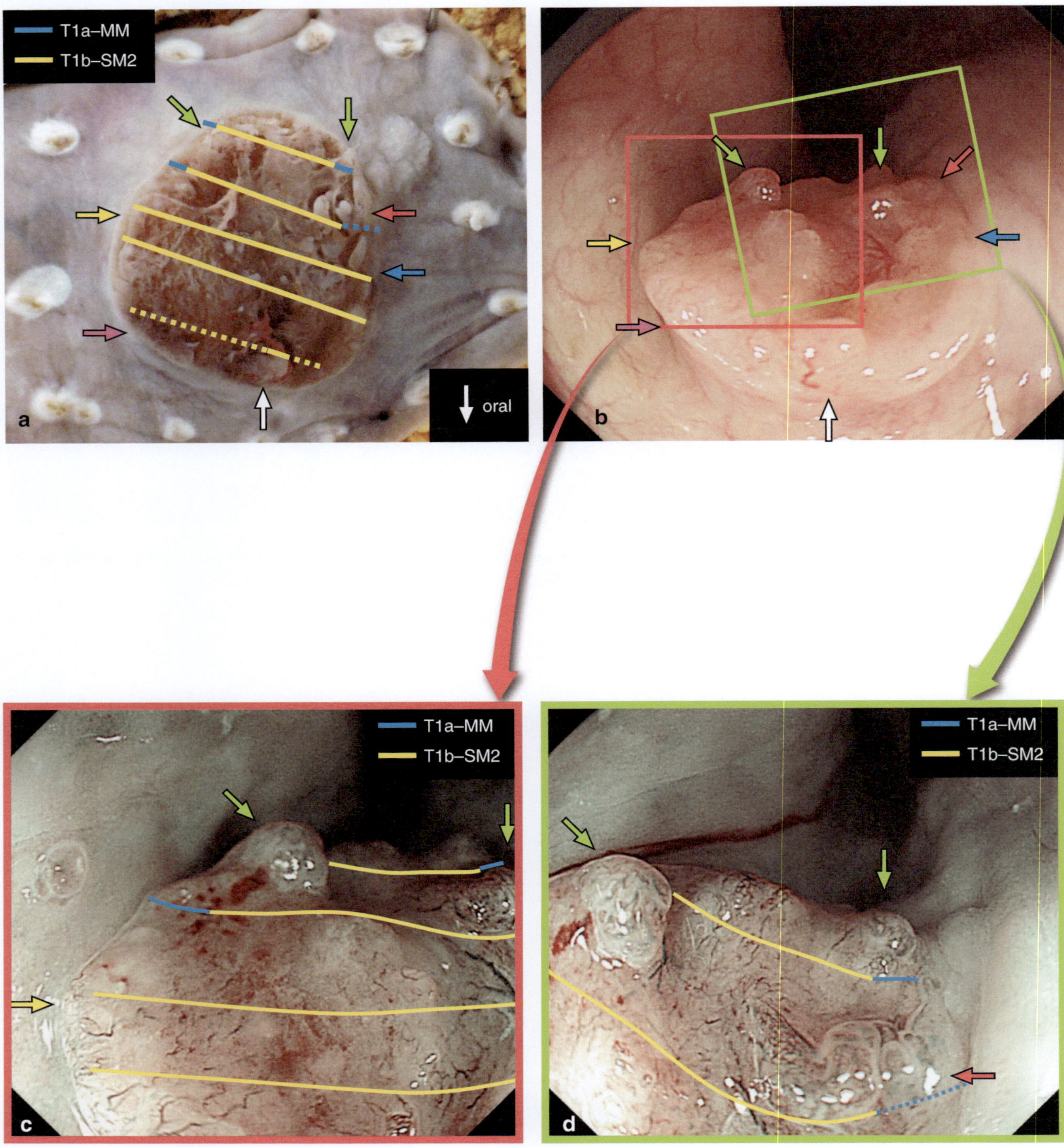

Fig. 24.7 Mapping of the cancer distribution projected on the fixed resected specimen. Comparison of the fixed specimen and the endoscopic image and NBI magnified endoscopic image of the lesion

- The areas with sparse vascularity, lost thickness of the depressed lesion, and lost SMT-like elevation at the base showed intramucosal cancer components.

Conclusive Diagnosis
Esophageal squamous cell carcinoma, poorly differentiated, 0-Is, T1b-SM2(4,000μm), INFa, ly(+), v(+), HM0, VM0, pR0, 14 × 11 mm, Mt, Lt.

Summary
Chemoradiation treatment (FP course, 59.4Gy/33Fr) was added after ESD, and the patient is surviving disease free for 3 years. This case showed at its base the circumferential SMT-like elevation and showed no intraepithelial extension by iodine dye staining or magnifying NBI observations, suggestive of a typical special-type esophageal carcinoma.

24.4 Answer

The correct histological type is (2) special-type esophageal cancer (poorly differentiated squamous cell carcinoma).

Question 10: What Is the Diagnosis?

25

Ryutaro Furukawa

R. Furukawa (✉)
Department of Endoscopic Medicine, Saku Central Hospital
Advanced Care Center, Saku, Japan

T. Oyama (ed.), *Endoscopic Diagnosis of Esophageal Carcinoma for ESD*, https://doi.org/10.1007/978-981-32-9030-3_25

Which Is the Correct Histological Type? (Fig. 25.1)

1. Esophageal carcinoma
2. Papilloma
3. Inflammatory polyp

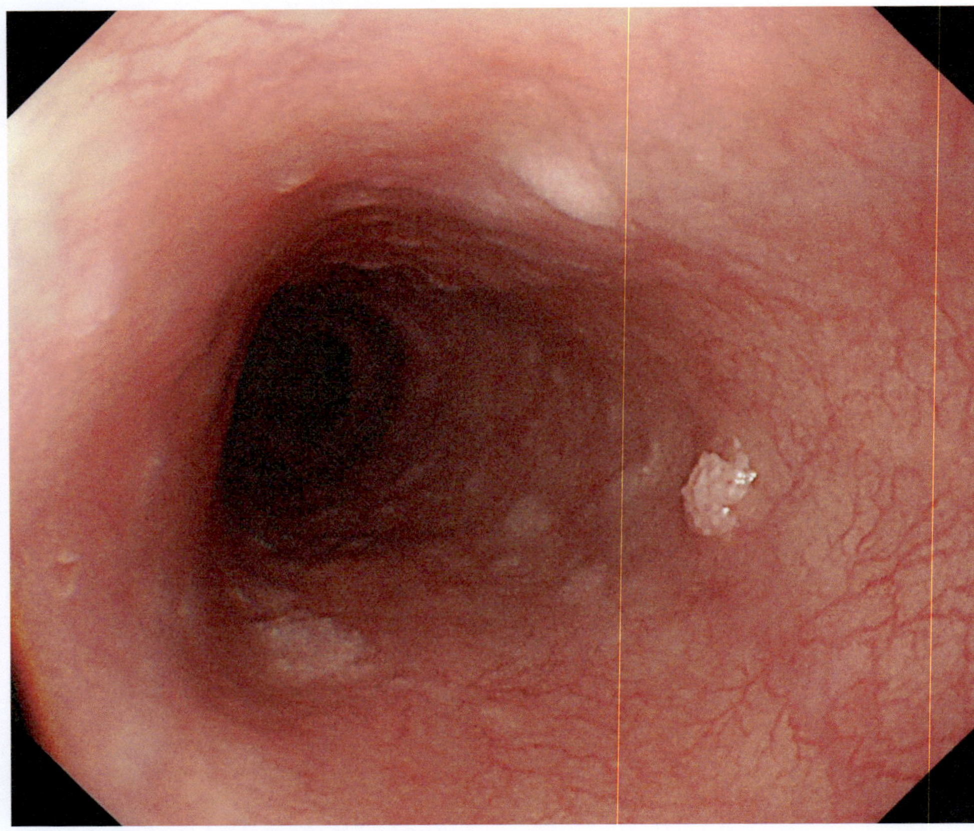

Fig. 25.1 What is the diagnosis?

25.1 Let's Look at These Six Images and Think (Fig. 25.2)

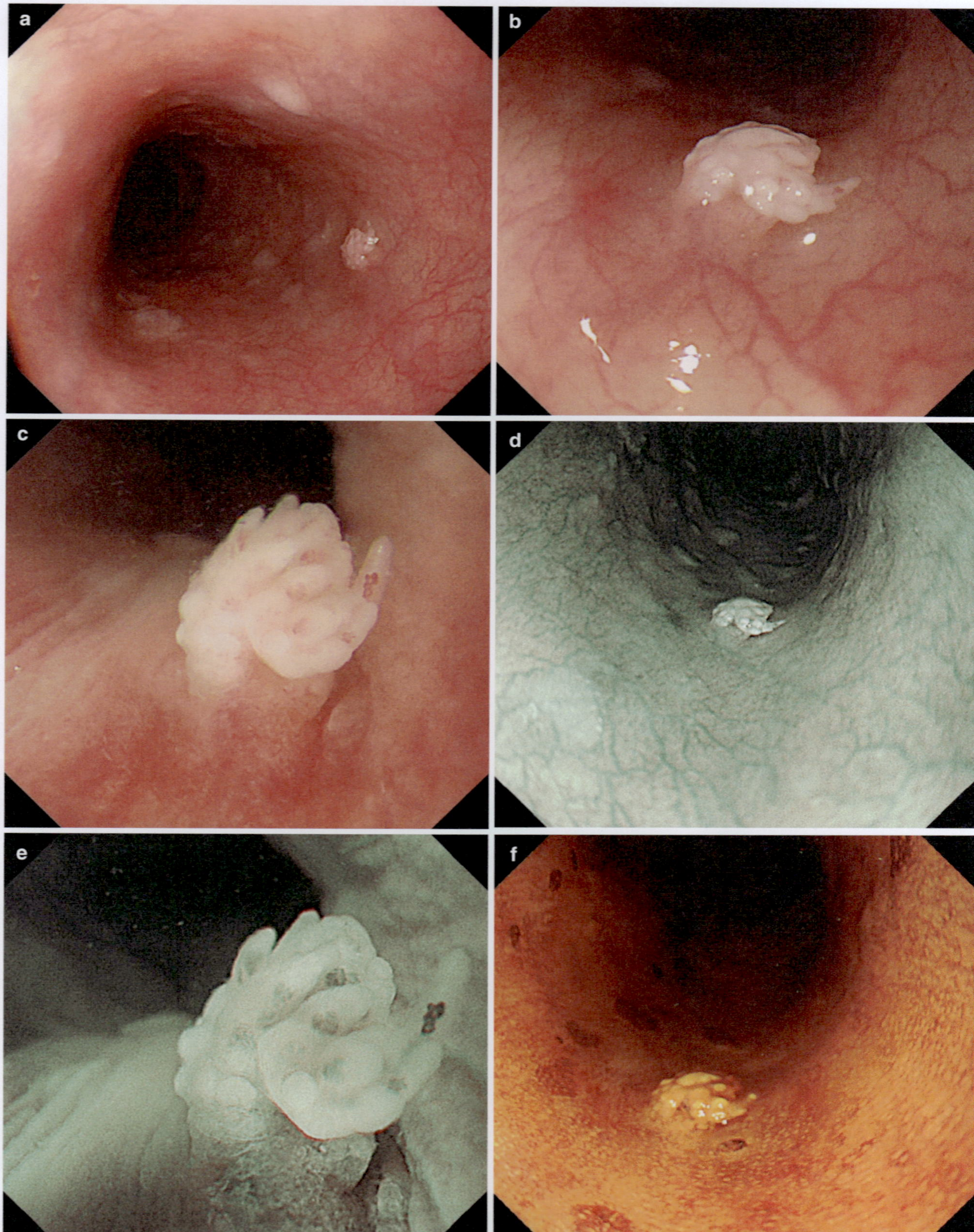

Fig. 25.2 Explanations start from the next page

25.2 Let's Observe the Following Six Images Carefully (Fig. 25.3)

Let's Observe Color Tone and Shape (Fig. 25.3a)

- There was a whitish raised lesion with clear demarcation noted at the right side of the mid-thoracic esophagus.
- The lesion can be differentiated from glycogenic acanthosis observed in the background by difference in shape.

Let's Observe Closely (Fig. 25.3b)

- On close-up observation, the lesion appeared to have mulberry-like form with nodular surface.

Let's Observe with Water Immersion (Fig. 25.3c)

- When observed with water immersion, the mulberry-like form became more distinct and appeared to have a stalk.

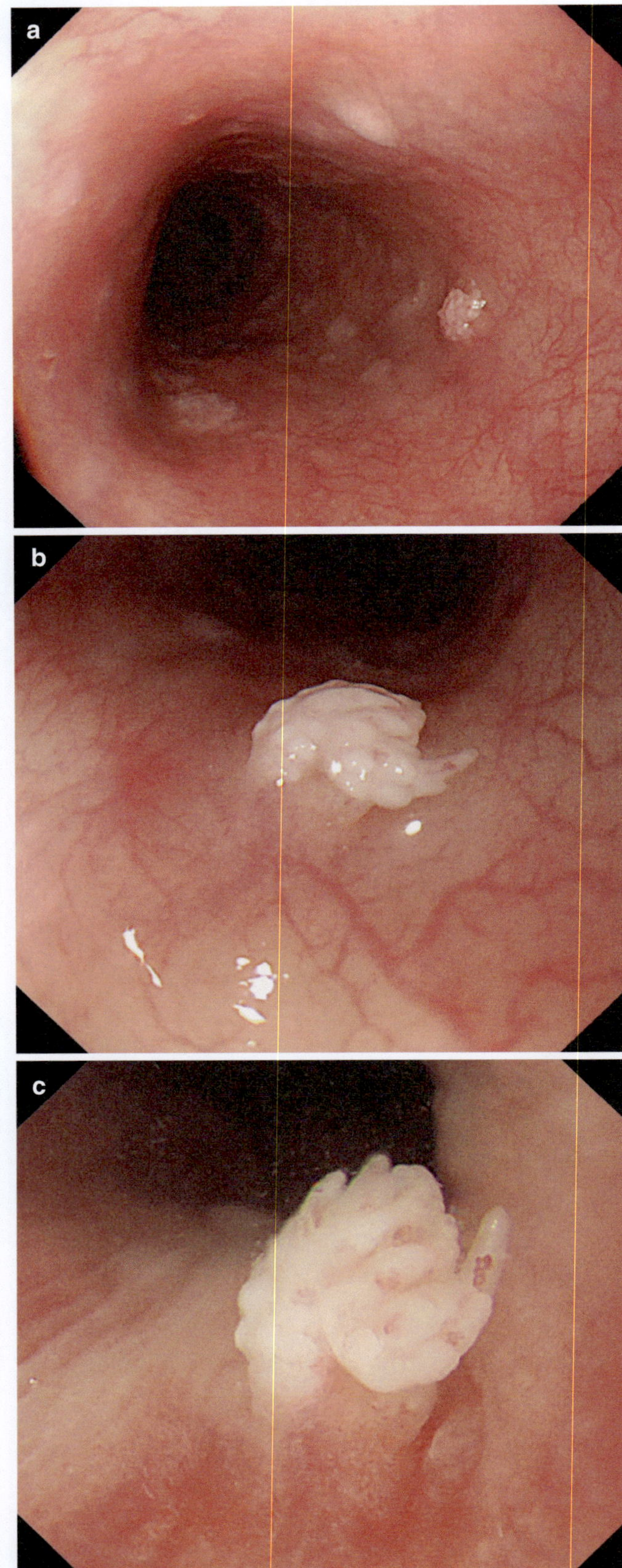

Fig. 25.3 Same images as Fig. 25.2

Let's Observe with NBI (Fig. 25.3d)

- Non-magnifying NBI showed a clearly demarcated whitish elevated lesion.

Let's Observe with Magnifying NBI (Fig. 25.3e)

- When observed with magnifying NBI, papillary protrusions showed microvessels with no irregularities.

Let's Observe with Iodine Dye Staining (Fig. 25.3f)

- The raised lesion became lightly stained with iodine dye.

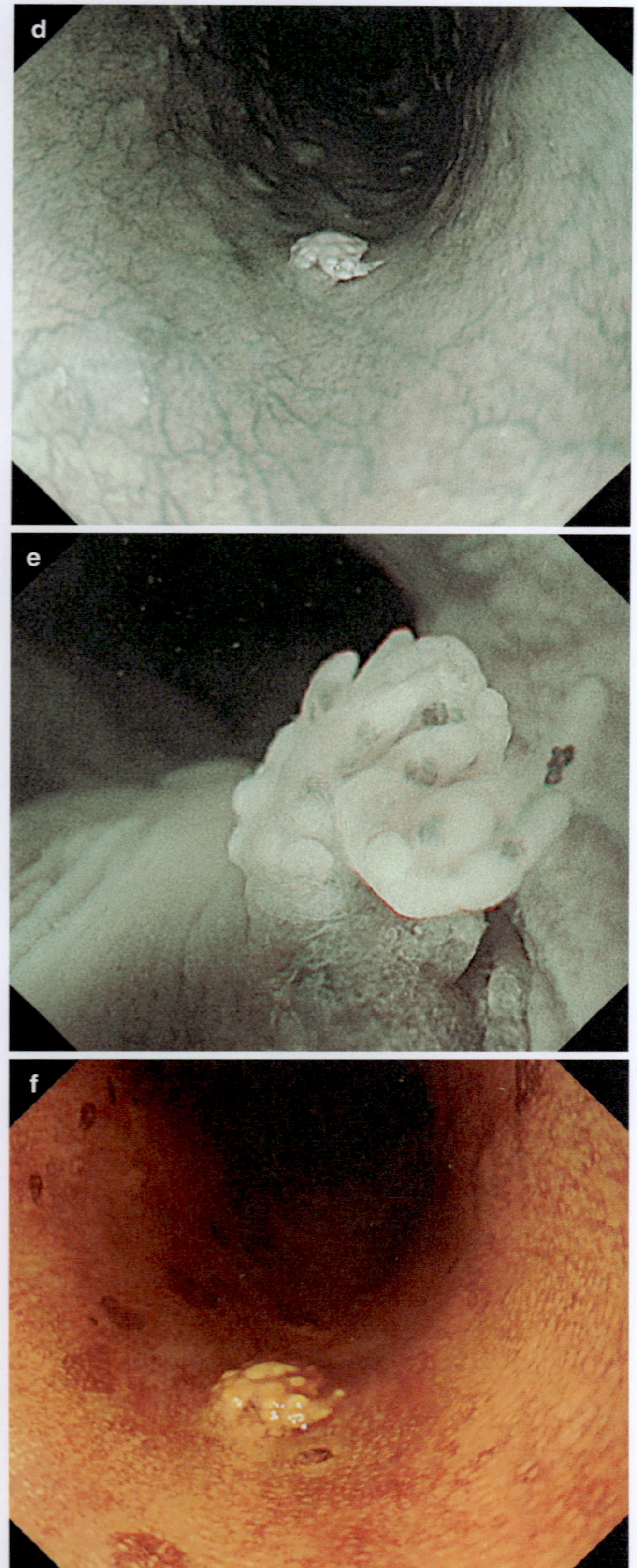

Fig. 25.3 (continued)

25.3 Let's Compare with the Resected Specimen Towards the Final Diagnosis

A biopsy specimen showed squamous cell epithelium without atypia, showing papillary growth around thin cores of interstitial structures including blood vessels (Fig. 25.4).

Conclusive Diagnosis
Esophageal papilloma

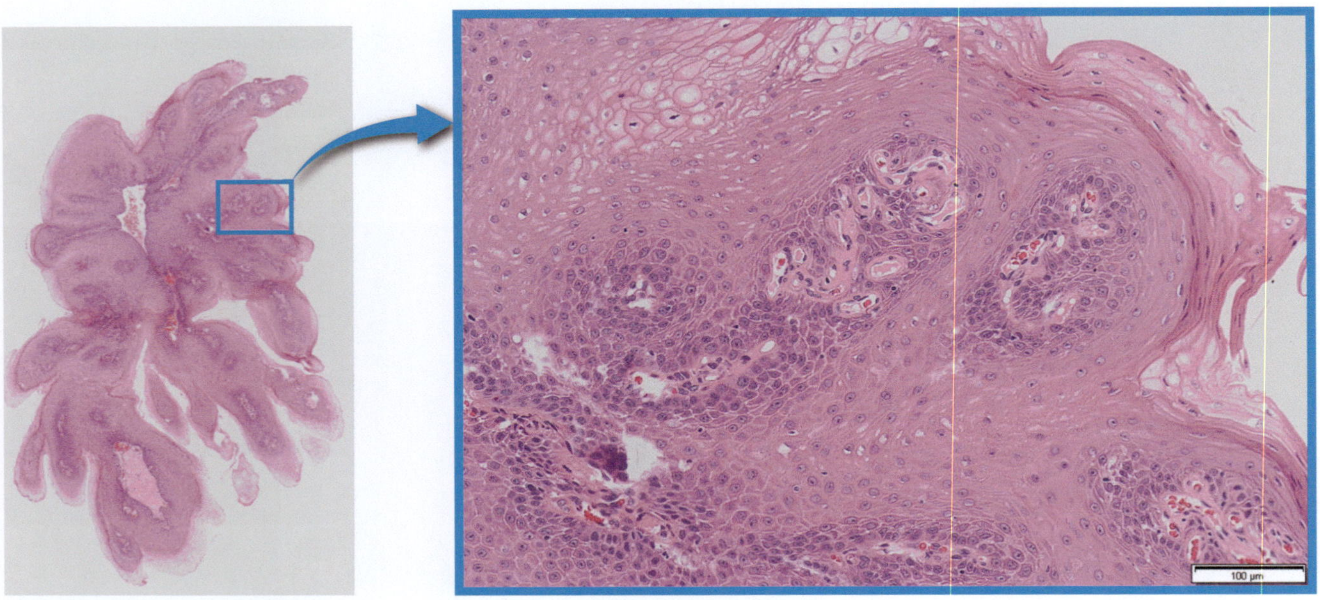

Fig. 25.4 The biopsy specimen of the lesion

25.4 A Reference Case

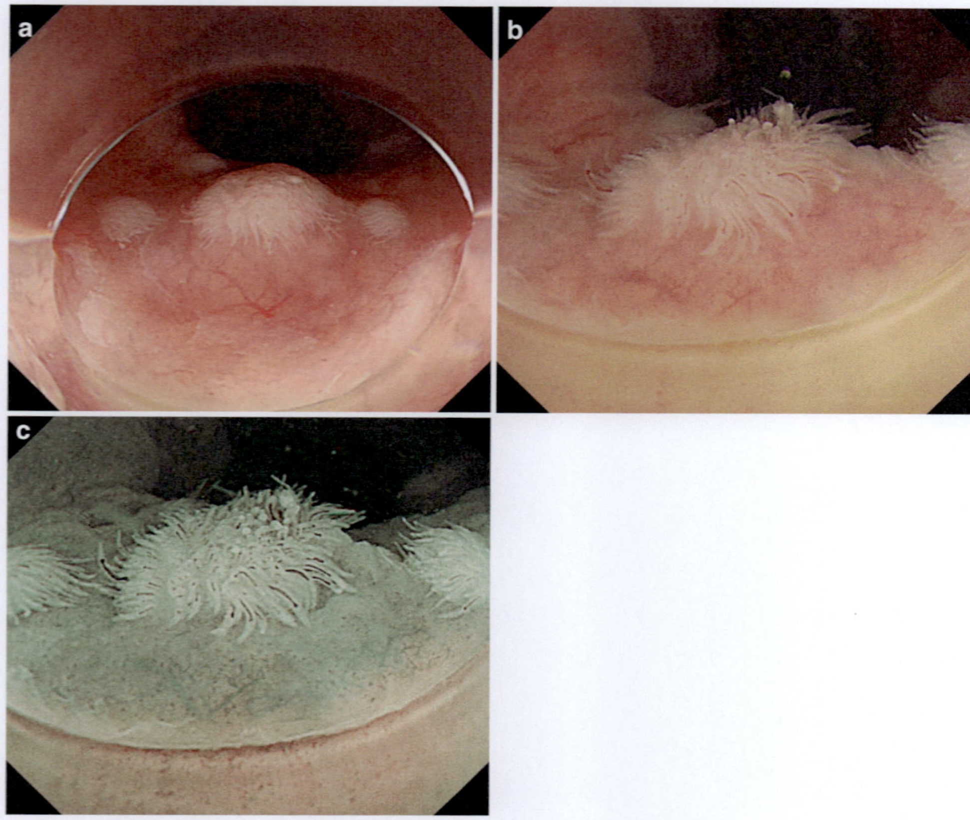

Fig. 25.5 (**a**) A woman in her 70s. Whitish elevated lesion of the esophagus. (**b**) Water immersion image showed a sea anemone-like appearance. (**c**) Water immersion magnifying NBI showed papilla with no vascular atypia

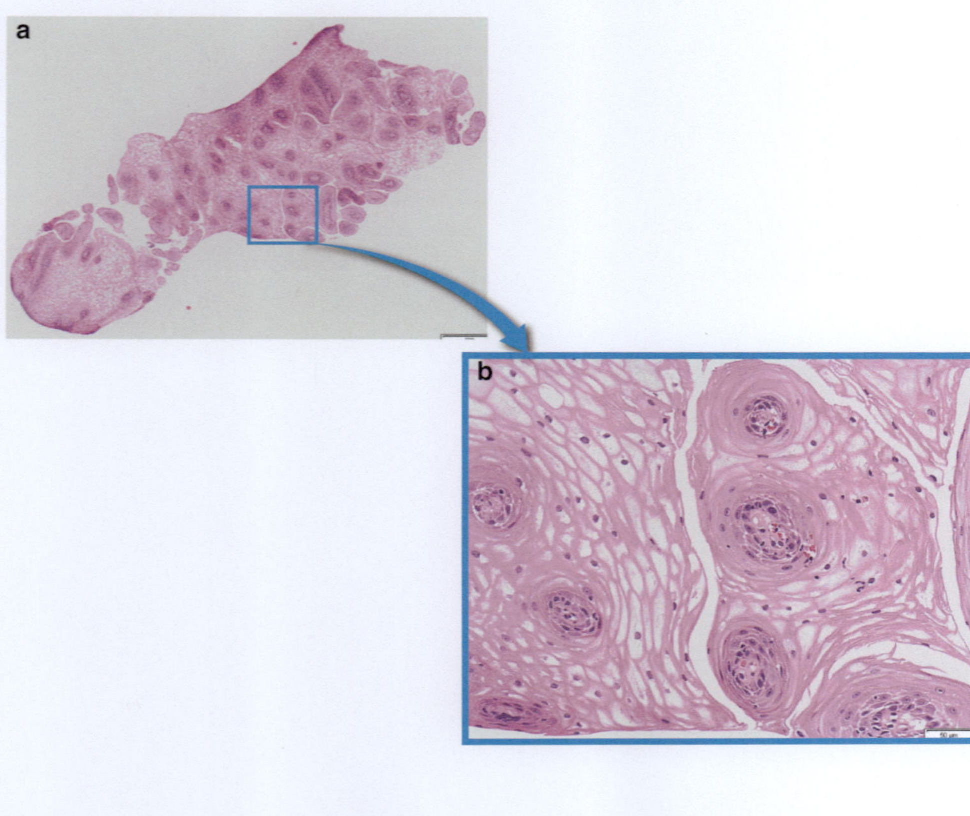

Fig. 25.6 Prominent papillary proliferations were observed, surrounded by thin squamous cell layers without cellular atypia

Summary

Papilloma has characteristic shapes resembling mulberry or sea anemone, making it relatively easy to diagnose. But occasionally, differentiation from esophageal cancer becomes necessary. In case of papillary squamous cell carcinoma, vascular atypia is found within papilla, opposed to papilloma without vascular atypia. It is important to observe carefully with magnifying NBI, considering iodine dye staining and biopsy for confirmation.

25.5 Answer

The correct histological type is (2) papilloma.

26 Question 11: What Is the Diagnosis?

Shinichiro Takeda

S. Takeda (✉)
Department of Gastroenterology, Matsudo City Hospital, Matsudo, Japan
e-mail: s-takeda@lilac.plala.or.jp

T. Oyama (ed.), *Endoscopic Diagnosis of Esophageal Carcinoma for ESD*, https://doi.org/10.1007/978-981-32-9030-3_26

Which Is the Correct Diagnosis? (Fig. 26.1)

1. Inflammatory polyp
2. Esophagogastric junctional adenocarcinoma
3. Squamous cell carcinoma

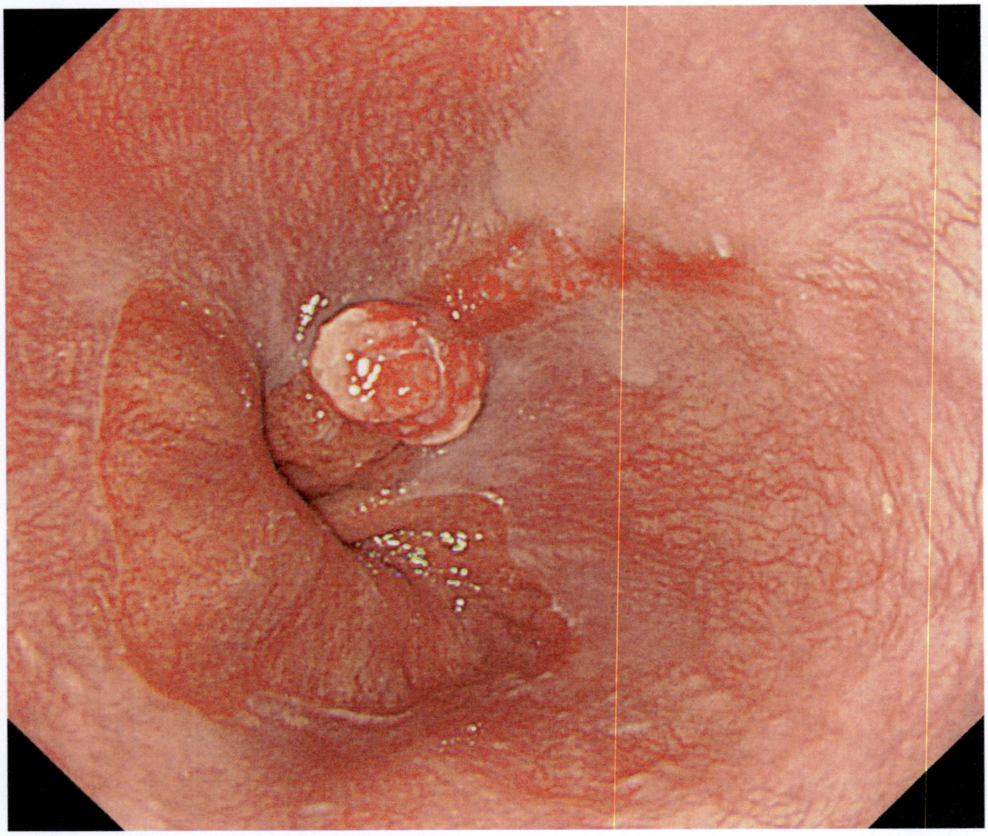

Fig. 26.1 What is the diagnosis?

26.1 Let's Look at These Six Images and Think (Fig. 26.2)

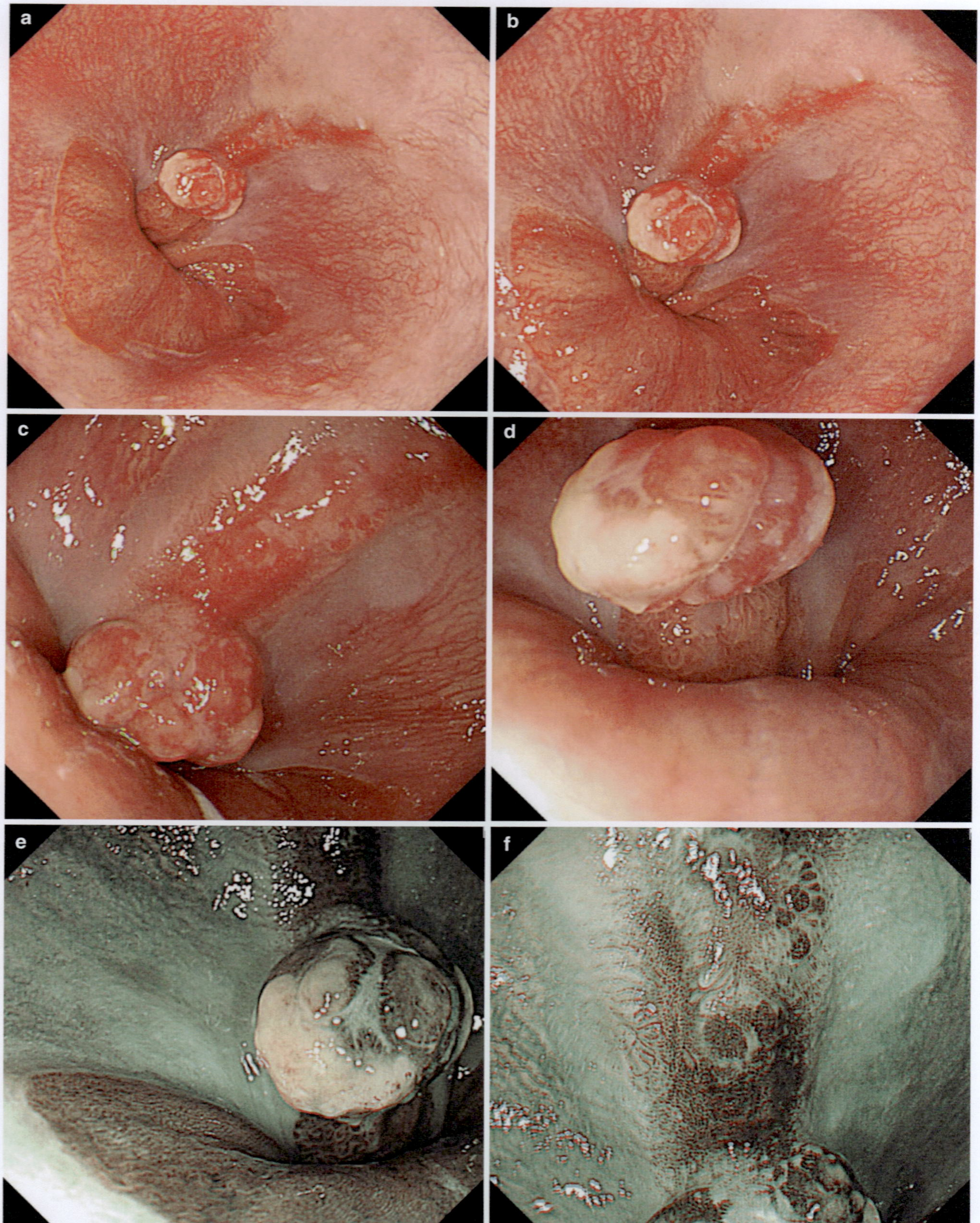

Fig. 26.2 Explanations start from the next page

26.2 Let's Observe the Following Six Images Carefully (Fig. 26.3)

Let's Observe with White Light Imaging (Fig. 26.3a)

- A reddish raised lesion was noted at the 2 o'clock direction within the squamous epithelium of the esophagogastric junction (EGJ), accompanied by a reddish longitudinal area extending orally.
- The oral side of the EGJ was noted with palisading blood vessels, making differentiation of an inflammatory polyp from esophagogastric junctional adenocarcinoma important.

Let's Observe the Palisading Blood Vessels (Fig. 26.3b)

- Palisading blood vessels were noted in the anal side of the squamocolumnar junction as marked by the yellow arrows (Prague classification C0.5/M1.5), confirming the diagnosis of Barrett's esophagus.
- This case was diagnosed as short segment Barrett's esophagus (SSBE), as the Barrett's mucosa was not 3cm or longer circumferentially.
- When observing for Barrett's esophagus, it is helpful to have the examinee to take a deep breath to move the SCJ orally.

Let's Observe Closely (Fig. 26.3c)

- By approaching closer to the lesion and observing with low-power magnification, a whitish patch of squamous epithelium was noted within the raised lesion. The oral side of the raised lesion showed some reddish mucosa, but with unclear demarcation without irregularity of the border.

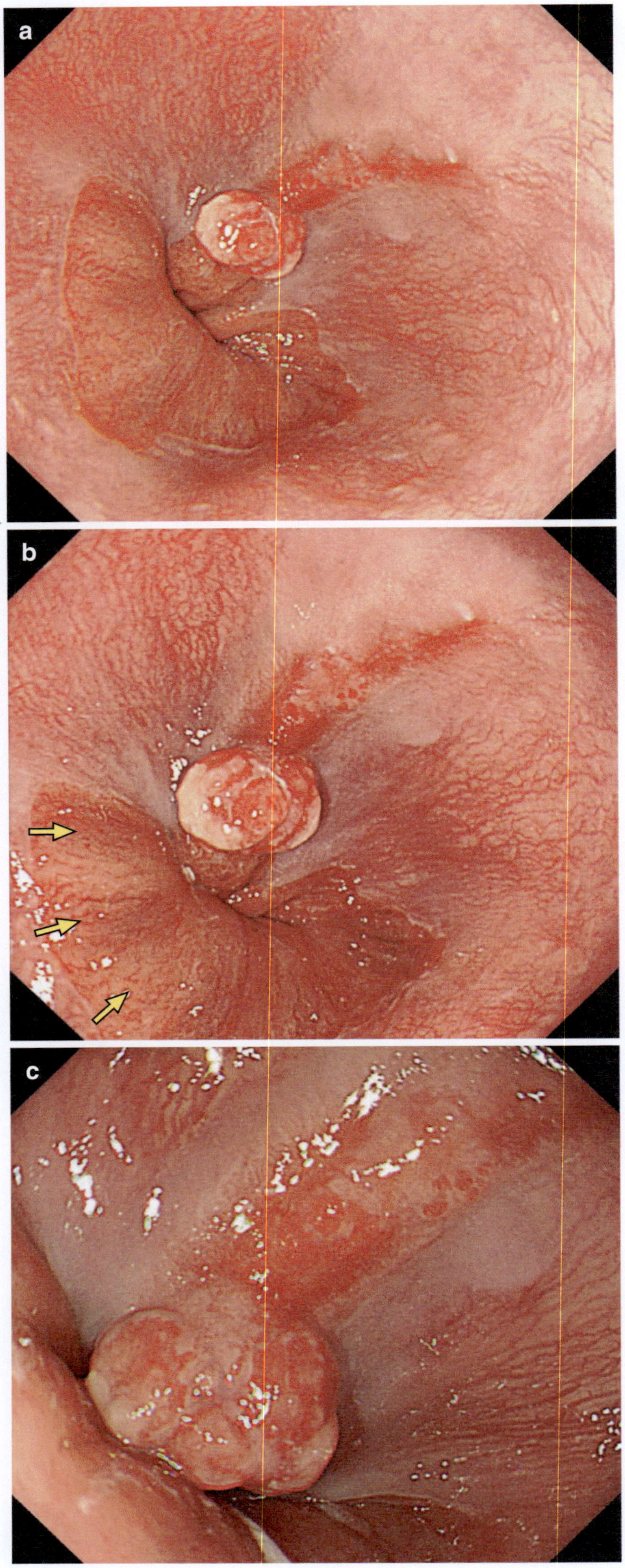

Fig. 26.3 Same images as Fig. 26.2

Let's Observe the Esophagogastric Junction by Adjusting Respiration (Fig. 26.3d)

- With the stomach deflated and having the patient take deep inspiration while expanding his abdomen, the EGJ was observed.
- The anal side of the raised lesion showed the gastric mucosa, allowing observation for the presence of redness, unevenness, and raised lesions.
- When using a magnifying scope, the use of low-power magnification brings close-up viewing in focus, allowing easier observation.

Let's Observe with NBI Paying Attention to the Vascular Structures (Fig. 26.3e)

- No abnormally dilated blood vessels were noted within the reddish area of the raised lesion.
- No abnormal blood vessels were noted within the remaining squamous epithelium by white light observation.

Let's Observe the Surface Structures with NBI (Fig. 26.3f)

- Dilated blood vessels were noted matching the reddish area, but the size of the blood vessels differed little.
- By magnifying NBI observation, the presence of abnormal blood vessels beneath the squamous epithelium must be looked for, since extensions of adenocarcinoma beneath the squamous epithelium could be observed at times.
- Differences between right and left sides of the areas covered by squamous epithelium were noted, and the surface structures of the slightly raised areas were observed in the gaps of the squamous cell epithelium as marked by the red arrow, suggesting possibility of cardiac glands of the esophagus.

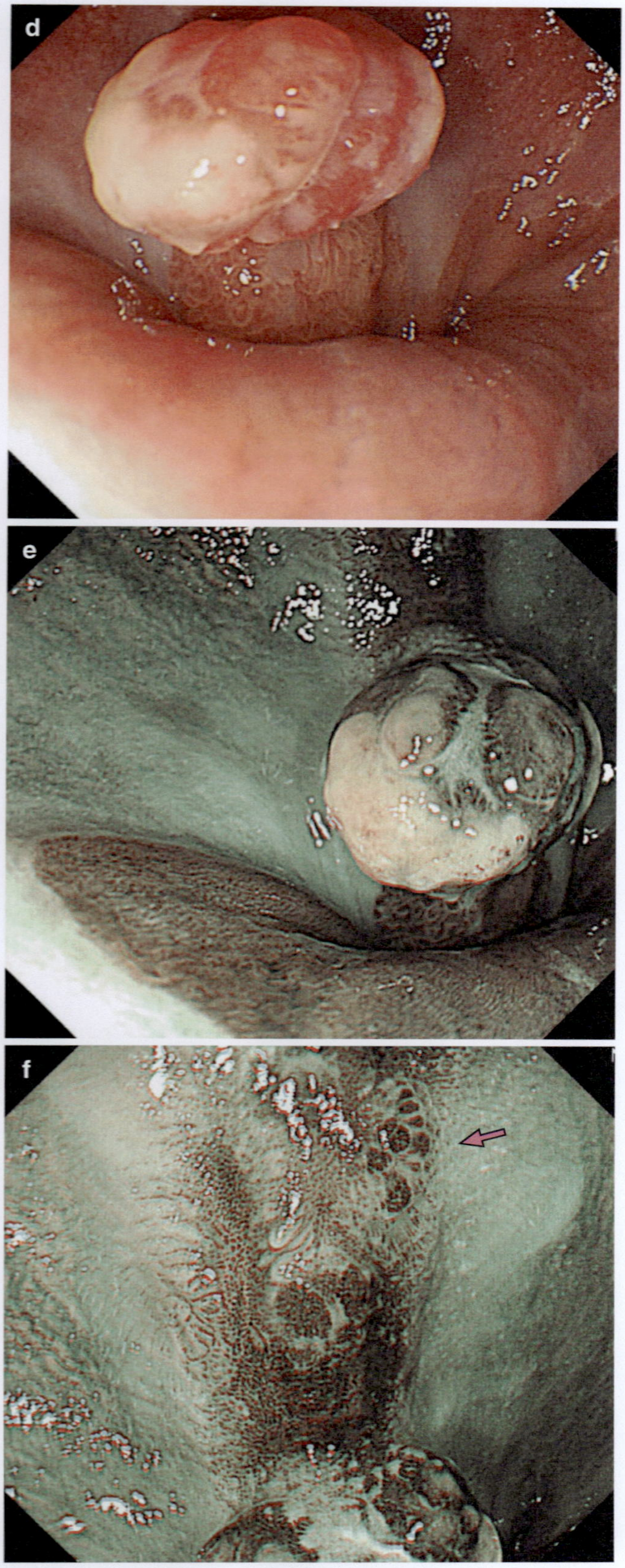

Fig. 26.3 (continued)

26.3 Let's Compare the Biopsy Specimen with the Endoscopic Images Towards the Final Diagnosis

Let's Observe the Surface Structure with NBI (Fig. 26.4a)

- The anal side of the lesion was noted with clear and similar villi-like pattern, with white zones of even width, without irregularities.

Let's Observe with White Light Imaging Before Obtaining a Biopsy Specimen (Fig. 26.4b)

- The oral side of the lesion was noted with clear and similar villi-like pattern, with white zones of even width, without irregularities.

Let's Make it Clear Where the Biopsy Was Taken from (Fig. 26.4c)

- It is important to leave an image documentation for future reference showing where exactly the biopsy was taken from.

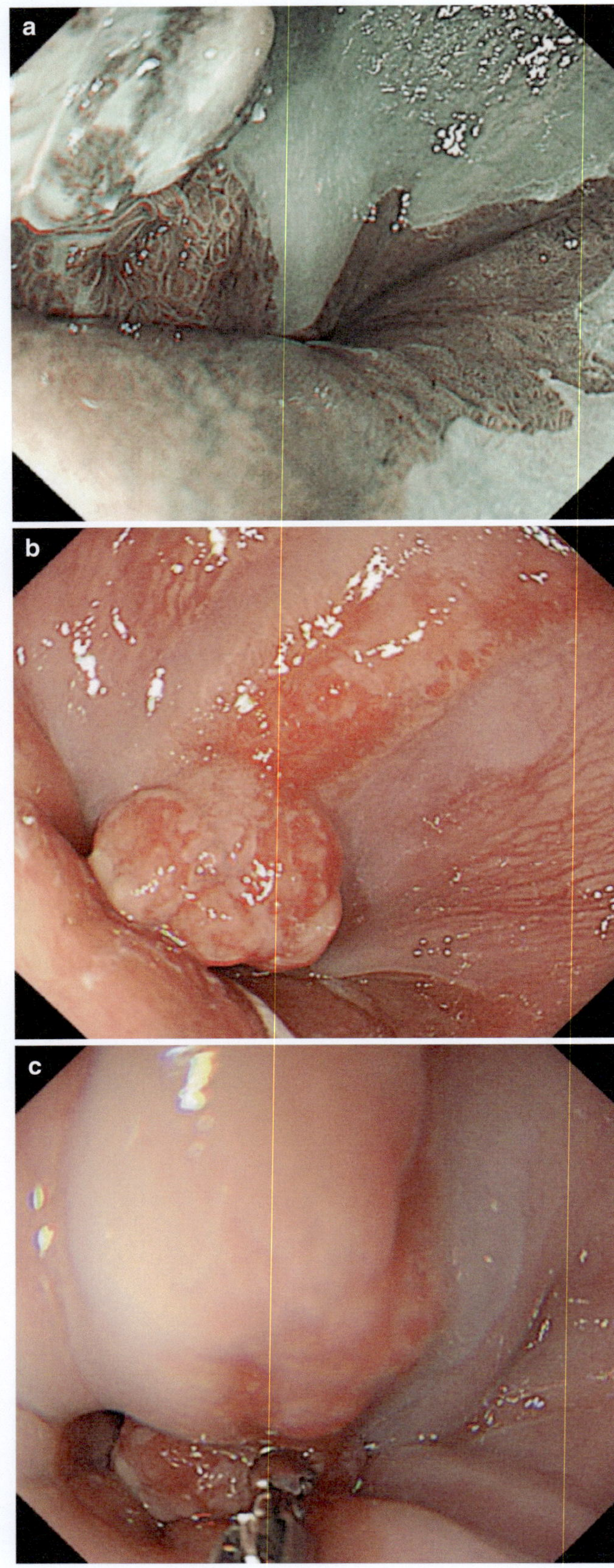

Fig.26.4 (**a**) NBI magnified image of the lesion. (**b**) White light image of the lesion. (**c**) Image to indicate where exactly the biopsy was taken from

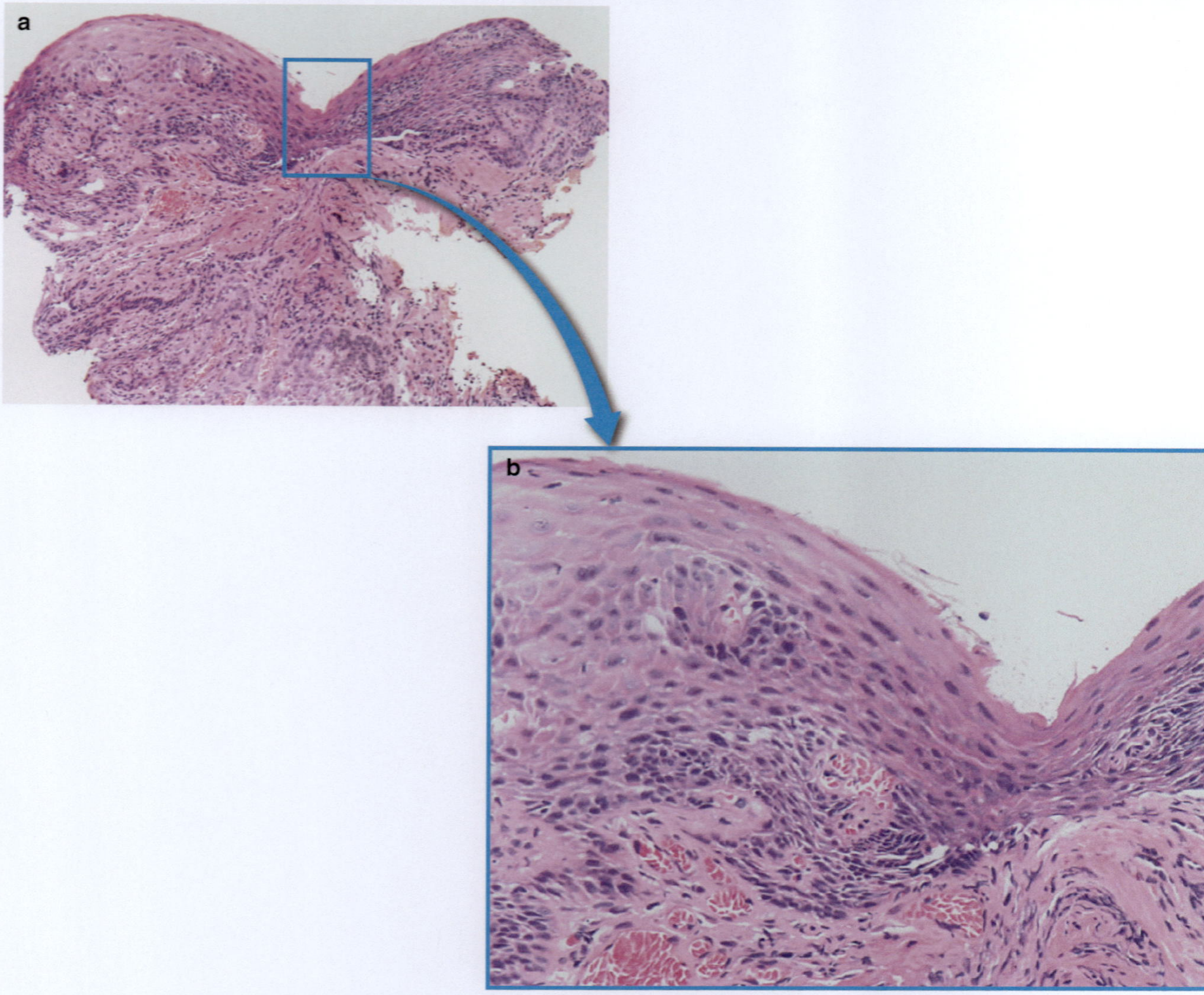

Fig. 26.5 (**a**) The biopsy specimen of the lesion. (**b**) Magnified image of the area indicated with the blue square

Let's Look at Histopathology of the Biopsy Specimen

- Hyperplasia of the squamous epithelium and infiltration of inflammatory cells were noted. The reddish raised area had disappeared post-PPI use in this case (Fig. 26.5a).
- Nuclear atypia was mild suggesting regenerative changes and denying epithelial malignancy (Fig. 26.5b).

Summary
Differentiating healing reflux esophagitis from esophagogastric junction adenocarcinoma could be difficult at times. It is important to reexamine after PPI treatment and if the lesion is found without healing to carefully evaluate for the presence of irregularities or atypical blood vessels.

Conclusive Diagnosis
Inflammatory polyp

26.4 Answer

The correct diagnosis was (1) inflammatory polyp.

27 Question 12: What Is the Diagnosis?

Nobukazu Yorimitsu

N. Yorimitsu (✉)
Department of Endoscopy, Saku Central Hospital Advanced Care Center, Nagano, Japan
e-mail: 99097ny@jichi.ac.jp

T. Oyama (ed.), *Endoscopic Diagnosis of Esophageal Carcinoma for ESD*, https://doi.org/10.1007/978-981-32-9030-3_27

Which Is the Correct Diagnosis? (Fig. 27.1)

1. Squamous cell carcinoma
2. Adenocarcinoma
3. Erosion (reflux esophagitis)

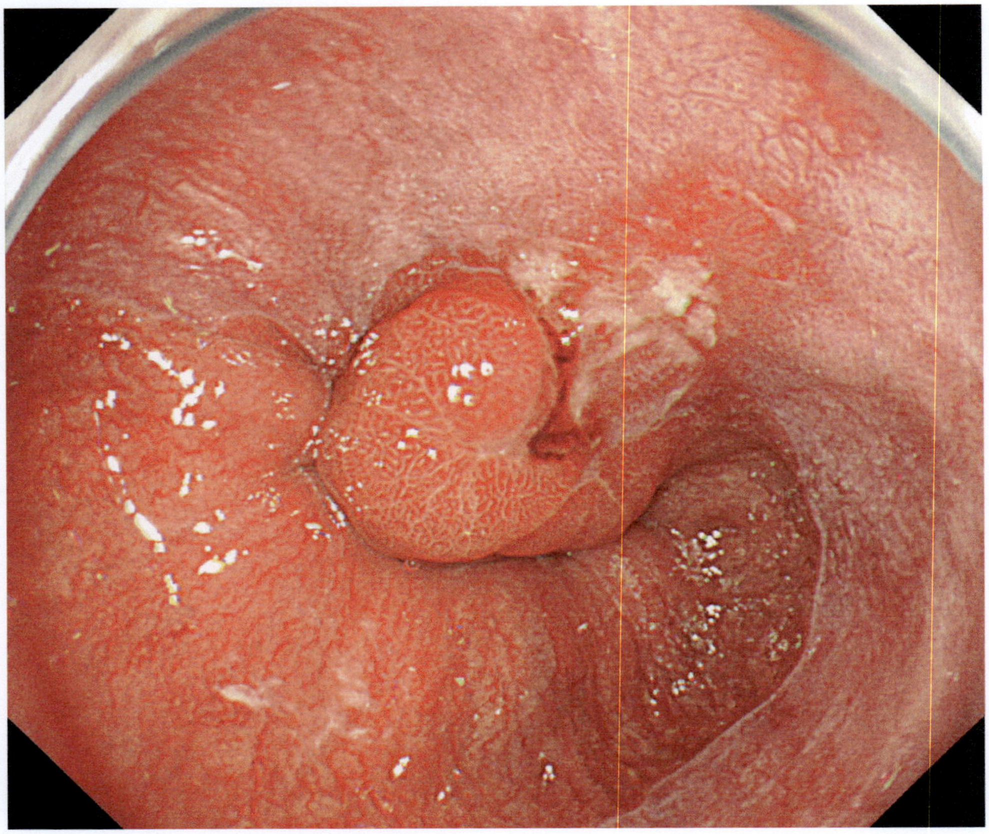

Fig. 27.1 Which is the correct diagnosis??

27.1 Let's Look at These Six Images and Think (Fig. 27.2)

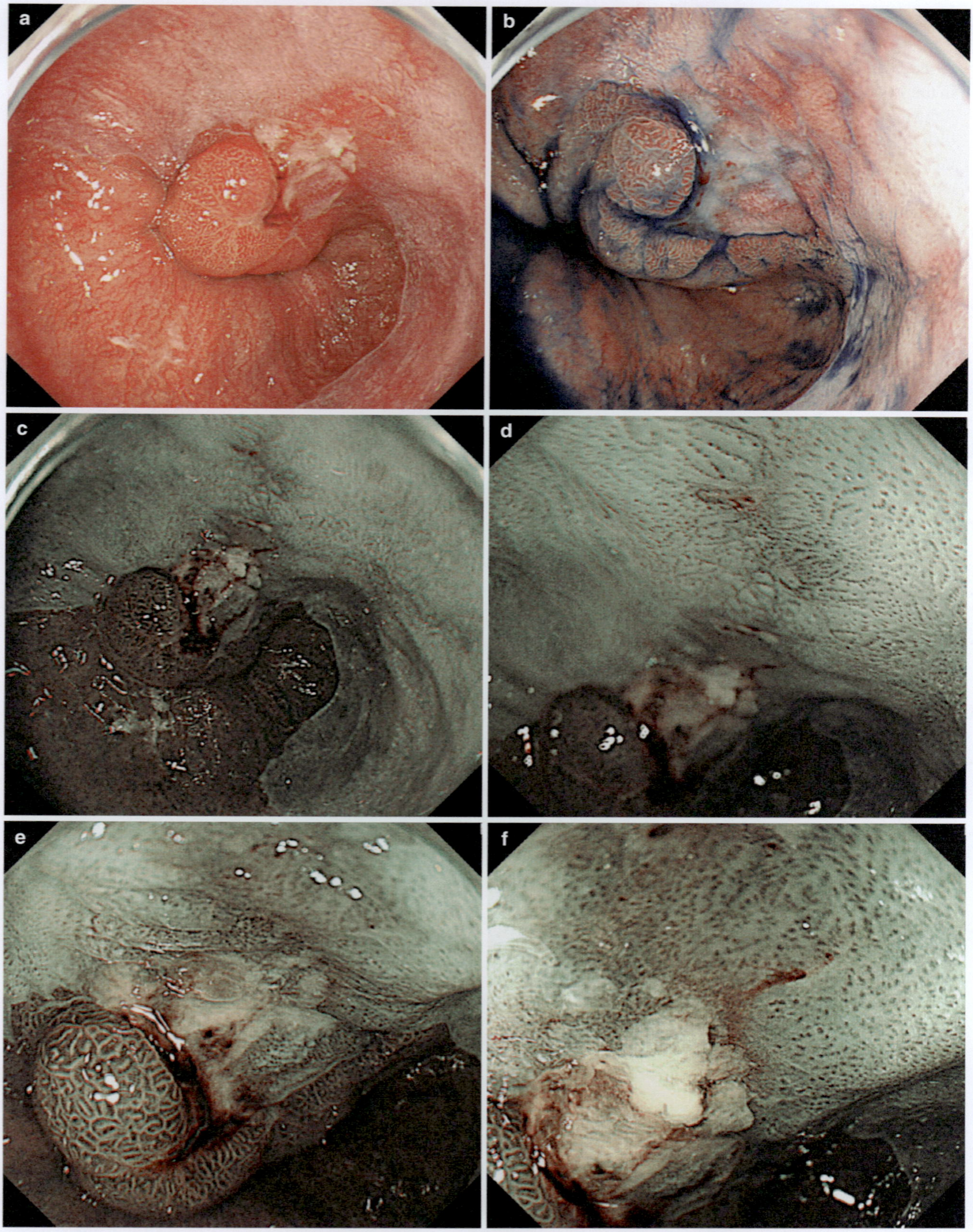

Fig. 27.2 Explanations start from the next page

27.2 Let's Observe the Following Six Images Carefully (Fig. 27.3)

Let's Observe with White Light Imaging (Fig. 27.3a)

- A reddish depressed area with white exudates was noted in the 1 o'clock direction at the oral side of the squamocolumnar junction. It was accompanied with a smooth reddish raised area on the anal side. The reddish depressed area was designated as Part A, the area of adherent white exudates as Part B, and the raised area as Part C as marked with the yellow arrows .
- Differential diagnoses included esophageal squamous cell carcinoma (SCC), esophageal adenocarcinoma, and erosion.
- Palisading blood vessels were noted on the gastric side of the SCJ in the 6 o'clock direction suggesting Barrett's esophagus, while the anal side of the reddish raised part could not be observed making it impossible to confirm Barrett's esophagus on the anterior wall side.

Let's Observe with Indigo Carmine (IC) Dye Spraying (Fig. 27.3b)

- While the oral side of the raised area (Part C) became clear with IC spraying, demarcations of the left wall side and the right wall side were unclear.
- Demarcations of the depressed area (Part A) and the area with white exudates (Part B) were also unclear.
- Demarcations of Parts A, B, and C were all unclear with IC spraying, showing no evidence of epithelial tumor.

Let's Observe with NBI (Fig. 27.3c)

- The depressed area (Part A) was noted as a weakly brownish area (BA) as marked by the yellow arrows, suggesting squamous cell carcinoma.
- The raised area (Part C) appeared to be with the same color tone as the surrounding mucosal epithelium with unclear demarcation, denying likelihood of epithelial tumor.
- No additional information was obtained regarding Part B.

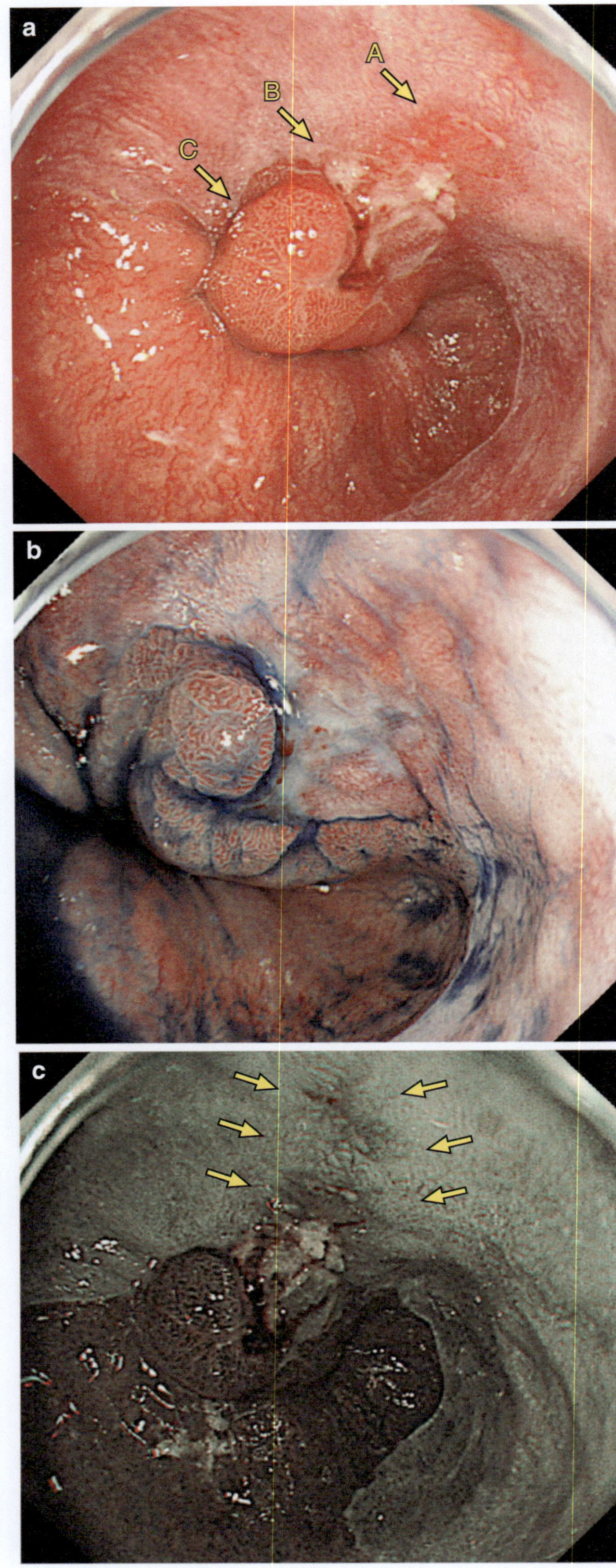

Fig. 27.3 Same images as Fig. 27.2

Let's Observe the Raised Area (Part A) with Magnifying NBI (Fig. 27.3d)

- The depressed area was noted as a clearly demarcated BA with dot-like dilated blood vessels.
- Vascular arrangements were regular with little atypia.
- There were no findings to suggest SCC, but the findings were thought to be consistent with inflammatory changes.

Let's Observe the Raised Area (Part C) with Low-Power-Magnification NBI (Fig. 27.3e)

- The raised area (Part C) showed somewhat enlarged evenly sized villi-like pattern, without irregularities and with low density of villi and white zones with even width.
- There were no findings to suggest epithelial tumor but were with findings to support hyperplasia.

Let's Observe the Area with White Exudates (Part B) with Magnifying NBI! (Fig. 27.3f)

- White exudates were adherently attached to Part B, and the area was thought to have erosion.
- The erosion was surrounded by BA with dilated blood vessels with little atypia. Blood vessels appeared regularly and evenly spreading, making it unlikely to be SCC.
- Due to firmly adherent nature of the white exudates, observation of the area attached with white exudates was difficult. To determine the nature of the erosion to be either cancer or inflammation, it was decided to reexamine after treating with PPI.

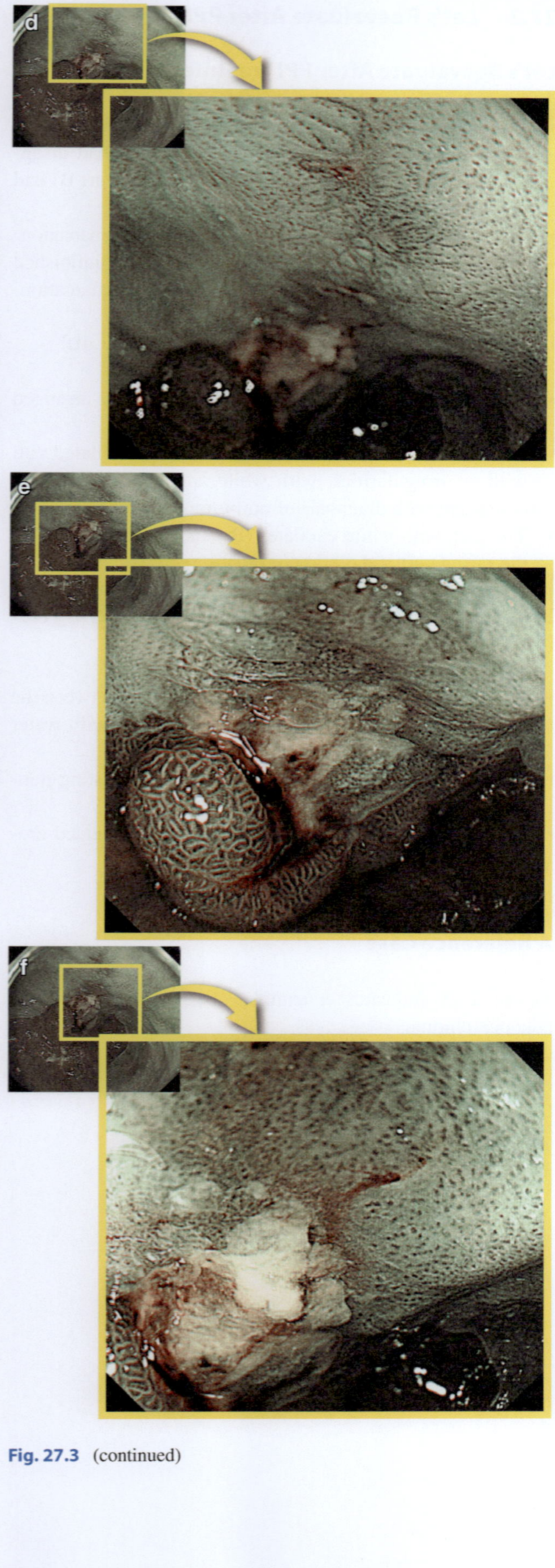

Fig. 27.3 (continued)

27.3 Let's Reevaluate After PPI Treatment

Let's Reevaluate After PPI Treatment (Fig. 27.4a)

- After taking PPI for 2 months, reexamination was performed. The reddish depressed area (Part A) had disappeared, and the erosion with white exudates (Part B) had turned into a reddish area.
- The surface of Part B was smooth with unclear demarcation.
- The anal raised area (Part C) had remarkably diminished in size, showing smooth surface and unclear demarcation.

Let's Observe with Magnifying NBI (Fig. 27.4b)

- The depressed area (Part A) showed regularly arranged dilated blood vessels.
- The surface of the raised area (Part C) showed dilated villi with no irregularities, with white zones of even width, consistent with diagnosis of non-tumor/hyperplasia.
- The area with white exudates (Part B) was shadowed by the raised part and could not be observed well.

Let's Observe with Water Immersion Magnifying NBI (Fig. 27.4c)

- Water immersion observation made the space between the depressed area and the raised area to spread with water pressure, allowing clear observation of Part B.
- Somewhat dilated IPCLs were observed suggesting non-tumor squamous epithelium.
- Based on these, the lesion was diagnosed as healed erosion caused by reflux esophagitis.

A Reference Case

Figure 27.5 indicates a sample of Barret's esophageal adenocarcinoma.

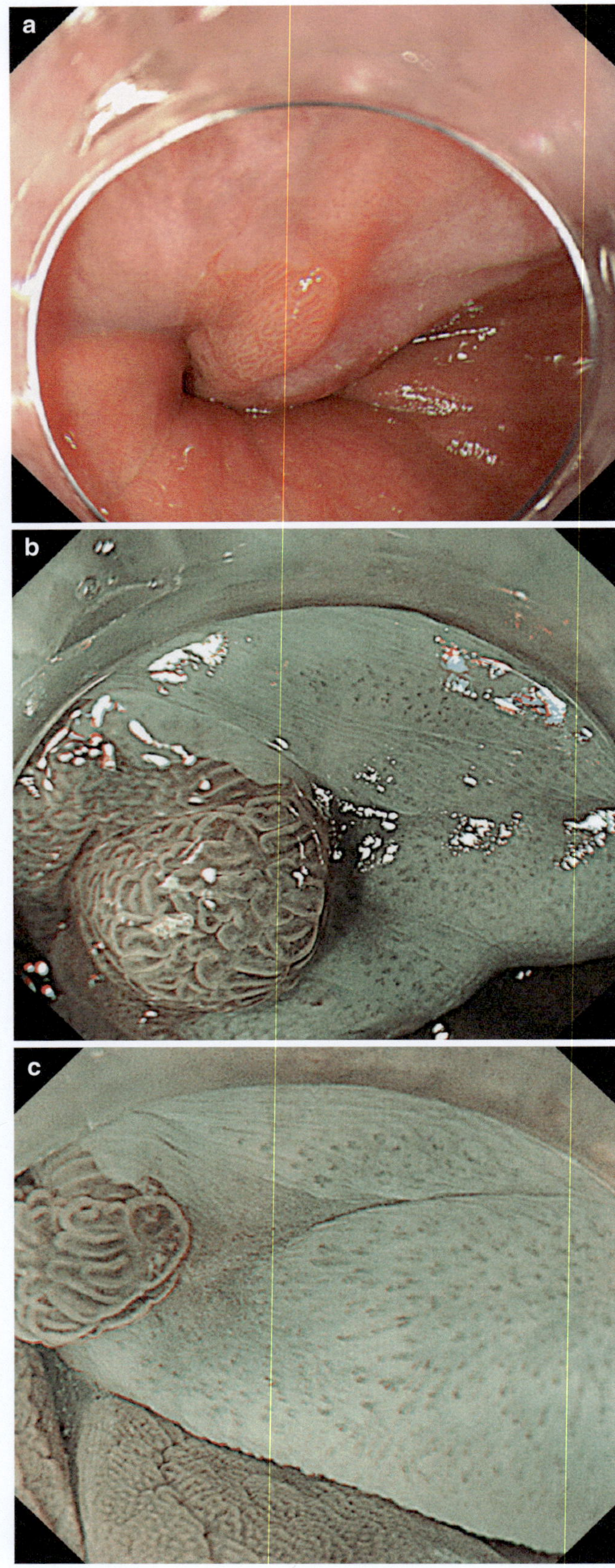

Fig. 27.4 (**a**) White light endoscopic image. (**b**) NBI magnified endoscopic image. (**c**) Water immersion image under NBI magnification

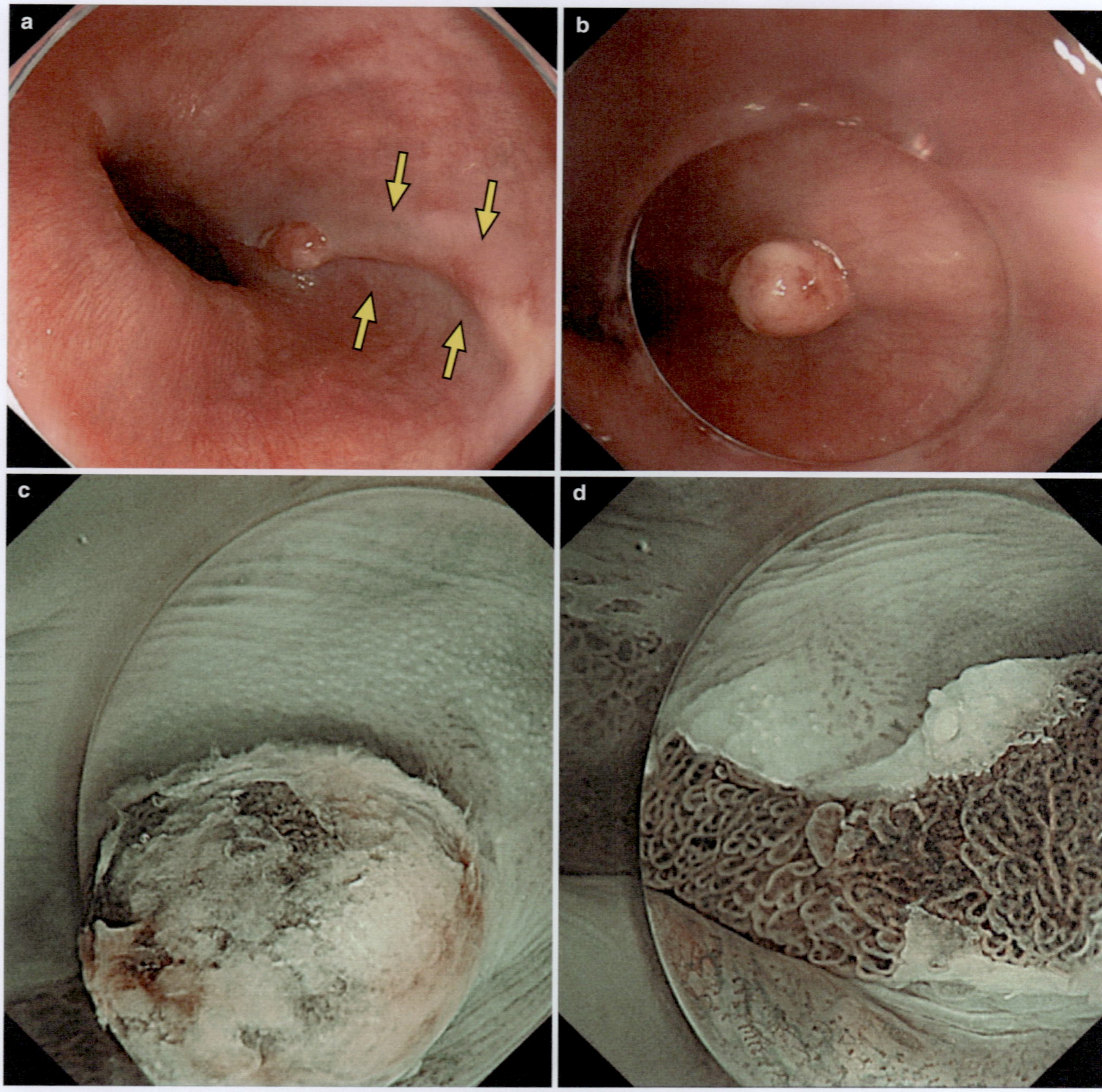

Fig. 27.5 (**a**) Before PPI treatment: A smooth raised lesion was noted at the SCJ accompanied by the oral linear redness marked by the yellow arrows. (**b**) Two months after PPI treatment: The linear redness had disappeared on reexamination, but the raised lesion remained. (**c**) Magnifying NBI observation (post-PPI treatment): The raised area was mostly covered with squamous epithelium and white exudates, making it difficult to allow evaluation of the surface structures. (**d**) The anal side of the raised area that showed irregular villi-like pattern of increased density was noted with diagnosis of tub 1, and the lesion was resected by ESD. The final diagnosis was Barrett's esophageal adenocarcinoma, 0–I+IIb, tub1, T1a-DMM, 9×5 mm

Conclusive Diagnosis
Erosion (reflux esophagitis + inflammatory polyp)

Summary
A depressed lesion with adherent white exudates at the SCJ was observed accompanied by reddish raised area on the anal side. Based on the location of the lesion and its background, SCC, adenocarcinoma, and erosion were considered as differential diagnoses. The depression and the raised area were both with unclear demarcation, and magnifying NBI showed no atypia of the surface and vascular structures, making epithelial tumors (SCC, adenocarcinoma) unlikely. But the surface pattern and the vascular structures were unclear; it was decided to be reexamined after PPI treatment. On the repeated evaluation, the erosion had disappeared, with diminished size of the raised area, showing no irregular surface structures or vascular structures, and the final diagnosis was confirmed as a healed erosion caused by reflux esophagitis. Reevaluation following treatment with PPI was helpful.

27.4 Answer

The correct diagnosis is (3) erosion (reflux esophagitis).

28 Question 13: What Is the Diagnosis?

Yoko Kitamura

Y. Kitamura (✉)
Department of Gastroenterology, Nara City Hospital Center for Digestive Diseases, Nara, Japan

T. Oyama (ed.), *Endoscopic Diagnosis of Esophageal Carcinoma for ESD*, https://doi.org/10.1007/978-981-32-9030-3_28

Which Is the Correct Diagnosis? (Fig. 28.1)

1. No lesions
2. Esophagitis
3. Esophageal carcinoma

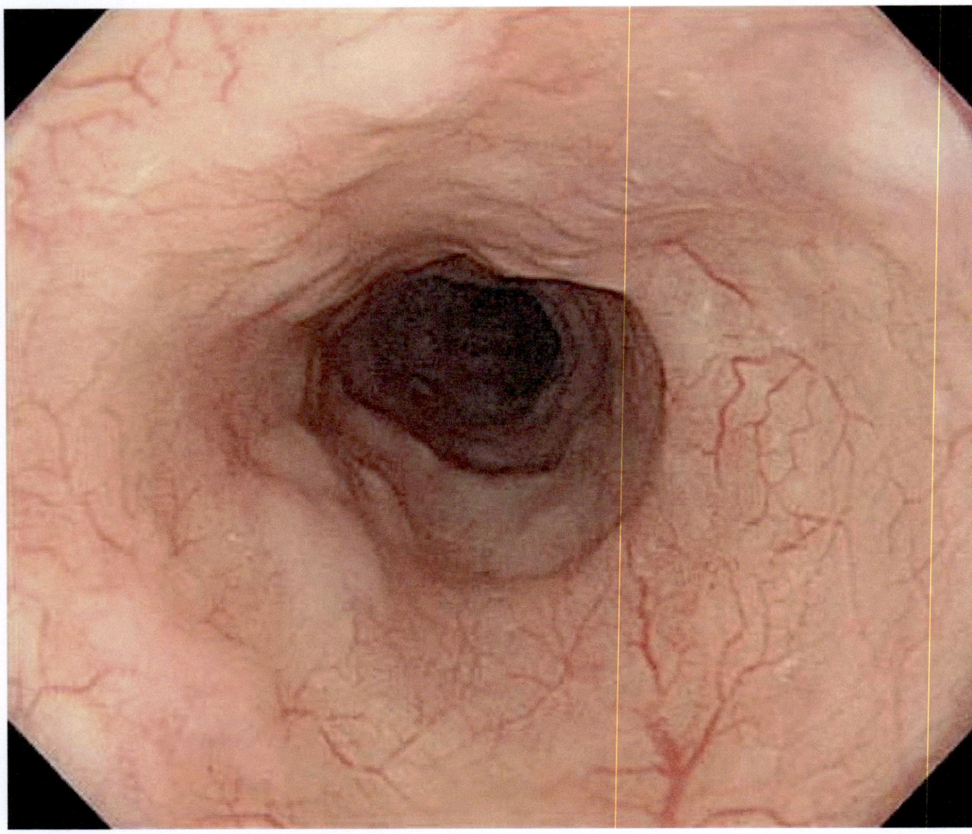

Fig. 28.1 Which is the correct diagnosis?

28.1 Let's Look at These Six Images and Think (Fig. 28.2)

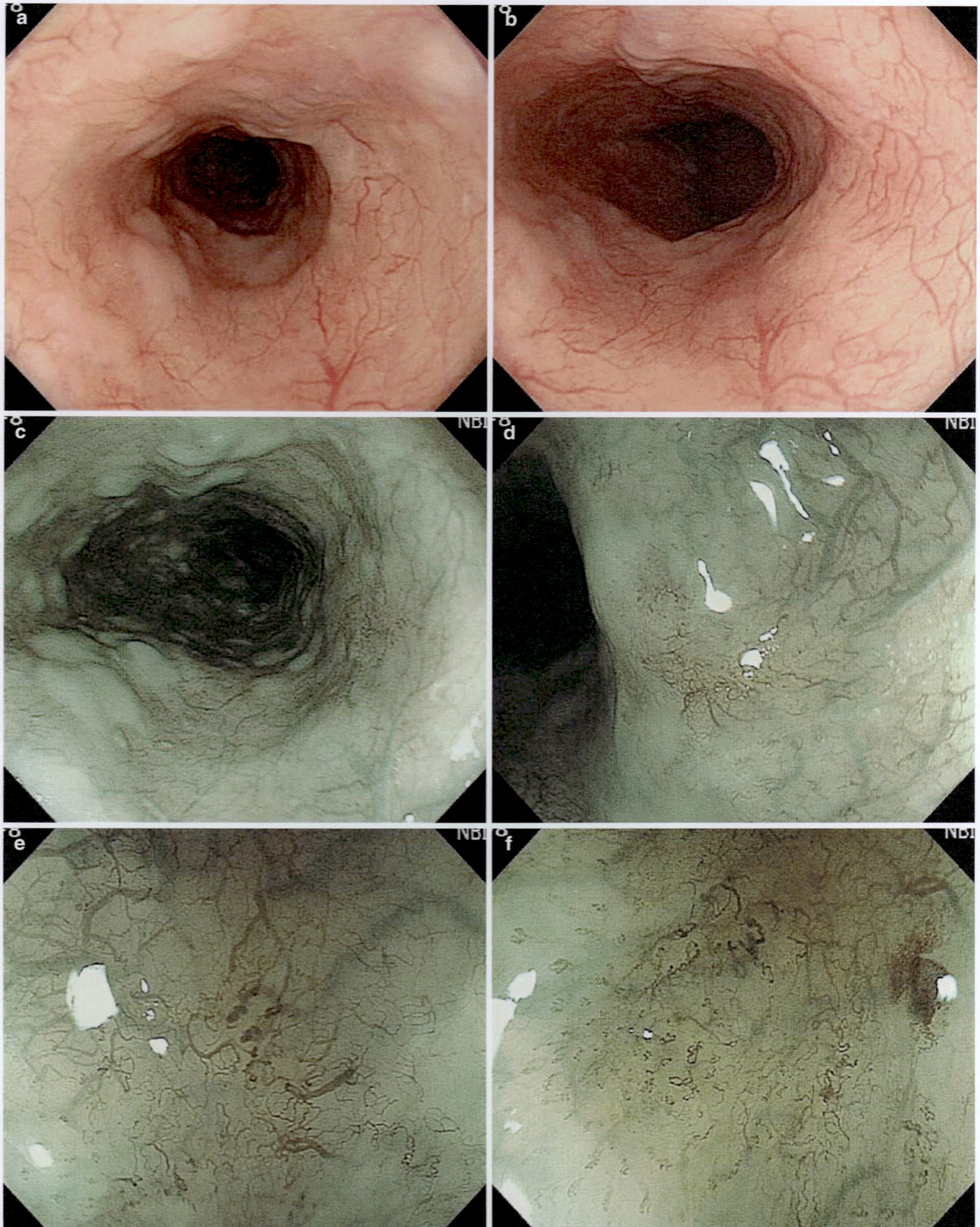

Fig. 28.2 Explanations start from the next page

28.2 Let's Observe the Following Six Images Carefully (Fig. 28.3)

Let's Note the Area of Disrupted Blood Vessels (Fig. 28.3a)

- There was an area of esophageal mucosa with disrupted blood vessels in the posterior right wall in the middle esophagus.
- However, demarcation was unclear, and the area of disrupted blood vessels was relatively obscure.

Are There Mucosal Height Differences? (Fig. 28.3a)

- Observation of the area with full air insufflation showed no mucosal height differences.

Let's Observe While Deflating Air (Fig. 28.3b)

- When air volume is adjusted by deflation, disruption of blood vessels become clearer, allowing the lesion to be identified as slightly elevated.
- With an identifiable domain, the presence of a neoplastic lesion was suspected.
- When observing esophagus, it is very important to use air adjustment.

Let's Observe with NBI (Fig. 28.3c)

- Although not a very clear brownish area, the lesion was identified as a slightly brownish area by non-magnifying NBI.

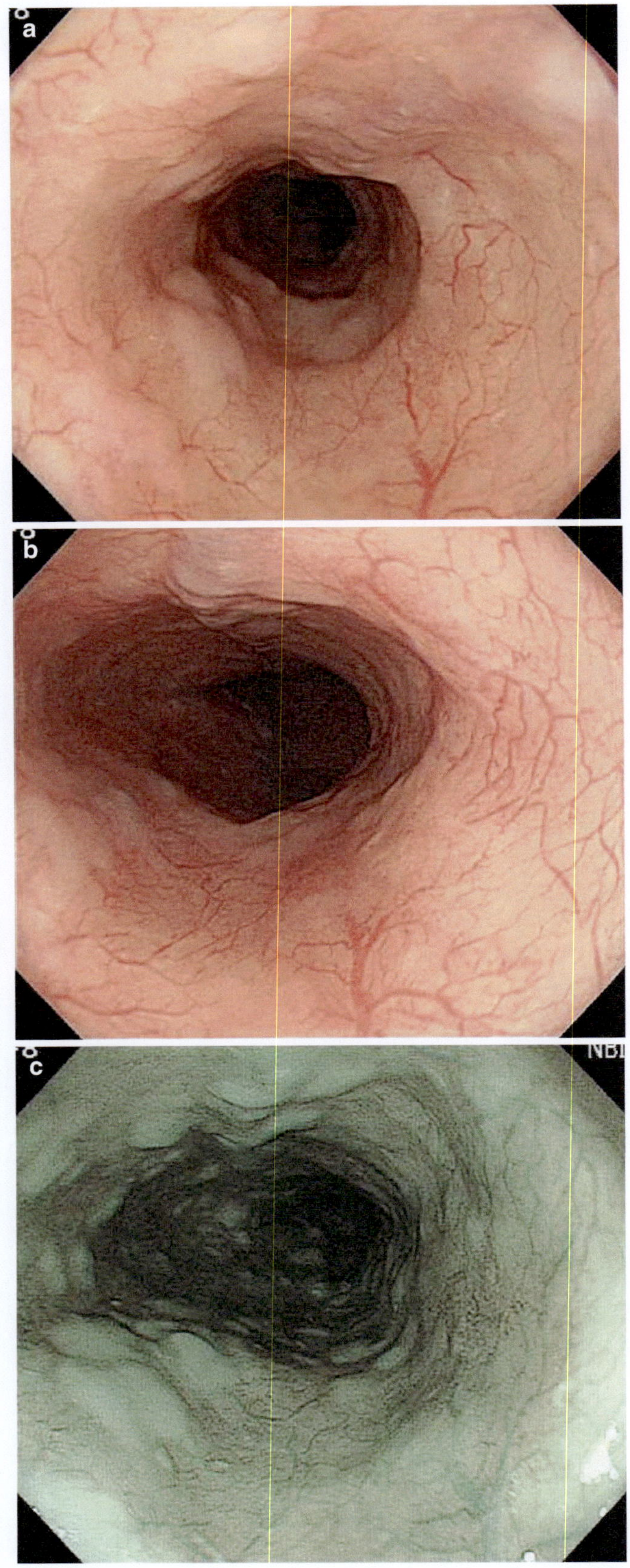

Fig. 28.3 Same images as Fig. 28.2

Let's Observe with Low-Power-Magnification NBI (Fig. 28.3d)

- With low power magnification NBI, the slightly brownish area showed increased blood vessels making the area appear brownish.
- It was apparent that the vascular pattern was not of the usual EP~LPM squamous cell carcinoma by low power magnification NBI.

Let's Observe with High-Power-Magnification NBI (Fig. 28.3e)

- The mucosal surface of the area of irregular blood vessels was shiny without irregular surface unevenness.
- There was no background coloration in the interstitial spaces between the blood vessels.
- Non-loop-forming blood vessels were noted partially in very fine network-like patterns (Type R).

Let's Observe the Entire Lesion with Magnifying NBI (Fig. 28.3f)

- The entire lesion was noted with the similar blood vessel pattern.
- Non-loop-forming blood vessels of the lesion were identified as Type R blood vessels.
- The main part of the lesion was LPM, and besides the small alveolar-forming LPM squamous cell carcinoma, differential diagnoses included endocrine cell carcinoma, basaloid cell carcinoma, and poorly differentiated squamous cell carcinoma.

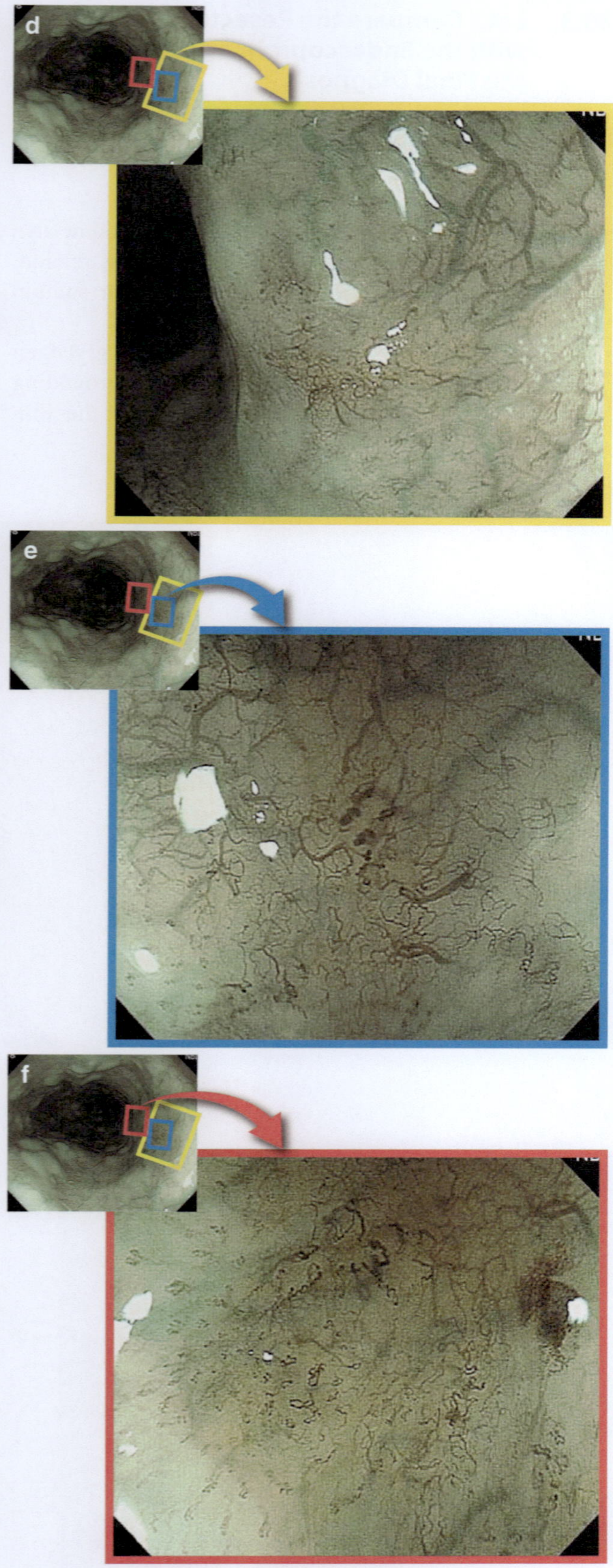

Fig. 28.3 (continued)

28.3 Let's Compare the Resected Specimen with the Endoscopic Images Towards the Final Diagnosis

Let's Observe After Spraying with Sodium Thiosulfate (Fig. 28.4a–c)

- The lesion did not remain unstained after iodine dye spraying and, although with unclear demarcation, showed pink color sign after spraying with sodium thiosulfate.
- This was due to differences in the amount of glycogen within the squamous epithelium of the surrounding thick healthy squamous epithelium and of the thin non-tumor squamous epithelium on the lesion's surface.

The yellow star mark in the image matches the yellow star marks in the iodine dye-stained fixed specimen (Fig. 28.4b, c).

Let's Observe the Fixed Resected Specimen (Fig. 28.4b)

- This is a formalin-fixed resected specimen. After formalin fixation, the lesion appeared somewhat faded colored than its surrounding and as an area with unevenness but with unclear demarcation.

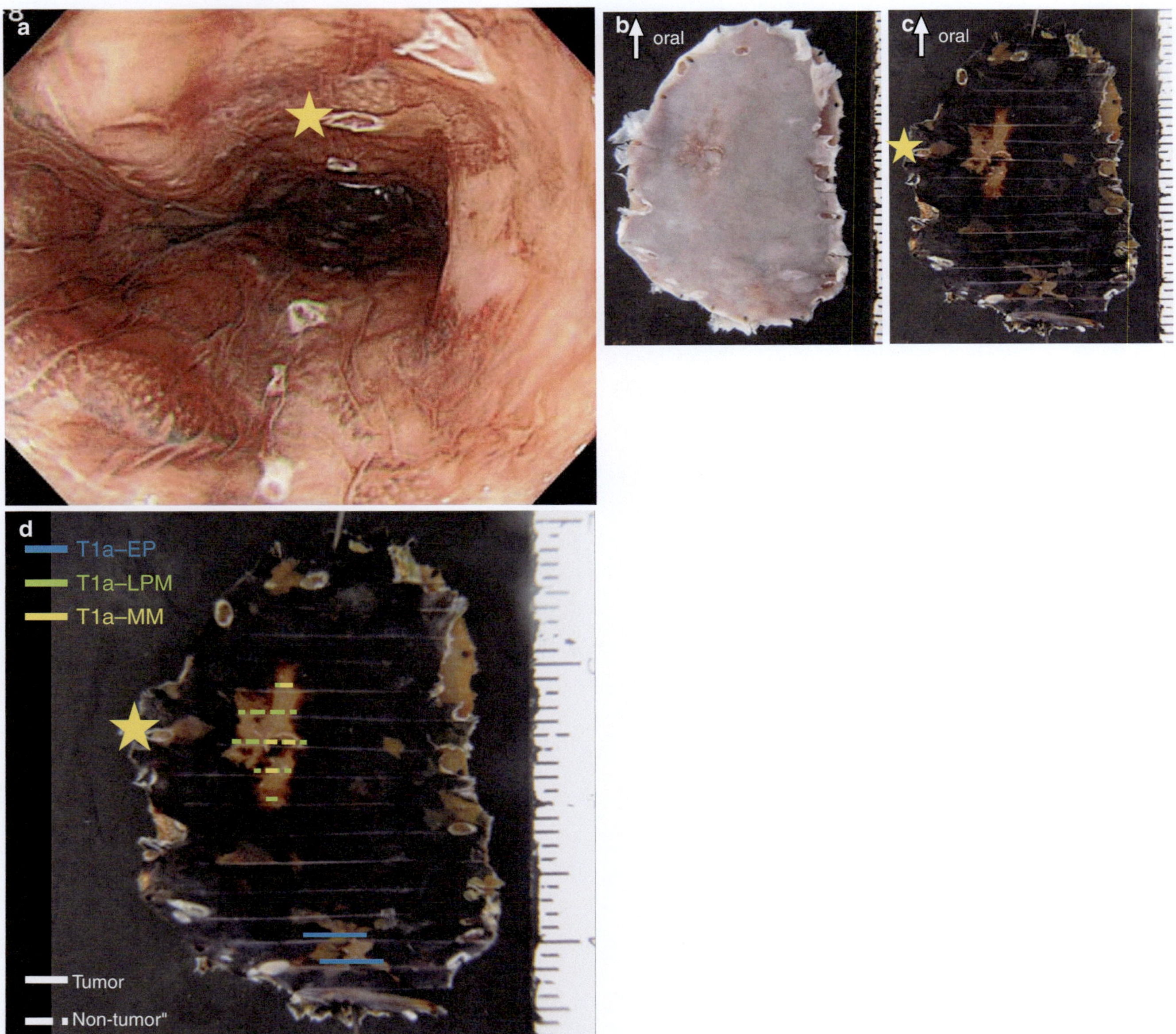

Fig. 28.4 (**a**) The endoscopic image after spraying with sodium thiosulfate. (**b**) Fixed resected specimen of the lesion. (**c**) The fixed specimen with iodine dye staining. (**d**) Mapping of the cancer distribution projected on the resected specimen

Let's Observe the Fixed Specimen with Iodine Dye Staining (Fig. 28.4c)

- An irregularly shaped unstained area was noted in this iodine dye stained formalin-fixed specimen.
- The specimen was sliced as to show the area of interest.
- After slicing the specimen, iodine dye was added, and sodium thiosulfate was sprayed making the lines of slicing appear very clearly.

Let's Compare with the Endoscopic Image

Figure 28.5 indicates comparison with NBI magnified image and histopathological images of the area.

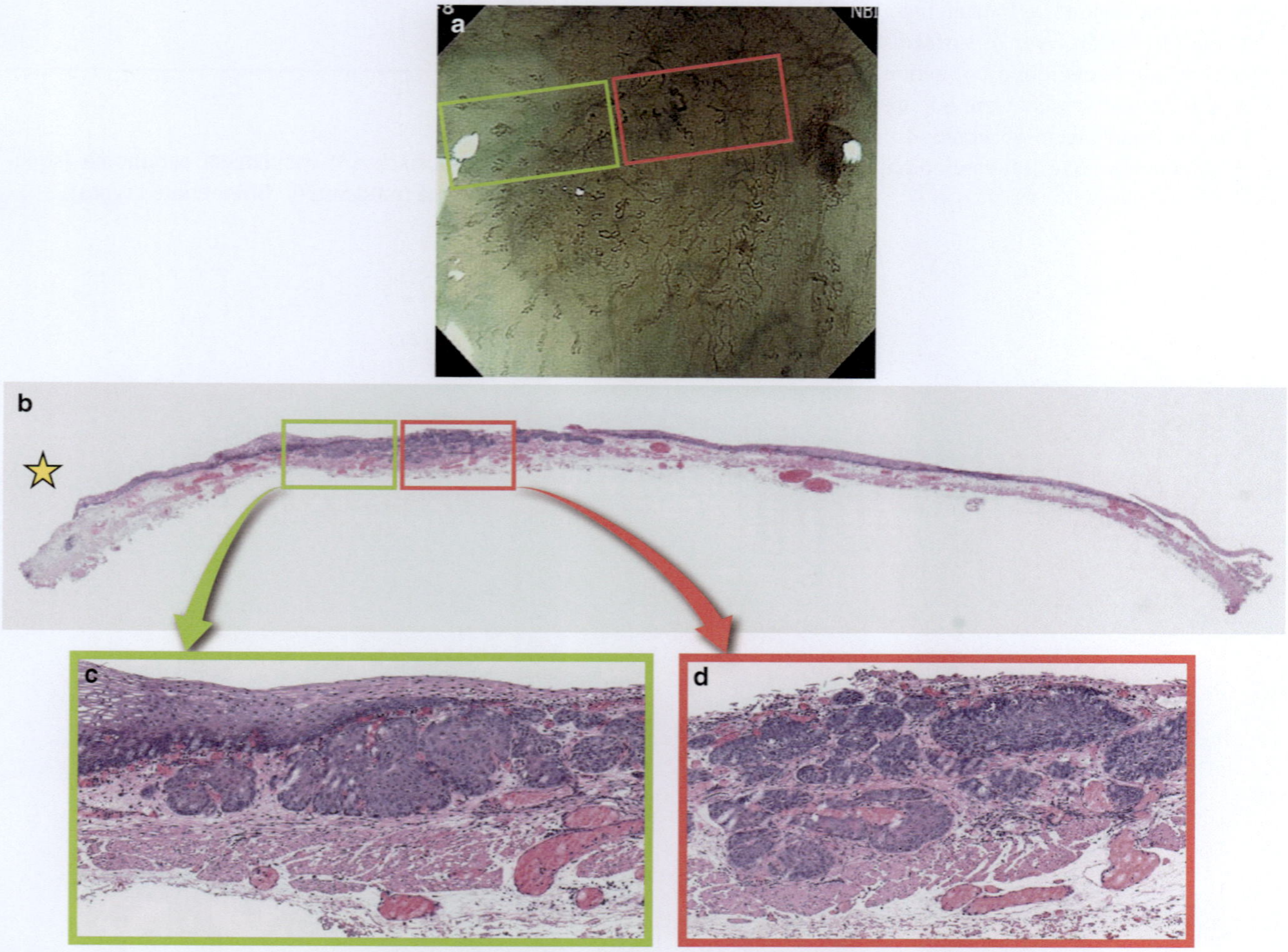

Fig. 28.5 (**a**) NBI magnified image of the lesion. (**b**) Histopathological image of area indicated with yellow star mark in Fig. 28.4c. (**c**) Within the lamina propria beneath the non-tumor squamous epithelium, alveolar-forming squamous cell carcinoma was noted. (**d**) Alveolar-forming squamous cell carcinoma was contacting the muscularis mucosa, and its invasion depth was diagnosed as T1a-MM. The surface of the tumor showed dense blood vessels thought to represent the non-loop forming blood vessels observed by magnifying NBI

Conclusive Diagnosis

Esophageal squamous cell carcinoma, moderately differentiated, 0-IIa, T1a-MM, INFb, ly(-), v(-), HM0, VM0, 12 × 4.5 mm.

Esophageal squamous cell carcinoma, 0-IIb, T1a-EP, ly(-), v(-), HM0, VM0, 4 × 4 mm.

Summary

Because the lesion was located mainly within the LPM covered by a thin layer of surface squamous cell epithelium, the background coloration was unclear, and Type B1 blood vessels were not observed. Since Type R blood vessels were observed, differential diagnoses including endocrine cell carcinoma, basaloid cell carcinoma, and poorly differentiated squamous cell carcinoma were listed, suggesting the presence of the invasive tumor near the surface. Since the shiny appearance of the lesion surface suggested a layer of non-tumor squamous cell epithelium, instead of using iodine dye staining for markings, it was necessary to perform markings outside of the area of irregular blood vessels using magnifying NBI and then perform iodine dye staining.

28.4 Answer

The correct diagnosis is (3) esophageal carcinoma [squamous cell carcinoma (moderately differentiated type)].

29 Question 14: What Is the Diagnosis?

Shinichi Furutachi

S. Furutachi (✉)
Department of Gastroenterology, Okayama Medical Center,
National Hospital Organization, Okayama, Japan

T. Oyama (ed.), *Endoscopic Diagnosis of Esophageal Carcinoma for ESD*, https://doi.org/10.1007/978-981-32-9030-3_29

Which Is the Correct Diagnosis? (Fig. 29.1)

1. Glycogenic acanthosis
2. Papilloma
3. Squamous cell carcinoma

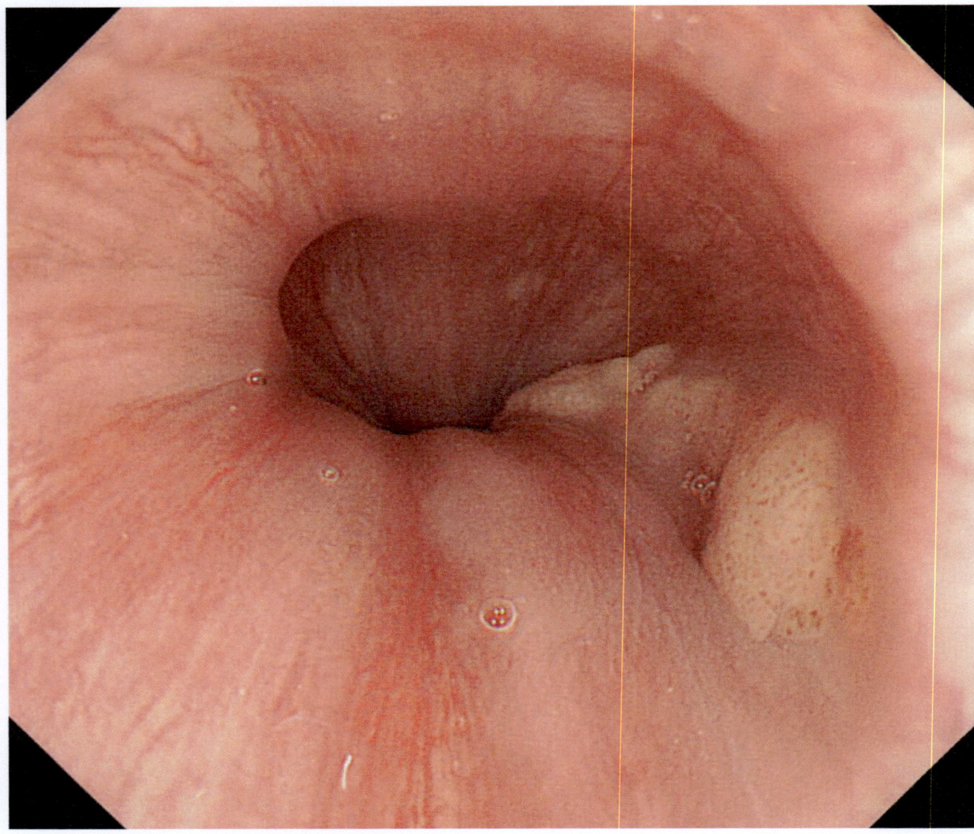

Fig. 29.1 Which is the correct diagnosis?

29.1 Let's Look at These Six Images and Think (Fig. 29.2)

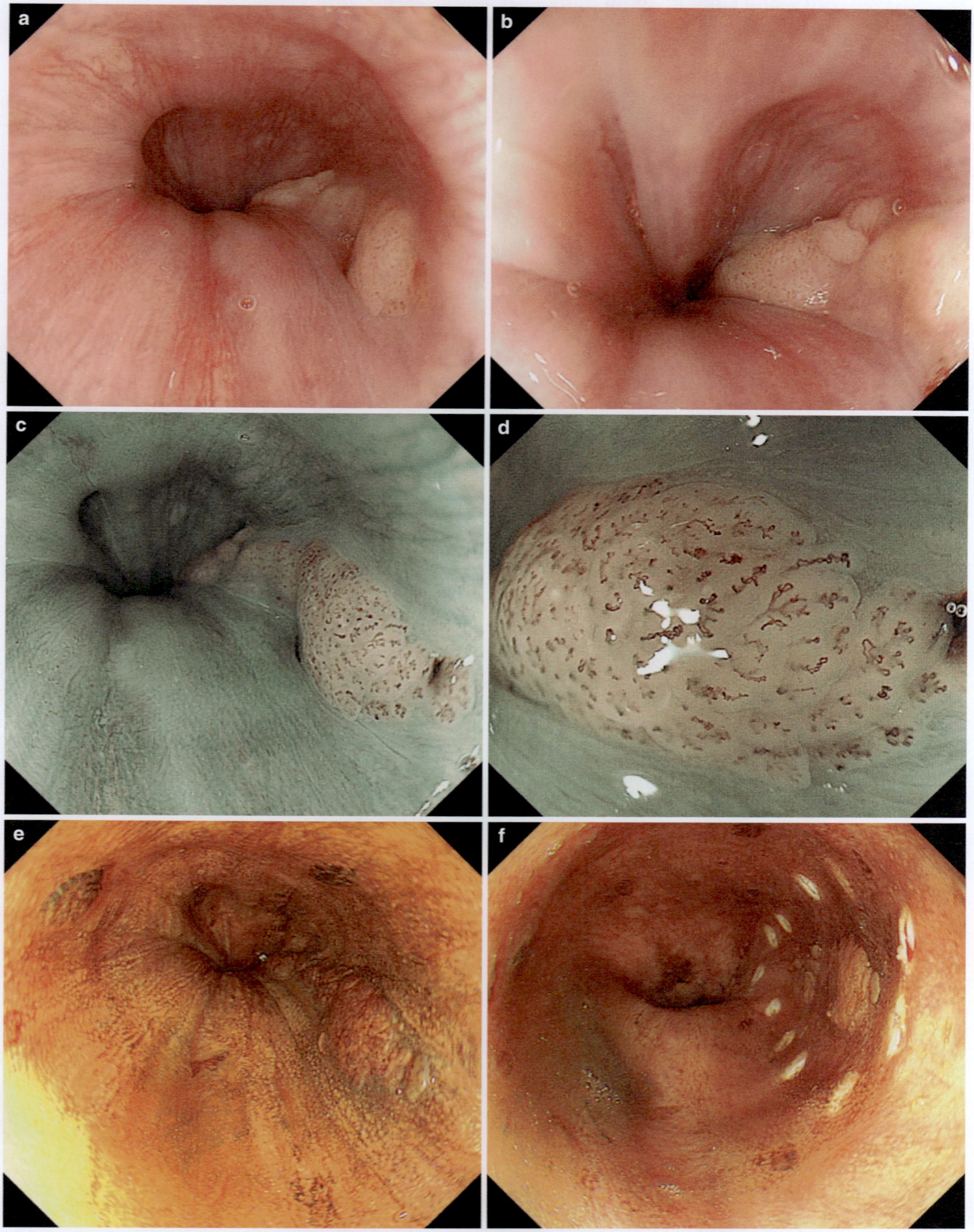

Fig. 29.2 Explanations start from the next page

29.2 Let's Observe the Following Six Images Carefully (Fig. 29.3)

Let's Observe with White Light Imaging (Fig. 29.3a)

- An elevated lesion was noted extending from the lower thoracic esophagus to the right wall of the thoracic esophagus, with faintly reddish color tone with clear demarcation, suggesting esophageal carcinoma.

Let's Observe the Anal Side of the Lesion (Fig. 29.3b)

- Observation from the central part of the lesion to the anal part showed narrowing of the width at the central part of the lesion due to biopsy by a referring doctor, and shape and color tone of the lesion were the same as the oral side.

Let's Observe with Non-magnifying NBI (Fig. 29.3c)

- The lesion was noted with slightly brownish background coloration of the surrounding esophageal mucosa. Also noted was proliferation of elongated dilated blood vessels matching the area of raised lesion.

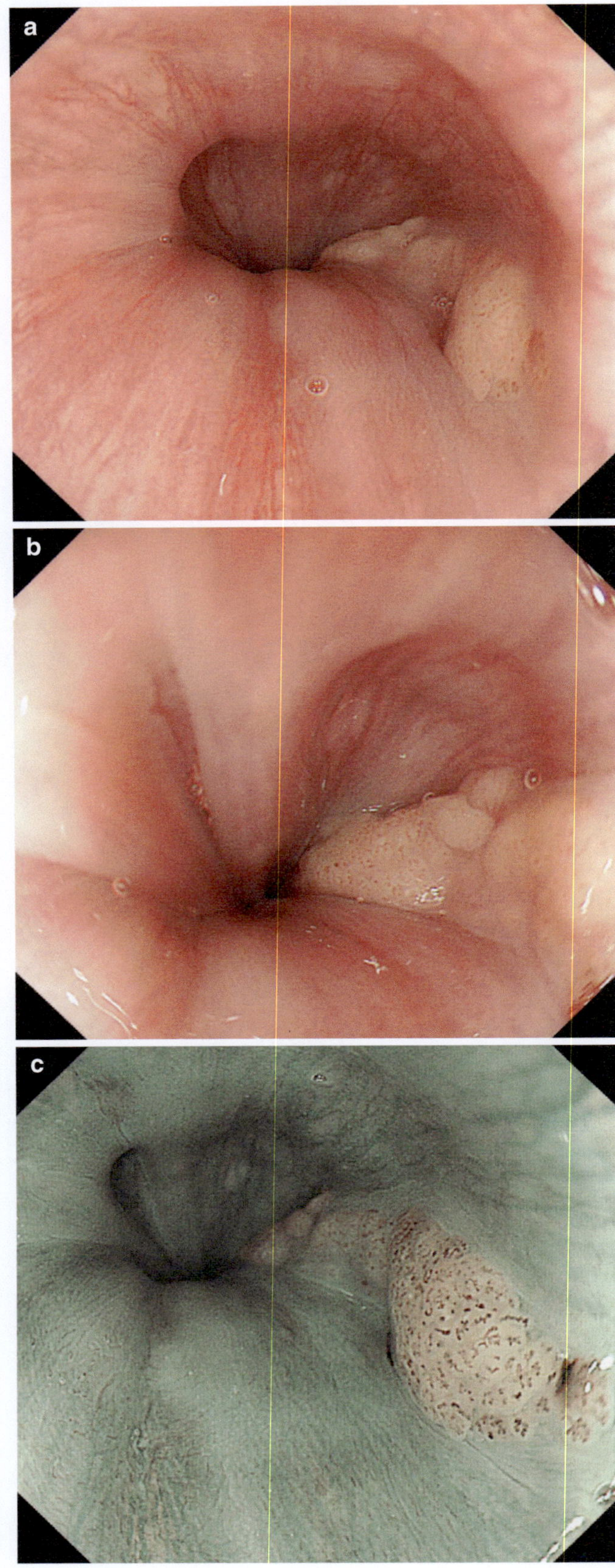

Fig. 29.3 Same images as Fig. 29.2

Let's Observe the Oral Side of the Lesion with Magnifying NBI (Fig. 29.3d)

- On magnifying NBI observation, the oral yellowish part of the raised lesion was noted with dilated, tortuous, irregularly shaped blood vessels of variable caliber, consistent with a diagnosis of squamous cell carcinoma.

Let's Observe with Iodine Dye Staining (Fig. 29.3e)

- Immediately following iodine dye staining, the lesion was stained with iodine dye.

Let's Observe Changes After Iodine Dye Staining with Time (Fig. 29.3f)

- This image was obtained after circumferential placement of the markings for ESD, approximately 4 min past spraying of the lesion with iodine dye. Observation with this timing showed the lesion as unstained.

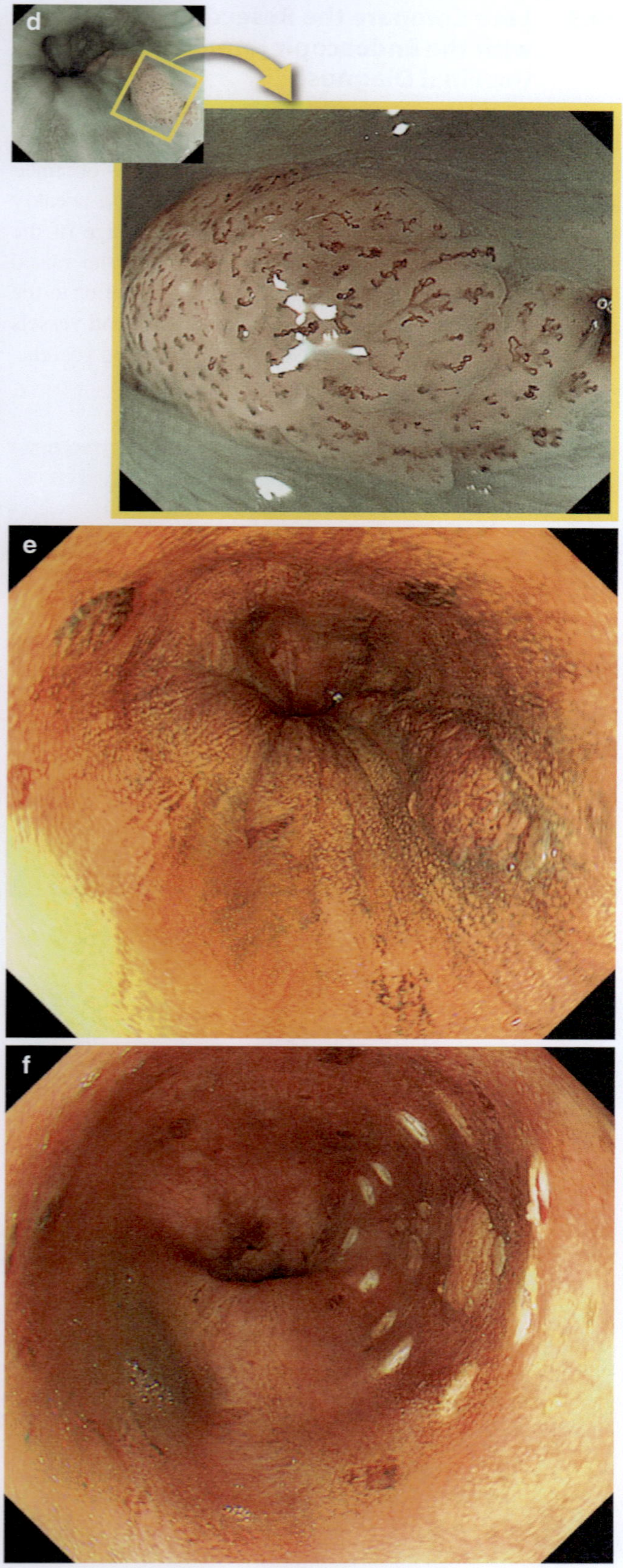

Fig. 29.3 (continued)

29.3 Let's Compare the Resected Specimen with the Endoscopic Images Towards the Final Diagnosis

In Fig. 29.4, the right side of the image is the oral side. Figure 29.4a is the stereoscopic image which was obtained after iodine dye staining, showing unstained to weakly stained area matching the raised lesion. The image of the freshly resected specimen (Fig. 29.4b) showed the raised lesion with clear demarcation except for the posterior to the anal sides with partially unclear demarcation. Blood vessels within the raised lesion consisted of Type B1 blood vessels.

Let's Observe the Histopathology Images (Fig. 29.5)

These are histopathological images of the section a marked by the red arrow in the top left section diagram of the resected specimen. The lesion shows upward growth as seen in the area marked by the red square and shows the full thickness of the mucosa replaced with enlarged nuclei as seen in the area marked by the blue square. The tumor was diagnosed as squamous cell carcinoma, without invasion of the lamina propria and with invasion depth of T1a-EP.

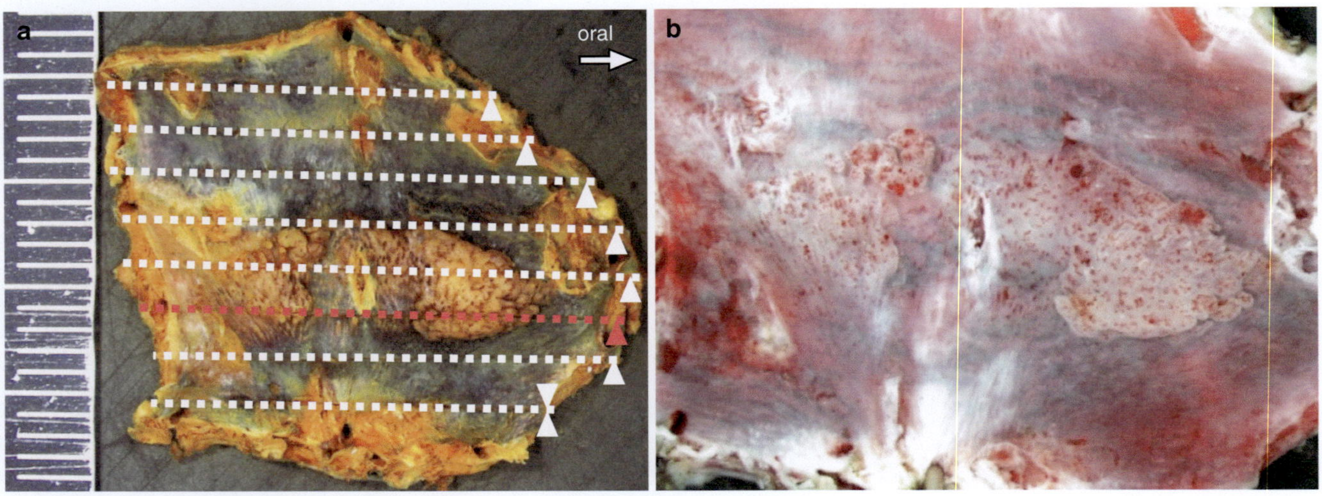

Fig. 29.4 (**a**) Stereoscopic image which was obtained after iodine dye staining to the resected specimen. (**b**) The freshly resected specimen of the lesion

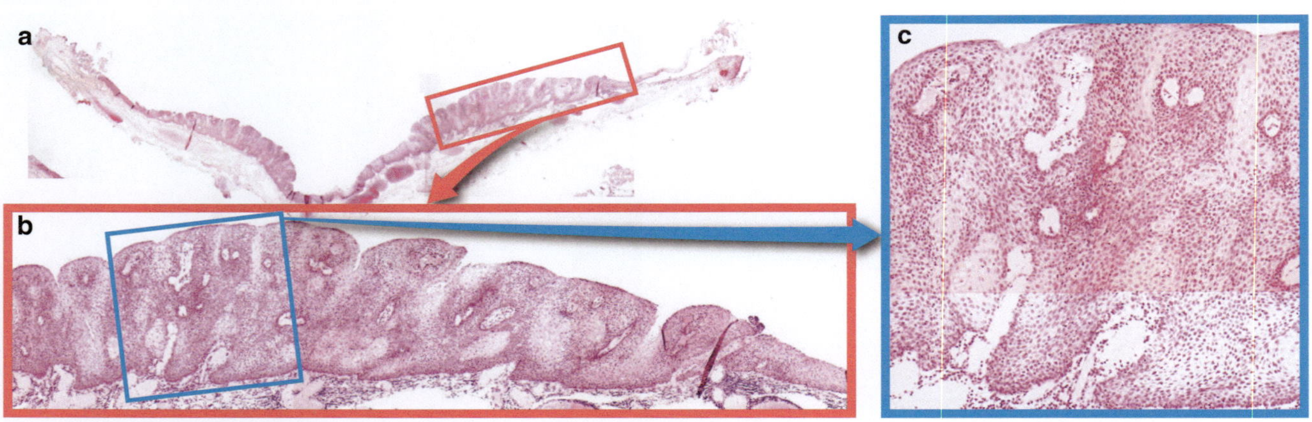

Fig. 29.5 (**a**) Histopathological image of the section a marked by the red arrow in Fig. 29.4a. (**b**) Magnified image of the area indicated in red square. (c) Magnified image of the area indicated in blue square in Fig. 29.4b

Let's Compare with Endoscopic Images (Fig. 29.6)

The white dotted line on this NBI image represents the section a. The histopathological image marked by the red square corresponds to the area slightly above this white dotted line. The elongated blood vessels noted within the surface of the tumor were thought to represent the blood vessels noted by magnifying NBI.

This Image Shows PAS Staining of the Same Section (Fig. 29.7)

As noted in the area marked by the red square, non-tumor part showed PAS staining positivity down to the middle mucosa, while the tumor part showed PAS positivity only at the very surface level.

As seen in the area marked by the blue square, the taller part of the tumor showed PAS positivity in part down to the middle mucosa.

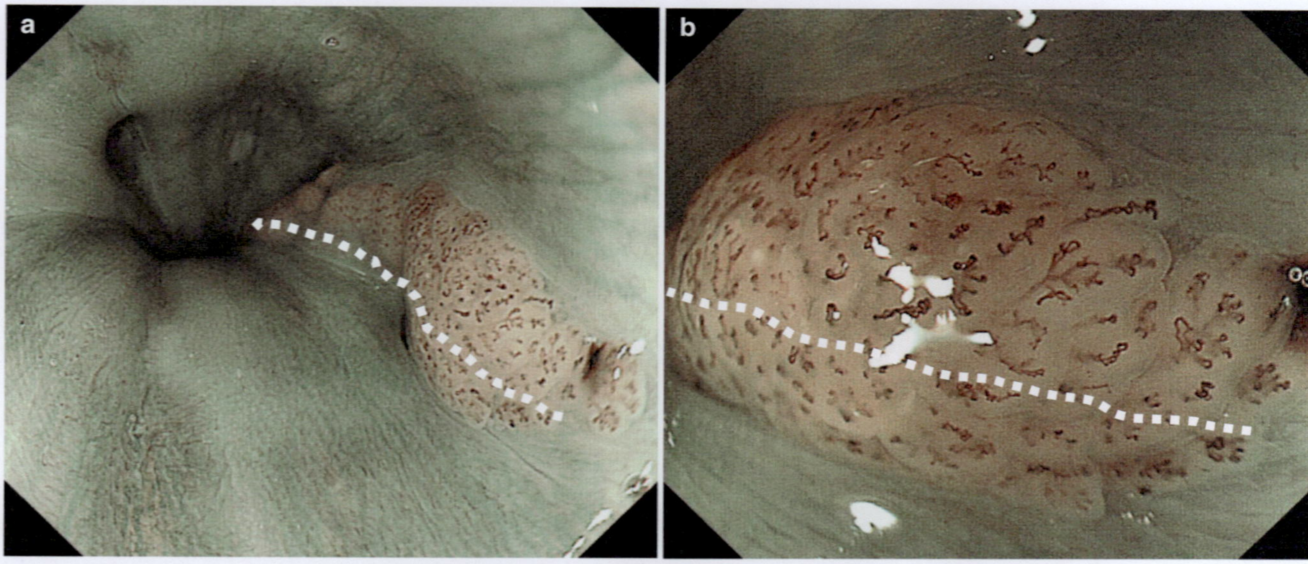

Fig. 29.6 (**a**) NBI image of the lesion. (**b**) NBI magnified image of the lesion

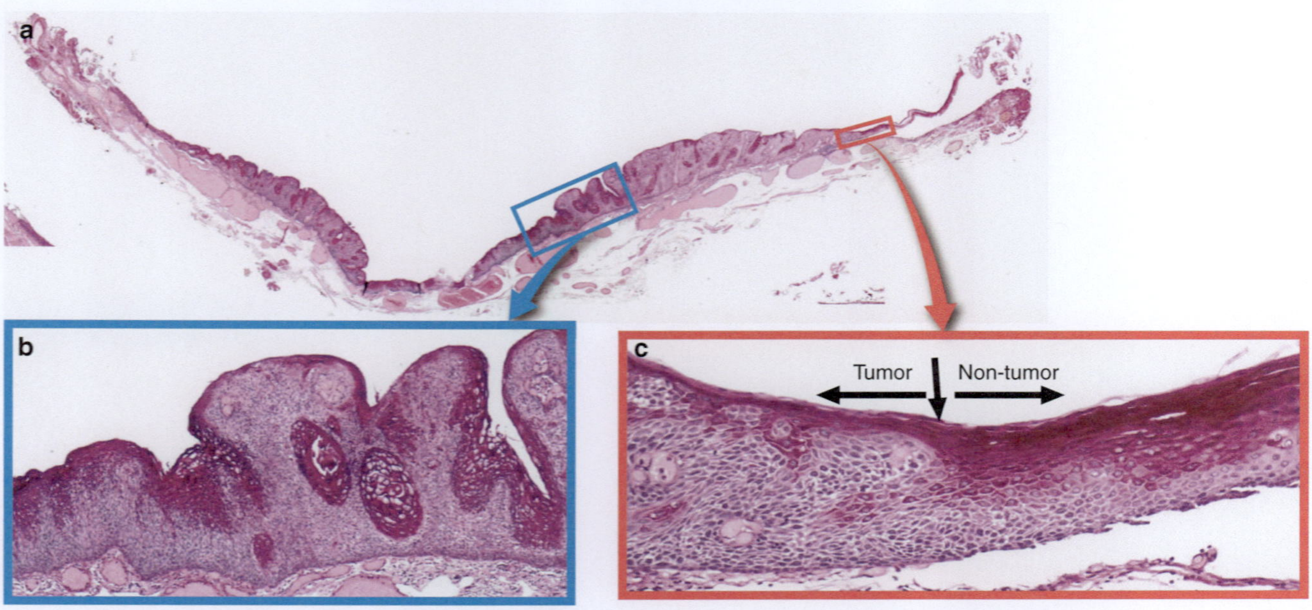

Fig. 29.7 (**a**) PAS staining image of the section a marked by the red arrow in Fig. 29.4a. (**b**) Magnified image of the area indicated in blue square in **a**. (**c**) Magnified image of the area indicated in red square in **a**

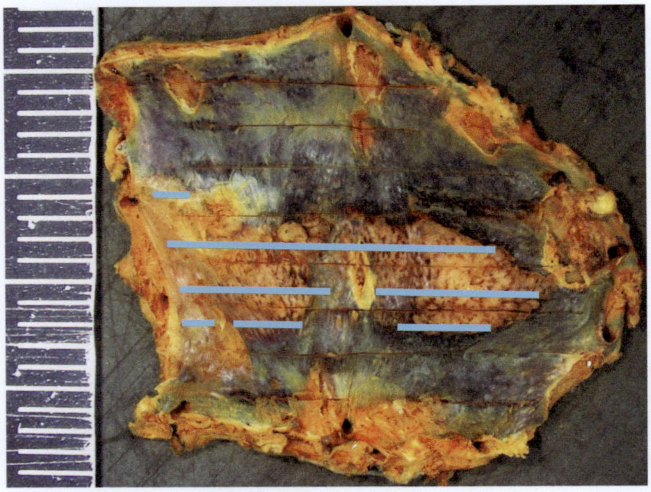

Fig. 29.8 Mapping of the cancer distribution projected on the resected specimen

Conclusive Diagnosis

Esophageal squamous cell carcinoma, 0-IIa, T1a-EP, INFa, ly(-), v(-), HM0, VM0, 17 × 6 mm, pCurA, Lt. (Fig. 29.8)

Summary

Although suspected of squamous cell carcinoma by white light observation or NBI observation, the lesion's response to iodine dye spraying differed from usual squamous cell carcinoma. Highly differentiated squamous cell carcinoma like this case while containing glycogen storage within the surface epithelium, the proportion and amount of glycogen containing cells occupy much smaller part compared with the non-tumor epithelium. Therefore, it is important to understand that highly differentiated squamous cell carcinoma shows iodine dye staining initially, but that it becomes unstained with time or becomes unstained with thiosodium sulfate spraying.

29.4 Answer

The correct histological type is (3) squamous cell carcinoma.

Correction to: Endoscopic Diagnosis of Esophageal Carcinoma for ESD

Tsuneo Oyama

Correction to: T. Oyama (ed.), *Endoscopic Diagnosis of Esophageal Carcinoma for ESD*,
https://doi.org/10.1007/978-981-32-9030-3

This book was inadvertently published with the incorrect copyright comment. This has now been corrected to Based on a translation from the Japanese language edition: ESD no tameno shokudo-gan jutuzen shindan by Prof. Tsuneo Oyama Copyright © Nankodo co., ltd., 2017 All Rights Reserved.

The updated online version of this book can be found at https://doi.org/10.1007/978-981-32-9030-3

T. Oyama (ed.), *Endoscopic Diagnosis of Esophageal Carcinoma for ESD*, https://doi.org/10.1007/978-981-32-9030-3_30